THE PLANDEMIC AGENDA

Be the master of your own destiny and not the evil elites that have created this Plandemic Agenda, I truly believe, it is to reduce the World's population to around 500 million by the year 2030. This is a book based on a truthful reality but also giving some hope for you all. But will they achieve that Sadly, I feel they will go very close in both with the vaccinated and unvaccinated of this Plandemic Agenda Spiritual War that we are all currently involved in. They are going to attack all of us from every front and aim to infect us all with Graphene Oxide and the mRNA (Spike Protein) through vaccines, water, and our food. The food chain is next on their Agenda with insects added to lots of our food products and mRNA added to all our livestock in 2023.

This book is not intended as a substitute for the medical advice of physicians so the reader should consult a physician in matters relating to his or her health and particularly with respect to any symptoms that may require diagnosis or medical attention and any alternative therapies mentioned in this book are only suggestions.

Some of the references in this book are specific to Australian Life and Times, but I do invite the reader to think about similar things, events and circumstances that are also happening in your own respective countries and habitats. I am dyslexic so book writing does not come easy, but I hope you find something of interest and after reading it gives you some hope.

Rainbow Harmonica Man

Dedication

My book is dedicated to the memory of Martina Batovska, who lived in Redcliffe Queensland, and tragically died on January 12th, 2022, and that may not have happened if it had not been for the Pandemic Covid 19. Also, to all the people around the World who have sadly died or have been injured because of this bioweapon.

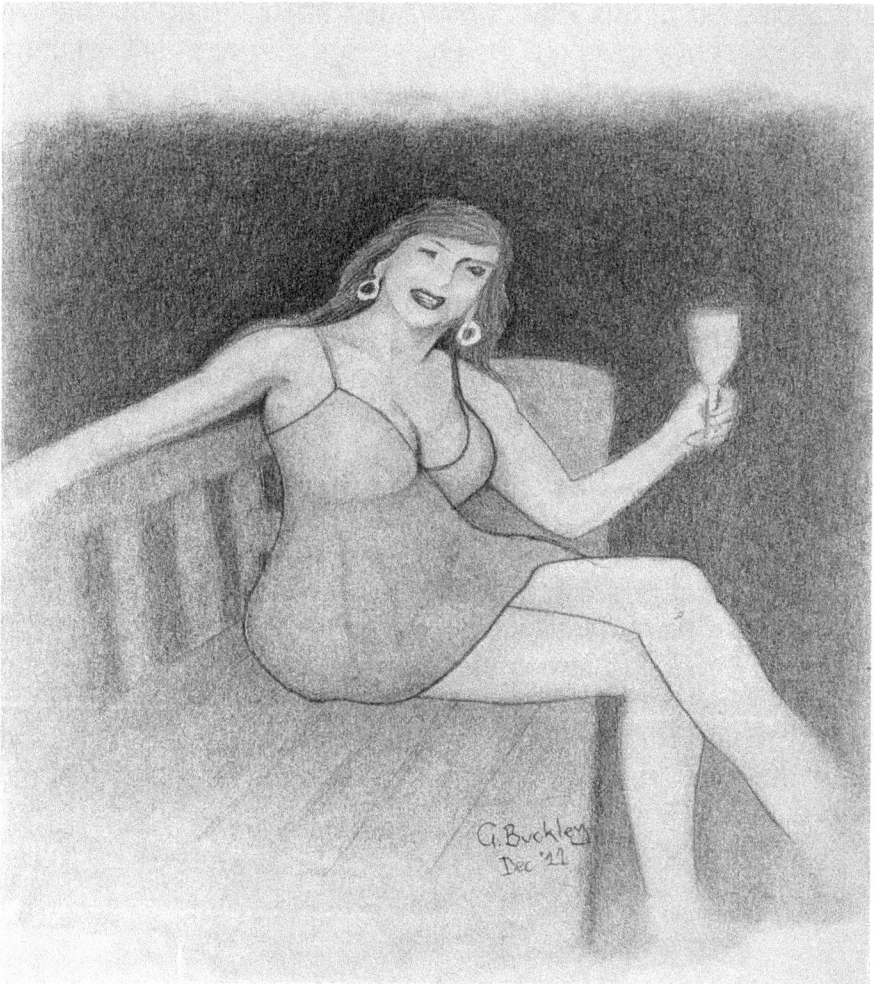

© G. Buckley

Background. Where I live on the Moreton Bay Peninsula, is a bay located on the eastern coast of Australia 14 kilometres from central Brisbane, Queensland and it is one of Queensland's most important coastal resources. The waters of Moreton Bay are a popular destination for recreational anglers and are used by commercial operators who provide seafood to market in the hamlet that I have lived in for many years, which is Scarborough Village Queensland, a coastal suburb of the Redcliffe Peninsula in the Moreton Bay Region, Queensland, Australia.

First published May 2023. Revised and updated December 2023.

Introduction

by Rainbow Harmonica Man

The awareness of this Plandemic started for me over 3 years ago when this so-called trumped-up virus Covid 19 was created in Wuhan China. Then sadly for me and for most of the World it has changed to be a total Mad-House. We have all had to endure Lockdowns, Mask Wearing, Checking In, PCR Tests and Vaccine Passports. Also, some of us have lost our jobs and sadly also the love of some of our family members, and our friends, due to our strong beliefs and our critical thinking that this was The Plandemic Agenda and out of the window went our free speech and the autonomy over our own bodies and: 'Our Body Our Choice'. By losing some of my friends that I have had over many decades as they truly believe "I Am a Nut Job" because I have critical thinking that they do not.

This has affected me mentally, because I have questioned, how can they be so Blind? I have been addicted to music for over four decades and have written two books about it which are (available on Amazon): John Warren ``Our Soul Music Journey" and John Warren "Our Soul Music Journeys", I have also, part-owned a record label "Red-Pants Records" with one my best friends Robert Paladino. But I had to sadly walk away from all of that, for my sanity because I cannot be around those people anymore. Sheepism is very endemic in the Soul music scene and especially in the Rare Soul Scene Worldwide. For many of you reading this will also have had to leave professions and career paths that you loved for similar reasons, simply because you would not comply and have any of these gene-therapy vaccines being put into your body. So, we all have had to endure our own "Yellow Star of David," moment but we have worn it with pride, and we are now affectionately called The Pure Bloods. This book is as truthful as I can compile it and holds back no punches.

4

It will shock, but also hopefully it will shock some of you back into reality and out of their "Matrix". We are all at war, with Good over Evil, and evil sadly has been winning for over three years; but they will not win if we all work together to defeat them, because they have tried these agendas before and have been planning this current Plandamic all based on Fear and Mistruths for a very long time. This spiritual war is the War-To-End-All-Wars and the control they plan for all is for our brains and ultimately our souls. This book is about giving Hope that Together we can reverse their plan to reduce the world's population to around 500 million, by the year 2030 and have us controlled and living in their (Not So) Smart Cities with its constant surveillance, eating the food they want us to consume, which include bugs and plant-based food and fake meat, mRNA injected into our livestock and plants, our bees and anything else they deem fit. And that's apart from our water supply with all its many added chemicals like Fluoride and Graphene Oxide etc.

These Experimental Vaccines are basically (Transhumanism), and mRNA will be in all the future vaccines that are produced and given to you from the day you are born. But you can say NO and take control over your own lives and your own bodies and finally get out of their Matrix. All the new cars will have kill switches in them, that are all part of the planned control over us and of what we eat, what we do, what we think and where we are allowed to go, living in their smart cities. If you are planning on travelling soon, I suggest doing it now and their power is all a 'Fear-Based Agenda' through the corrupt media that they own and control in what we are told is the truth. It always has been an illusion that's been started so many times before: for instance, with the Robert Kennedy assassination, the Titanic and more recently here in Queensland Australia, with the sad demise of two police officers and three citizens for reasons very clear to most of us? If you are Awake, you will not all die of these gene therapy mRNA vaccines even if you are vaccinated or because of the shedding of the vaccinated. There are so many ways to reverse the damage caused by this evil that they have been injecting some of us with Toxins like Graphene Oxide (GO). I have devoted a whole chapter on this and how to detox it out of your body along with all the other introduced chemicals through their Cloud Seeding Programs and all the poisons being added into our food chain. But it is so very important to eliminate this, as it is the Conductor that the (GO) needs to self-assemble in your bodies through their 4G and 5G networks, which is why they needed to put in all our bodies for it to work? and then to ultimately help achieve their Plandemic Agenda 2030.

Sadly your brains are being microwaved on a daily basis because of it, causing Zombism, Brain Fog, Alzheimer's etc, and this will be the new norm as it is currently with conditions like "Long Covid" which is basically caused by these vaccines and there will be many other conditions that be released like 'The Marburg Variant'. The Spike Protein is a lot harder to eliminate but you all need to start trying, and I will talk about ways in attempting to achieve that aim. The few writers in this book have been carefully chosen and that I probably would not have met if it was not for this C19 pandemic. They have since become my friends and have shown no fear and have all written with love and honesty and writing truthful books against this pandemic agenda come with inherent risks, but we must all try to 'End This World Tyranny' because our children and grandchildren's futures are very dependent on what we do today, and in the very near future. If you are not awake yet, hopefully reading this book will finally 'Wake You Up to Finally Turn Your TV Off'. To all the other freedom fighters around the world who have fought this great fight in the last 3 years of this tyranny against mankind, please take a bow. I am very proud to walk among you, but I feel the road to victory is going to be a very long one and maybe several years away, but victory will eventually be achieved and 'We Will Win' because we are stronger and have so much more to lose and we are so many, and our number grows stronger by the day. The elite's ultimate plan is to vaccinate all of us by stealth through our food and water and so we have to out-think them.

But there are many other conditions that will be released like 'The Marburg Variant' the one they will hold back until they need to when they will set the panic button and then just watch how the vaccine addicts (Sheeple) will react. We are smarter than them with some of them needing sexual gratification with our children, also some of them are not human, maybe clones and reptilians amongst them that enjoy eating bugs, but without GOD they are nothing but Evil and the Devil will always lose.

AGENDA 2030

The Great Reset
One World Government
Fourth Industrial Revolution
Technocractic Corporatocracy
Total dependency on the state
Social Credit system
Carbon Footprint Survaillance system
Universal Basic Income for compliant citizens
Programmable Central Banking Digital Currency
Depopulation
Mandatory Vaccines for all ages
Controlled fertility and reproduction
Radical assisted suicide and abortion laws
100 % Genetically manipulated food and soil
Ban on all natural remedies and treatments
Robot workforce
Internet of Things & Internet of Bodies
Microchips & implantable brain interface technologies
Constant exposure to non-native EMFs and RFs (5G, 6G, 7G)
Destruction of genders
Destruction of motherhood and fatherhood
Rationing of energy and all natural resources
Restriction on "non-essential" air travel
Smart Cities
Drones, facial recognition cameras, movement sensors
Abolishment of private property
Control and surveillance of nature and wildlife
Restricted access to wilderness (human free zones)
"Sustainable development" of the New World Order

IS THIS THE WORLD WE WANT FOR OUR CHILDREN?

There Agenda and Marburg will be next so prepare.

Content's

Chapter 1

THE START

How did we get here in this mess? Well, we will have to go back over 100 years to the Spanish flu, another contrived and Control-Based Plandemic created by the Elites.

WHERE DID THE SPANISH FLU BACTERIAL PNEUMONIA OF 1918-19 REALLY ORIGINATE? When the United States declared war in April 1917, the very small pharmaceutical industry had something they had never ever had before: a very large supply of human test subjects in the form of the US military's first draft. Pre-war in 1917, the US Army was 286,516 men. Post-war in 1920, the US army disbanded, and had 296,069 men. During the war years 1918-19, the US Army had ballooned to 6,050,020 men, with 2,060,000 men being sent overseas. The Rockefeller Institute for Medical Research took advantage of this new large pool of human guinea pigs to conduct vaccine experiments. Does this not all sound too familiar? which has all been pre-planned and is their Plandemic Agenda. Between January 21st and June 4th of 1918, a report was produced on an experiment where soldiers were given 3 doses of a bacterial meningitis vaccine. Those conducting the experiment on the soldiers were just giving dosages of a vaccine derived from a serum in horses and very ironic, considering the fact they have banned Ivermectin as a treatment for Con-Vid 19, explaining this Nobel prize-winning medicine was only for horses. The vaccination regime was designed to be 3 doses. 4,792 men received the first dose, but only 4,257 got the 2nd dose, and only 3,702 received all three doses. What truly happened to these soldiers? Were they shipped east by train from Kansas to board a ship to Europe? Were they ever in the Fort Riley hospital? Reports are that Several of the men in that experiment had flu-like symptoms: coughs, vomiting and diarrhoea after receiving the vaccine.

These symptoms were a disaster for men living together in barracks, travelling on trains to the Atlantic coast, sailing to Europe, and living together and fighting in the trenches. The unsanitary conditions at each step of the journey were an ideal environment for a contagious disease like bacterial pneumonia to spread. They had injected random dosages of an experimental bacterial meningitis vaccine into soldiers. Afterwards some of the soldiers had symptoms which "simulated" meningitis, but a doctor advances the fantastical claim that it wasn't actual meningitis. The soldiers developed flu-like symptoms bacterial meningitis, then as now, is believed to Mimic Flu-Like Symptoms. How did the "SPANISH FLU" spread around the world so quickly? and there was the element of a perfect storm in how the bacteria spread. WWI ended only 10 months after the first injections and sadly for the 50-100 million who died, those soldiers injected with horse-infused bacteria moved quickly during those 10 months.

In 1918. "Spanish Flu": Only the Vaccinated Died.

Autopsies after the war proved that the 1918 flu was NOT a "FLU" at all. It was caused by random dosages of an experimental 'Bacterial Meningitis Vaccine', which to this day, Mimics Flu-Like Symptoms. The massive, multiple assaults with additional vaccines on the unprepared immune systems of soldiers and civilians created a "Killing Field". Those that were not Vaccinated were not affected. The parallels between then and now are so very similar and there is conjecture that Bill Gates grandfather Dr. Frederick Gates was the creator involved? It kind of makes sense, with Bill Gates being the creator of this bioweapon causing this current Pandemic. And remember back then there was no mRNA, Graphene Oxide and EMFS from the 4G and 5G networks to help them succeed; but they did understand that 'LIFE' and everything is 'Vibration, Energy and Frequency', and with Mind Control they can achieve anything and they have. People even wore masks back then and understood with fear they could conquer all and then achieve their 'Agenda to Depopulate'.

The first official cases of C19 were recorded on the 31st of December 2019, when the World Health Organization was informed of cases of pneumonia in Wuhan, China, with no known cause. On the 7th of January, the Chinese authorities identified a novel coronavirus, temporarily named 2019-nCoV, as the culprit. Weeks later, on the 30th of January 2020, the WHO declared the rapidly spreading C19 outbreak as a Public Health Emergency of International Concern. It was not until the following month, however, on the 11th of February that the novel coronavirus got its official name: Covid 19. Nine days later, the US Centers for Disease Control and Prevention (CDC) confirmed the first person to die of C19 in the country. Covid 19 was declared a pandemic; but it was really a total Plandemic all based on fear and deception. In the first months of C19, global health authorities, government agencies, and the public were unsure of how the disease would spread and how it would impact everyday life. When in reality all you actually were doing was destroying your own 'Innate Natural Immunity'. I wrote about this in my book John Warren "Our Soul Music Journeys" published on Amazon in 2021, calling it out then as a Plandamic and wrote about some of the above nonsense.

All the Unvaccinated (The Pure Bloods) who are currently mostly healthy, happy and very proud that our critical thinking has since been proven to be correct because I do not know of any 'Unvaccinated Who Have Died of C19" but we all are sadly aware of so many who have died through suicide and due to these Vaccines (Bioweapon) and it has sadly divided nearly everyone's families worldwide as they had intended in their 'Divide and Conquer' mission that was always based on fear and so many miss-truths. But we all must feel for some of those who did take this poison to keep their jobs and provide for their families because I suspect some will be very angry and have not been very well since they were vaccinated. We are all aware of the massive amount of unvaccinated deaths and injuries from this "Poison" and it's beyond sad.

But for those of you who took this to go into a pub, music event, sporting event or to travel you were simply plain stupid and you will reap what you have sown into your bodies especially if you do not try to reverse the damage it will have caused to your body. This was always a genocidal plan, and it was clear that the initial restrictions were not enough to stop the spread of C19. What a surprise. Quickly, restrictions in most regions became harsher, with the UK enforcing a stay-at-home rule on the 26th of March 2020 and many European countries had to implement their own national lockdowns around this time so by the 2nd of April, total global C19 cases had already shot up to 1 million. The true seriousness of the plandemic came into light with this trumped up figure and Governments did what they could to postpone the spread of this virus before a vaccine could be declared safe for use. On the 6th of April, the WHO released guidance on mask-wearing, as more evidence began to highlight the role of aerosols in the spread of the disease. But new variants changed the course of this plandemic over the summer and many countries saw an actual drop in cases, deaths and hospitalizations, due to the restrictions their citizens had endured to prevent the spread of the virus.

However, towards the end of the summer, in August of 2020, the Lambda (Sheep Variant) was first discovered in Peru and a month later in September 2020, the Alpha Variant was first identified in the UK. The discovery of these variants was very significant; it showed that the virus was evolving as they had planned and as a result, symptoms and disease outcomes were changing so evidence was shown, for example, that the alpha variant may pose a heightened risk of poor C19 outcomes. With the emergence of these new variants, cases of C19 began to rise again in many countries and by the 29th of September 2020, there had been 1 million C19 deaths. vaccines? which was later to be proven false? On the 9th of November, trials demonstrated the Pfizer and BioNTech vaccines to be over 90% effective (Again Proven to Be False), and the Moderna vaccine was also proved to be effective just a week later 16th of November and another week later, on the 23rd of November the University of Oxford and AstraZeneca C19 were also shown to be effective and amazing if truthful that "Three Safe Vaccines" could be created in record time then shortly after, in December, the Delta variant was first discovered in India. Concerns over the potential increased transmissibility of the variants ('Were More Lie's as The Vaccines Don't and Never Did Stop Transmission') that was fuelled by a rise in cases in some countries such as the UK, which forced many governments to once again enforce lockdown measures to some extent.

Finally, on the 31st of December 2020, the WHO issued its first emergency use validation for a C19 vaccine, making the Pfizer/BioNTech vaccine the first to be available for use; and history has since proven it is not safe and is a genocidal-weapon and all was pre-planned.

The next step was towards making C19 vaccines globally available, a necessary step to ending the plandemic. So, when you read that and "Join the Dots" how could you have been hoodwinked into this "Scamdamic Plandamic Agenda" and if you were a "Believer" you must truly believe in the tooth fairy and their mantra was "2 Weeks to Flatten the Curve" and here we well over three years on and it sure is not flattened. But sadly, it has murdered a lot of people and sadly many more to come. Much can be learned from the story of the C19 Plandamic, and the many lessons learned will prepare the sheeple and the vaccine addicts for future planned infectious disease outbreaks and how easy the NWO can plan for potential future Pandemics.

Then, the Moderna vaccine and the Oxford/AstraZeneca were approved for use and national vaccine rollout initiatives began in full force. Astrazeneca was banned in March 2023 in Australia and "we did warn you". The rest will be banned at some point in time. A week later, on the 23rd of November the University of Oxford and AstraZeneca C19 were also shown to be effective and they have already released Monkey-Pox, which was a very silly name to test how daft you were in your response? They still have their dreaded 'MARBURG' up their sleeve for when they want to escalate this Plandemic Agenda to the next level. On April 19, 2023 Virax Biolabs Group Limited, an innovative biotech company focused on the detection of immune responses to and diagnosis of viral diseases, announced today that it has entered into an agreement for the distribution of Marburg Virus PCR testing kits. This has always been their plan and if you are not vaccinated you have nothing to fear.

Disaster looms as the Marburg Virus may have already been released through Co-Vid19 vaccine payloads. The Marburg Virus disease (MVD), formerly known as Marburg hemorrhagic fever, is very severe and often a fatal illness in humans with a fatality rate of up to 88 percent. In my humble view, the whole pandemic was to see how we would react to a common cold-style virus and then see how we would comply and so many have currently taken this bio-weapon gene therapy for basically a cold and are now termed 'Vaccine Addicts' and seem very eager to get their next clot shot which is currently vaccine number 5 here in Australia.

Bill Gates "Has just warned Australia in January 2023, to brace itself for The Next Pandemic" which will be man-made and be far more lethal than the Covid Virus" (Yes, Bill, We Are on To You). We know that Marburg is not particularly contagious, but it has a very high rate of fatality. We also know the mechanism by which this will be released, and that is from inside the lipid nanoparticles in the shots that people have already received as inside the hydrogel particles there exist pathogens that have not yet been released. Those pathogens are chimeric and include E. coli, Marburg, Ebola, Brewer's Yeast and Staphylococcus among others. We also know that when they broadcast an '18 Gigahertz Signal for One Minute from the 5G System', three different times as a pulse, it will cause those lipid nanoparticles to swell and release these pathogenic contents, thereby causing a Marburg epidemic that they have already spent their money on developing.

Covid vaccines install Marburg "payloads" in human victims and a 5G broadcast signal will activate this bioweapon, unleashing the next raging Pandemic and why I so strongly advise you to remove the Graphene Oxide (GO) which is the conductor for the 4G and 5G out of your bodies. To eliminate the (GO) and understanding that this is paramount, you need to continue to keep it out of your body as much as humanly possible. For those of you who are unvaccinated you do not need to fear Marburg, but we need to Fear that this will be the excuse used to force the 'Unvaxxed' into Quarantine Camps where Kill-Shots will be administered". The Zombie Apocalypse preparedness program is already in place because The Federal Emergency Management Agency has already put out Zombie Commercials and ConOps (Concept of Operations) before in case of a zombie apocalypse. "Callendar agreed and cited Conplan 8888 Stratcom, which was put out in 2011. He said it was all about five different types of zombies and a zombie apocalypse.

He added that every National Incident Management System-compliant state already had their zombie apocalypse preparedness training. The Colorado-based lawyer noted that the Centers for Disease Control and Prevention has a zombie apocalypse preparedness website up and running for the past five years. For those of you who are truly Awake will all have witnessed so many bizarre incidents that you might never have seen before? and because I ride a bike in Queensland Australia for hours every day, I notice so much more of these kinds of zombism. Such as, people who seem to be awake "But nobody is at home." We all have noticed strange events lately in the news? like helicopters crashing into each other in broad daylight and a lot more car crashes as though the driver is asleep? or distracted like never before. People also have been drowning in larger numbers and maybe it is because they don't have the motor skills, awareness and fitness they once had. They do tests for alcohol and drugs on a driver and maybe soon there will be a need to do a vaccine test and that would become more relevant in explaining the sleepiness and zombism of some of these drivers.

So, as such, they do not fulfil the medical term and or the legal term of a Vaccine? So, mRNA therapy does not satisfy public health measures directives on that basis in my humble opinion? Why was it ever mandated? We all understand the reasons why and this would hinge on whether it should ever be accepted as a vaccine and since mRNA therapies do not render the immunised persons are immune, and do not inhibit the transmission of the virus; they surely cannot qualify as a public health measure capable of providing collective benefit that supersedes individual risks and therefore logically cannot be mandated. Mandating it for the great good of the community and your little old granny was a total "Falsehood" and all of us the unvaccinated have heard this total rubbish such as " You're Not Protecting Yourself And Members of The Community," and by not complying, we were being victimised by the guilt trips put on us by some of our family members and are so called friends which has done lasting mental damage to some of us.

The total lack of human trials is also under question and most of you reading this are aware Pfizer wanted to suppress the information of the 'trials they had rigged' for 75 years for obvious reasons, and since they have had to release them, it has become abundantly clear that it was all a facade based on lies and mistruths. Gene Therapy is classed as an experimental technique that uses genes to treat or prevent disease and gene therapies generally are used for diseases that have no other cure well because C19 was never isolated in a laboratory; it does not technically exist and with the miracle that the flu and common colds disappeared magically overnight. Is this a variant of a cold or flu? It is all conjecture but a lot of you are aware there were other much safer treatments like Ivermectin and Hydroquinone available but them being cheap, big Pharma was never going to allow the truth about these therapies being beneficial to be revealed. How many people have died unnecessarily? In a future chapter I will talk about the "UK's End-of-Life murder in hospitals and old people's homes" with the use of drugs and especially **Remdesivir.**

Understanding mRNA and that they are snippets of a genetic code that instructs cells to produce proteins, mRNA C19 therapies deliver genetic instructions into your cells triggering your body to produce spike proteins of the virus (The Spike Protein) Covid. Basically, in layman's terms, the mRNA vaccines are gene therapy as they fulfil all the definitions of gene therapy and none of the definitions of them being a vaccine. C19 could never have been described as a disease because it is a giant umbrella of clinical symptoms that was used to associate with influenza and other febrile diseases. Is a virus a disease? So, what is all this gene therapy doing when it sends the strand of synthetic RNA into a human being and is invoking with our human body's the creation of a pathogen. A vaccine is supposed to trigger immunity and it's not supposed to trigger you to produce a Toxin. Drug companies understand the legal definition of vaccine versus gene therapy because with experimental gene therapy it does not come under the financial liability shielding, but Pandemic emergency use vaccines do.

This is one of the reasons they used the C19 State of Emergency which we would all describe as a cold, was so that the drug companies and those applying this gene therapy into our bodies were insulated from legal immunity from being sued. This is going to end very badly for them worldwide and so it should for all those hospitals and medical practices, doctors and nurses and anybody who injected this experimental gene therapy into a lot of you reading this, that they could be legally sued. Medical practices are starting here in Australia, to remove bulk billing so are they possibly preparing for the onslaught of legal claims against them? Ironically, they made you sick by destroying your innate natural immunity, triggering some of your dormant cancers to wake up and other illnesses. This sadly has happened to my own mother in the UK after her second injection, and now you must pay upfront to see those same doctors? when they got paid very well to inject that poison into your body and some of you are a lot sicker because of it?

In the Aboriginal communities here in Australia I currently have a friend currently teaching in them near Alice Springs who is not unvaccinated, who informed me the Aborigines were offered high cash inducements of up $500-$750 to take these clot shots. This is history repeating itself in many ways from when the English put glass in their food in Tasmania, in the days of the colonies to exterminate them. The class actions are already beginning from the amount of people who have died and are injured from these vaccines and in my book John Warren "Our Soul Music Journeys" published in 2021 on Amazon.

I had highlighted the graph of vaccine injuries from all the vaccines that have been introduced worldwide compared to the Covid 19 vaccine and up to the 12th of November 2021, it already showed **2,457,386 injuries** and new data coming out are showing according to official figures published by the UK Government institution, the Office for National Statistics (ONS), by the 1st of June 2022, 1 in every 73 Covid-19 vaccinated people in England had sadly died. But during the same time frame, only 1 in every 172 not-vaccinated people had died and more alarming is a study conducted by scientists from several respected institutions across Germany & Switzerland have discovered that 1 in every 99 Covid-19 vaccination children aged 5 and under found that the risk of children requiring emergency care or hospitalisation following Covid-19 vaccination was 117% higher than the average.

This Horrific Disparity compared to all the other vaccines explains a lot and surely this should have been enough for the many governments around the world to deem this bioweapon gene-therapy poison Not Safe? In 2023 we have sadly seen the devastating effects even more and yet it is still an "Emergency Approved Only Vaccine" for a Non-Emergency. The Media Worldwide for 'obviously monetary reasons' have always promoted this gene therapy as safe? and all their reporters should hold their heads in shame in the complicity of their actions in this planned Genocide.

The churches around the world have also played a big part in this total Plandemic and especially the Catholic Church.

"Pope Francis of the Roman Catholic Church has indicated that he believes all people everywhere should get Vaccinated".

'Evil is as Evil' does Pope Francis and Hell Awaits You. The Catholic church has defended some of their children loving priests for decades and it's time you were all made accountable. It is ironic when the churches come down on the side of evil and yet there are some priests who have been ostracised for not taking this poison; and where I live in Qld Australia there is a breakaway church in the Moreton Bay region where in sermons by "Jon," who is an incredibly passionate priest, he has talked about the dangers of this gene therapy. His passion and honesty and integrity should be a real Christian lesson to all those other priests who truly are not christian but satanic. This breakaway church that is doing God's work is growing faster than the "Mushrooms in The Rain" that we've been getting here in 2022-2023 here in Queensland due to another part of their Plandamic plan through their Bio-Engineered (Cloud Seeding).

This Agenda proves the point of 'Mind Control' and of belief systems which I will also explore more in a further chapter because mind control is how this nightmare has been achieved so very much so soon. It was many decades in the making but sadly got us to where we are now. I truly believe there is Hope for you all and especially if you only had two injections of these so-called vaccines there is a 'Big Chance' that you were given a Placebo because if the person injecting it in you had basic morals and understood the implications of what they were doing? and truly believed in the mantra "Do No Harm" they might have chosen especially in healthy patients in giving them a placebo. We truly pray and hope so, and you all would have been aware that some of these vaccines had to be kept at very low temperatures and that would have helped them to deliver these vaccines in a way that would make them null and void on that basis. If vaccines are not kept strictly at the right temperature, they do not work. 'You Have to Have Hope'. Some of you reading this would be naturally very worried of the implications of your actions and would regret it immensely, but if you only had two vaccines you might have dodged a bullet?

But sadly, the **Booster** is a different story as I hear this so much: "I was alright taking the first two vaccines, but when I took the booster, I had a serious adverse reaction and have not been well since." It is easy to spot people who are so brainwashed and that are so far down the rabbit hole, they will never ever come up again for air and are sadly doomed by their own actions. This is their own "Walk into The Gas Chamber" and they will never admit they were wrong and will continue to take these toxic poisons till it kills them. Most of the brainwashed I find have had three plus injections and their brains are being zombified.

You are truly wasting your time trying to educate them, sadly because they will never, ever listen and when you hear so many did it to go into a pub or attend a music event like some of my friends who went to a soul music night, it truly baffles me why people can be so very Stupid? and why they did not do some basic due diligence on an experiment where you were all the 'Guinea Pigs'. The music scene that I've been involved with for over four decades, it is accepted that some people are still taking stimulating drugs to dance and to stay awake all night to enjoy the music, and it's easy to see a correlation there when taking this drug so willingly. Some of us who did not take these toxic poisons have been ostracised by them and been labelled conspiracy theorists and I have had this done to me many times and they were very vicious on social media especially "Evil Book" where I get banned a lot for my honest views. It truly is a Badge of Honour to be banned on an evil site owned by a Satanic Worshipper. One my "Trolls" even commented on Facebook a lad originally from London, UK who lives now lives in Buderim, Queensland that "That Covid Would Kill Me."

Well, suck eggs old chap, because you always were going to be wrong, and I am happy to name and shame them. We need to show them up, as their actions in encouraging others is a crime against humanity because sadly some took their advice and will now be sick and have their lives shortened by listening to them. Had they erred on the side of caution as I and some others had strongly encouraged them to do so, they would not be sick now and have compromised immune systems. So, Barry Slimes in Adelaide, John Wankland in Western Australia, Graham Mouse in Sydney, and Phil Prick in the UK, please take a bow. The world is now aware of your actions which I had warned you about and you must be made responsible for your own actions. The power of the media and peer pressure all based on a total scam of fear and pandemic mistruths and with the sheeple like I have named above quickly has got us to where we are sadly today with the very high vaccination rates here in Australia.

Mass Hypnosis is everywhere and is alive and well, especially in Australia, with some people in such a state of paranoia that some are still wearing face masks and still believing this poison worked. They say they had five jabs and yet they admit having also had C19 up to five times; and they simply will not ever work out that the vaccine does not, and the vaccines never did work, and when asked the reasons 'why they respond with comments like this "because I would Have died if I got C19'. Well in a word you are already brain dead and what is the definition of madness is continuing to do the same thing expecting a different result, like the vaccines might work one day.

There is no hope for them "Dumb and Dumber" and simply speaking, this always was Agenda 2030, an evil plan created by the New World Order; and that C19 is a political cover up causing the greatest genocide and financial collapse in the history of the World. Even in small countries like Norway they have reported deaths 18% above the usual averages in 2022, and this has only just started and once they have started to achieve this population reduction, which is already happening and you will be subjected to live in lockdown conditions due to their Climate Lockdowns in their not Smart Cities. When you compare the deaths above the average, the once bad boy Sweden now has the lowest excess deaths from Wuhan coronavirus (COVID-19) among many nations worldwide because it did not impose lockdowns and kept schools open.

So, stand up together and say NO, we have all had enough, and so many of us are aware that they want to eradicate most of us because they class us all simply as 'Livestock'. They satanically plan to have complete control of individuals through brainwashing and fear and with the destruction of private enterprise and the abolishment of constitutional protections, they will also outlaw guns and demolish Religion, as the NWO do not believe in God because they worship only Satan.

This excerpt is taken from the 1981 book by Bilderberger Jacques Attali, then an advisor to François Mitterrand, and is an example of their mindset: "The future will be about finding a way to reduce the population. We start with the old, because as soon as they exceed 60-65 years, people live longer than they produce and that costs society dearly. Then the weak, then the useless that do not help society because there will always be more of them, and above all, ultimately, The Stupid. [So, are you the stupid?]

Euthanasia will be targeting these groups, euthanasia will have to be an essential tool in our future societies, in all cases. With TeleHealth Queensland you can book an appointment to discuss Euthansia and it is another part of the Agenda you do not need to commit suicide anymore they will help you legally. Of course, we will not be able to execute people or build camps [sadly he got that wrong, with our wellness camps here in Queensland and around the world]. We will get rid of them by making them believe that it is for their own good as overpopulation, and mostly uselessness, is something that is too costly economically and socially as it is much better when the human machine comes to an abrupt stand still than when it gradually deteriorates. Neither will we be able to test millions upon millions of people for their intelligence, you bet that and sadly reading that to me it is as clear as mud we were basically always "Livestock" to dispose of when they wish, dependent on their own levels of critical thinking. There is a saying that you truly are the master of your own destiny and intellect does not necessarily mean you are smart, especially if you have attended those brainwashing universities, that set you up for a life of complying and doing as you were told but not all who attended university are compliant and thankfully, some I am very proud to call my friends. So, I'm going to try to end this chapter on a high note which is Vibration and the seven things that can affect your vibration frequency from the point of view of quantum physics. Vibration in quantum physics basically means everything is energy and we are vibrant beings on certain frequencies, every vibration is equivalent to a feeling and in the World, there are two species of vibrations: Positive and Negative and any feeling makes you broadcast an agitation; it's a vibration that affects their zombified brains. Which is why occasionally I get physically attacked but more often on a daily basis I get the usual rude finger, a sign that they are not happy with the sound of my harmonica and maybe the state of happiness I am in also noticing it with some children, which I did not notice when those children were not vaccinatedIt's all because of vibration and the (GO) plays a part in of the above, some days when I play the harmonica it can be hard to get a "Smiley Face" especially in the elderly, but when I do and then start a conversation with that person and will often find that they are a pure blood (unvaccinated) or they are unaffected by the toxic vaccines that they have had. Sadly, it is only going to get a lot worse as the levels of (GO) in the bodies of the vaccinated are increased and the 5G frequency is turned up. Many normal, healthy people are full of vitality, and because we do look healthy, we really do stand out. We are fitter, you will notice we are laughing and seem very happy, and people have also mentioned to me that they always seem to be yawning and tired and go to sleep like they are elderly although some are still very young.

The personality changes can be very alarming, especially when they are a family member or close friend and recently, we had some doctors speaking at an event in Sandgate, Queensland at a brave warrior establishment and it was very noticeable that the vaccinated public were not a bit interested as they walked past listening to information that might help save their lives.

I have attempted to write this book for those who are still asleep after 3 years and waking them up is going to be extremely hard but I truly feel I must try because to see young people who were very healthy before going into decline health wise, since there were vaccinated especially when there is a person you know well, family member or friend, it is extremely distressing and not admitting that they were wrong, and just say I am sorry and regret being so gullible and then we can help them. A common theme in this book is repetition of keywords like: **Graphene Oxide (GO), 5G, Marburg, Spike Protein, Zombism, Agenda 2030 and Covid-19 (C19).**

I have done this on purpose simply because those few words are the ingredients for your early demise and I have spoken to few doctors who agree and you got to remember that these doctors are people who have walked away from big salaries because they believe 100% that their beliefs are and will be proven correct, and that is unless you really work hard to try to fix some of the damage that has been done and especially after 3 vaccines or more then the chances of your natural survival for long will be greatly limited.

Over three years on we have all seen all this play out exactly as it was intended and nations leaders around the World are culpable in this 'The Final Solution' as history always repeats. Writing this comes with the responsibility it does carry but I will not try to sugar coat it as it's tragic watching this play out and not one person who is a pureblood reader wants to be correct that this nightmare we predict will ever come true and that critical thinking is saving us from the future you who were not so prudent will not have. Often, I would say how very lucky that I was to be born in times of no wars like my forefathers, and how wrong was I that this is the biggest 'War' that mankind has and will ever face: the Spiritual War, Good over Evil, God against the Devil, so when this is finally over what side of history do you really want to be talked about.

Do you want to be spoken in centuries to come as the one who sat on your hands while "The World Burned" because I see it especially in the younger generation who maybe we spoiled too much but is it also because of a lot of one parent upbringing? if I sound very harsh good because for many generations real men stood and fought in many wars like the Boer War, W.W1, WW2, Korea, Vietnam, Iraq and more recently Afghanistan and were away for years fighting for the greater good of mankind and paid the ultimate sacrifice and are now living in graves far, far away, or coming back with injuries physically and mentally. You might think you look tough with your tattoos and piercings when walking your tiny dogs but you're very mentally weak, so if there is a flicker of bravery in you wake up then stand up and fight alongside us then the future race will not judge you accordingly like the cowards you currently are. For me it has always been about the children because we all dust so what happens to me is not important but to give them a future is paramount in the scheme of things. Stand Up for Freedom Today. And Free **Julian Assange**, a real Australian Hero and not those cowards in Government who could have helped him but sat on their hands for very obvious reasons.

Chapter 2

Graphene Oxide - The EMF Conductor

I have been fortunate to have been around the music industry for over four decades as an DJ, Entertainer and currently a bike-riding, harmonica playing clown. Music is so powerful that if you listen about death and destruction it will interfere in what you are thinking, and it will lower your Vibration. Remember you are what you think because of your setting "Intentions". Life is all frequency, and in all frequencies, it is so very important in understanding about the 4G & 5G agendas and how it conducts through the (GO) that is in the Vaccines for reasons that should be very clear by now. This will be the basis of this chapter but please smile and be happy, and you will understand that it makes logical sense when you're in a good mental place and understanding of this life will be much easier. It is so important to understand that for this Plandamic Agenda to work they need you to have this 'Gene Therapy Toxins' in your body, because the Graphene Oxide is the conductor for the EMFs to be able to work, especially when they turn on their 5G towers and turn up the frequencies.

These 5G towers are popping up everywhere and even my local hospital in Redcliffe, Queensland, has three of these 5G evil towers on the roof. Graphene is a single layer of carbon atoms, tightly bound in a honeycomb lattice. Graphene is a single layer of carbon atoms, tightly bound in a honeycomb lattice. It's an allotrope of carbon that was discovered in 2004 when researchers at University of Manchester isolated a single plane of graphite (Graphene) using a kind of scotch tape. This 2D material revealed properties that lend to several applications in electronics, remote sensing, medicine, quantum computing. It is stronger than a diamond yet more flexible and transparent. Graphene conducts heat and electricity and is super tough, so much so that it is used for

Bio-devices, Biosensors, Human Tissue Scaffolds, Drug delivery and Gene Therapy Vectors. Does that not ring some Alarm Bells? and if it does not? Then you really do and will have a big problem because your health and your family's health are at stake. Graphene Oxide (GO) is the main ingredient used in Hydrogels developed by DARPA and used in all the Covid Vaccines. Graphene Oxide was first added in the flu vaccines in 2019 and are in all vaccines currently being made which all your loved ones will be subjected to and why would you ever put any vaccines into a newborn when you truly understand about their innate natural immunity. They have created a two-dimensional nanomaterial which is graphene oxide nanoparticles) and found that it displayed potent adjuvant (immunoenhancing) effects on influenza vaccines that are delivered intranasally.

They also claim that (GO) is the chemical of the future, and it is going to be in everything, in all our Foods and Water, also (GO) has a direct effect on human neurons, and they can be controlled from the outside with a magnetic field apparatus. Graphene technology, using external fields to self-actuate in the body, makes it prone to over-stimulate then inflame the body due to background EMF radiation (4G LTE and 5G cell towers and IoT gadgets). " This is a mass, uniformed, without consent global experiment. They never been able to get this into humans on an experimental basis before and no human subject review board would ever approve of protocols with this stuff in it." Dr. Jane Ruby mentioned they were conducting tests on (GO) and its effects on human cells and specifically, it was a dose-finding study to see how much (GO) they can put in a human body before it becomes Toxic.

This is a direct correlation to what Karen Kingston, a former Pfizer employee and current analyst for the pharmaceutical and medical device industries, discussed on the Stew Peters Show when referencing (GO) and Covid Vaccines. 'This (Covid Vaccine Campaign) is essentially a dose finding study. They rushed this thing out to see how much of this they can put into people before they die.

Remember we're supposed to get the (GO) boosters every six months to see how much they can build up in our system. Graphene Oxide is everywhere in all the paper masks and in all the PCR tests and according to many reports by very well-established members of the science community that are becoming more apparent in number and the corona vaccine contains at least 98% Graphene Oxide (GO), Lipid Carriers and a piece of viral DNA that is supposed to be used by our own cellular machinery to produce viral proteins for a proposed immunity.

But right now, the corona vaccine is causing **'Blood Clots'** resulting in strokes and fluid retention in the lungs causing death and people who have taken the vaccines and the unvaccinated need to start to remove the (GO) from their body as it is incredibly dangerous and inflammatory. So, it is very important to get this Toxin out of our bodies, because it is inside all of us, vaccinated or not vaccinated and in another chapter on detoxes I will explain how. Now, our biggest concern regarding the ingredients in the vaccines is the Graphene Oxide (GO), which along with the Spike Protein is causing death, while there is a potential for an even greater threat as (GO) absorbs radiation from cell phones and Wi-Fi rendering it more oxidative, destructive and deadlier. Graphene Oxide is magnetic and conducts EMF, (GO) is a semiconductor.

Published information has discussed the fact that (GO) readily absorbs 0.5 to 40 gigahertz EMF, which covers all the 4G, 5G, Wi-Fi and microwave wavelengths and once (GO) absorbs the EMF, it becomes more oxidative and forms more free radicals, increasing the need for Glutathione to be used more as an antioxidant to protect cells and less as a chelator. So, in other words, once (GO) gets into your system, it creates conditions that prevent it from being excreted and Mercury in the human body does the same thing by damaging the organs responsible for excreting it from the human body, the liver and kidneys.

We have listened to many first-hand accounts discussing how (GO) transforms the body into a conductor of EMF (electromagnetic fields) and this can be measured with an EMF metre, and everyone should have one and test their houses and environments. Further to this, I have noticed the EMF increase when vaccinated people grab on to an insulated electric cable, you can test the accuracy of (GO) that causes vaccinated bodies to become magnetised by placing metal objects on people and watching how the metal sticks to human bodies that contain (GO), like a magnet to a fridge. Then see how the EMF field increases and decreases when (GO) loaded people get closer and further away from sources of radiation like Wi-fi and electrical fields and insulated electric cables. I have several different EMF readers and I use them a lot to determine where it is safe for me to enjoy a meal in a restaurant or coffee shop ect. Because if I don't, the effects of the emfs will make me feel very tired and also remember because I am not vaccinated, and because I detox frequently from (GO) it would be very minimal.

So, I will talk more about the ways to reduce it out of your body with NAC because the good news: Now that (GO) has been identified as a contaminant, there are ways to remove (GO) from our bodies and help restore our health. But you need to do this regularly because it is everywhere in our food and water, and you don't have to be vaccinated or have complied with the mask wearing and PCR tests that also have (GO) in them to be affected.

Glutathione is a substance made from the amino acids: glycine, cysteine, and glutamic acid and it is produced naturally by the liver and involved in many of the processes in the body, including tissue building and repair, making chemicals and proteins needed by the body, and for our immune system. We all have a natural glutathione reserve in our bodies, and this is what gives us a very strong immune system but when glutathione levels are high in the body, we have no problems and our immune system functions very well.

But when the amount of (GO) in the body exceeds the amount of glutathione, it causes the collapse of the immune system and triggers a terrible cytokine storm. The way that (GO) can rapidly grow to exceed glutathione in the body is by electronic excitation simply meaning the EMFs that bombard the Graphene to oxidise it, rapidly trigger the diseases. So can you see why I am like a long-playing stuck record, talking about the same two things repeatedly which are. Graphene Oxide and EMF'S. It will only take these two monsters to bring your health down very quickly as you will have seen in some of your friends and family members.

By the age of 65. Glutathione levels fall drastically in the body and this would explain why the population most affected by these Covid-19 bioweapons are the elderly with glutathione levels which are very low and in people with pre-existing health conditions such as diabetes, obesity, etc. Likewise, glutathione levels are very high in infants, children and some athletes so this could explain why C19 has not affected these people as much, it makes simple common sense but sadly so many do not seem to get it. Sadly, there is always a day of reckoning for all our actions, and five minutes of due diligence in researching these vaccines on sites like Yandex.com would stop you from adding even more of these poisons into your bodies. So, many of us have spent so much of our time simply because we love humanity to try to educate you but in return we were labelled 'Conspiracy Theorists' but we did TRY and will continue to TRY as we really care about YOU call it "Cruel Love" when I use very strong words and statements that I truly believe in 100%. I don't give up on anybody if they simply admit they were wrong and say "Please Help Me John" and then I will even if they have been cruel to me in the last three years, so love and blessings to all you for who am I to judge. Graphene Oxide when oxidised or activated by specific EMF frequencies overruns the body's ability to create enough glutathione, which destroys the immune system and causes the illness you are currently experiencing (such as Covid symptoms and all the "Variants").

Ricardo Delgado stated that these antioxidants eliminate the Graphene Oxide and when you understand that this is paramount, you need to continue to keep it out of your body as much as possible. He has personally helped people affected by magnetism after inoculation. This is in people with just only two doses of Pfizer who have become magnetic and after these supplements they no longer have this symptom. We are all surrounded by EMF radiation from Mobile Phones, TVs and Wi-Fi and many areas around the World are turning on their 5G and there have been investigations showing the correlation between the 5G networks and the Covid outbreaks in a certain area and to best protect yourself from (GO) poisoning and the activation of (GO) in your body it is necessary to do several things to limit your EMF exposure.

Some of the suggestions on how to do this include: do not live in a city with a lot of towers if you can help it, which is becoming nigh on impossible, turn off your Wi-Fi at night, and stay away from smart metres and other smart devices. If possible, put your mobile phones on aeroplane mode especially when they are near your body. I also strongly recommend you use EMF protection products such as orgone energy devices, to help transform the EMF radiation to mitigate the harmful effect Anti-Radiation Stickers for 4G phones Quantum Shields are not expensive and do the job but for 5G, you will need a Shungite sticker (costing around $8). I have been testing these products for about two years and also sell a lot of EMF readers and I would strongly recommend everyone to have one and get used to using them.

Your life could depend on it. They can be expensive and the easiest one and best value I find is Erick hill RT 100 available on Amazon for $100 but are a lot cheaper in the US, and this metre simultaneously measures and displays Magnetic Field, Electric Field. The Measurement and the measurement types are expressed in units of electrical and magnetic field strength and power density. Also, this metre is ideal for EMF measurements of power lines, electrical appliances, industrial devices, cell phones, base stations, and microwave leakage and this device is shipped fully tested and calibrated and, with proper use, will provide years of reliable service. This metre is used to indicate radiated electromagnetic fields wherever there is a voltage, current, electric (E) or magnetic (H) field. Examples include the electromagnetic fields from radio broadcasting, TV transmitters and power lines. Electric Field Strength This is a field vector quantity that represents the force (F) on an infinitesimal unit positive test charge (q) at a point divided by that charge. Electric field strength is expressed in units of volts per metre (V/m). The Electromagnetic fields propagate as waves and travel at the speed of light (c). The wavelength is proportional to the frequency. λ (wavelength) = c (speed of light) Near-field is assumed if the distance to the field source is less than three wavelengths. For far-fields, the distance is more than three wavelengths.In the near-field, the ratio of electric field strength (E) and magnetic field strength (H) is not constant, so measure each separately. In the far-field, however, it is enough to measure one field quantity, and compute the other accordingly.

It could explain the brain fog when you wake up and remember if you are vaccinated you are at much higher risk due to the higher levels of (GO) build-up in your bodies, which I have tried to explain and the obvious reasons why, then I would also suggest moving your bed if there is a power source close by. But there are also options such as Grounding Pillow Cases which I have had for a while. You plug them into your power source and ground the pillowcase because protecting your brain is paramount, there are also grounding sheets and grounding mats.

I would recommend checking them all out to protect you and your family's brains. I use a lot of Shungite, which is a great EMF blocker, and have a large piece on my bed, and near the front door, and I am permanently wearing shungite necklaces and bracelets and I also wear a Harmony protection pendant, some of you might be wearing different products like Tesla. They all are very beneficial in stopping the attempts to **'MICROWAVE YOUR BRAIN'.** This is such an Important Topic: I cannot stress enough the dangers of EMF combined with (GO) and the reason why I am doing a whole chapter on this attempt to zombify us all and how to eliminate it out of our bodies, but the best Emf blocker and so very special that I personally buy so many kilos of it is called Shungite. It is important to test the shungite with a multimeter to see if it is real because there is a lot of fake shungite as it can only be obtained from the Karelia region of Russia and is it not ironic that Russia is fighting this evil agenda with us all. In 2017 research also suggests that a fullerene-based compound within shungite has an antioxidant and anti-inflammatory action against UVB-induced skin damage.

What Is Shungite? shungite is a black, lustrous mineral that is made of more than 98% carbon in elite shungite; it was first discovered in the Karelia region of Russia near the Shunga village; shungite was first given the name in the late 1800s. I will also speak more on this very important topic in another chapter as it is very complex understanding the 3 types of this carbon and its benefits. Many crystal shops stock it at around $5 for the more common shungite, a small piece to put in your purse or wallet which I strongly recommend. There is also elite shungite which is very rare and a lot more expensive and I will also talk about making Shungite Water. All these topics I will cover in more detail in the detox chapter as I actively treat my own body daily and we are not spiritually old till we are 100 but if we are to get there living on this "Hell on Earth" then we must help ourselves. **Please note all the natural therapies I recommend in this book are suggestions only, I am thankfully not a Compliant Doctor but someone who is very cautious about what I put into my own body.** Some of you reading this when I talk about spirituality and who do attend a church and take the bible literally will probably not understand the ''Proof of Existence'' and will have closed minds on this subject. In fact, last year at a local church, I was told I was not welcome because I spoke about these subjects, and I was reminded that I was worshipping the devil. Oh, those of closed minds when unvaccinated religious /spiritual people like me who are judged and not welcome in some churches simply because they discriminate against us who are spiritual and who believe in the power of a high force. Ironically you were judged by your own churches when you were not vaxxed, masked or would not check in and then you judge me. I often pray to the universe, and it rarely lets me down and I truly feel a higher force is guiding me to write this book and there is a Len Barry song "The Moving Finger Writes" and as I am not a natural writer, it is not my calling, but we can only try.

If just one person reading this is saved then I have achieved something, as Schindler wrote "You Save One Soul You Save The World" and I hope that soul is you. Over forty years ago I lived on 'Kibbutz Beit Guvrin' formed by Turkish holocaust survivors. It was a non-religious kibbutz, and they did not believe in God. I learned a lot in my six months there and visiting Yad Vashem, the holocaust museum in Jerusalem. It has taught me history does repeat, some of them had no choice when walking into the gas chamber and being poisoned but you do? There is a distinct correlation between Zyklon B and these Poisons and it is basically the "Final Solution" because nations are bankrupt and they can't have you living to a great old age.

So it is very logical to understand the agenda that there as to be a "Final Solution" and that all the useless bottom feeders the old, the infirmed, the aborigines and the mentally deranged needed to be gotten rid of and what better way was there but to cause a Pandemic and use all there tools in their tool box. Which are the Governments, Churches, TV and Media just to name a few and it's working just watch the death rates above the average climb year on year. We did warn you, but we are not Conspiracy Theorists which is actually wrong. Try instead using the words "Truth Seekers" and everything we predict will come to pass as Agenda 2030 is plain to see it's right under your Nose.

Chapter 3

The Spike Protein

The Spike protein present in the Wuhan coronavirus C19 vaccines is one of the most bioactive and potentially the most damaging substances known to mankind. It penetrates the blood-brain barrier, cell nucleus and even affects your DNA replication. The spike protein appears to reprogram the immune system in a very strange way as the BNT162b2 mRNA vaccine against the C19 virus has been shown to reprogram both adaptive and innate immune responses. When it penetrates the cell nuclei, the free-floating spike protein inhibits DNA repair and if any mutations to the spike protein of the Covid virus occur in the future, the vaccinated will be even more vulnerable and may possibly be unprotected due to their inability to produce the N antibody. I have talked about this in my book published in 2021 John Warren "Our Soul Music Journeys" on Amazon. So meanwhile, the unvaccinated would have much better immunity to any mutations due to their ability to produce both S and N antibodies after infection." First, These Vaccines Mis-Train' the immune system to recognize only a small part of the virus [the spike protein]. Variants that may differ, even slightly, in this protein are able to escape the narrow spectrum of antibodies created by the vaccines," Secondly the vaccines create **'vaccine addicts'** meaning people who become dependent upon regular booster shots because they have been vaccinated only against a tiny portion of a mutating virus. The Spike Protein was always going to be a major issue and, in my chapter, later in detoxing I will explain how to attempt to do this, but like anything this is evolving so very rapidly with so many vaccinated getting sick and if you had more than two vaccines it is naturally a lot harder to fix the damage that the Spike Protein has been created in your body, but you will do anything if you're unwell enough, so do not ever give up.

Cancer's return is very prevalent and happened with my own mother Lilian living in Rushden, Northamptonshire UK. Her cancer had been dormant for decades but returned with a vengeance after her second vaccine of AstraZeneca which has just been banned in Australia in March 2023 and to say I am angry and upset would be an understatement and I am sure so many of you can relate similar stories of your loved parents and so many of you may have your parents with you today if they maybe had listened to you and that is so tragically sad when often because you were unvaxxed you were not even allowed to even say "Goodbye". I will talk about this more in a later chapter because of the high incidence of cancers today that are being diagnosed, many of them sadly are stage four and are classified as Turbo Cancers.

Vaccinated individuals have also encountered many immune problems and reinfections and these conditions, dubbed VAIDS (or Vaccine Acquired Immune Deficiency Syndrome), have been very concerning as they could be damaging to individuals. "Professor Luc Montagnier, a Nobel Prize winner for medicine for his discovery of the human immunodeficiency virus (HIV) said himself that those who received the third dose of Co-Vid19 vaccines should go to the laboratory and take an AIDS test, then sue their governments. The legal cases will mount as this calamity on mankind unfolds as Pfizer itself has a long list of possible adverse events from its vaccines, with nine pages of side effects and illnesses which are barely scratching the surface.

Understanding Immune Deficiency New York-based physician Dr.Vladimir "Zev" Zelenko warned that anyone with immunodeficiency can die from a common illness like a cold. Vladimir sadly passed away in 2022 from Lung cancer? aged "If someone has an immune deficiency, then yes, they can die from a cold. And they're going to die in a moment. Some of you reading this will not understate the importance of our innate immune system and how our body recognizes things and can fight them off.

I personally don't have any medications in my body or any vaccines like the flu vaccine and I rarely get sick with a cold or the flu. But we all get sick occasionally and five years ago I was diagnosed with Aspergilloma, a 'Fungus Ball' which was a fungus in my lung, and it was very daunting coughing sometimes tablespoons of blood. I had to have two bronchoscopies at Prince Charles Hospital in Brisbane, to look at doing a partial lung removal. But I then took control of my own body and destiny, and I then took Cbd Oil and exercised my lungs for up to 4 hours a day whistling and playing a harmonica and my lungs have finally recovered but it took several years, to the point the lung specialist has recently discharged me in October 2022.

When I had mentioned how I had achieved it, the specialists were not interested in alternative therapies and because I was not wearing a mask in the hospital, they could not wait to get rid of me. I am sure many of you reading this also have not trusted the traditional medications and have taken non-traditional medicines instead. So, returning to VAIDS, Doctors are calling this phenomenon 'immune erosion' or 'acquired immune deficiency,' accounting for elevated incidence of Myocarditis and other post-vaccine illnesses that either affects the vaccinated more rapidly, resulting in death or more slowly, resulting in chronic illness,"and it is a major concern for countries like Australia and New Zealand which are "Prison Islands" with are very high vaccination rates. I was always aware that we had a lot of sheep here and that were exported to the world for decades, and when I was a child living in the UK, we often enjoyed New Zealand lamb. But the Sheepism has been very contagious amongst a lot of you all and what has happened to the Anzac Spirit? Surely over 100,000 that died for our freedoms, must sadly be turning over in those graves in far-off lands because of a lack of moral fibre in some of the vaccinated. I will talk more about the "Freedom Movement" in the next chapter as we all saw the incredible scenes from the Canberra rallies and it's just a shame a million freedom fighters.They had to do the heavy lifting for the rest of you sitting home warm and cosy watching your TV'S while so many of us are fighting for your children and our grandchildren's futures are not gone forever.

Shedding sadly, this topic affects all of us, the vaccinated and the unvaccinated, and has put a strain on many relationships? and there will be many who are reading this who have banned their partners from their bedrooms? due to the concerns about their health being affected by shedding. I truly believe they are correct and in fact I have publicly spoken about the non-sharing of body fluids, and I practise what I preach, and have been celibate for several years as the words throat, tongue and cervical cancers will be on many people's lips in the near future. Mens sperm samples collected from three fertility clinics in Israel show that Fauci Flu shots fight against men's reproductive capacity, rendering them impotent and in some cases sexless which was always one the Agenda's. So, is unvaccinated seamen the new bitcoin?

Evidence also shows that vaccinated adults are more likely to transmit SARS-CoV-2 infection to their children who live in the same household. Researchers from the University of Colorado detected the presence of SARS-CoV-2 specific IgGs and IgAs in swab samples taken from children who live with fully vaccinated parents. Children who live in unvaccinated households are less likely to have SARS-CoV-2 specific antibodies in their nasal passageways and saliva. This evidence also shows that children who are unvaccinated could be developing specific immune responses to the spike proteins that vaccinated people are shedding through their skin and into the air. This could be the reason for the uptick in SARS-CoV-2 specific antibodies in nasal passageways and the saliva of children. Traditionally in vaccinology, this non-consensual process of transmission is referred to as "Viral Shedding." In Pfizer's own study design documents, researchers were concerned with the possibility of "occupational exposure" and warned that caretakers and close contacts of the recently vaccinated could be exposed to the spike proteins that are translated and synthesised in their cells. These toxic nanoparticles circulate throughout the body, cause damage to organs, and may shed through the skin. Unvaccinated children could be affected by this shedding process, and the SARS-CoV-2 specific antibodies in children could be evidence that they were previously by the heavily vaccinated adult population.

This leads us to the topic of a **Placebo** as we are all aware they used them in the clinical trials but is it not possible? that they were used in the actual vaccine centres? We all can surely hope so because most of my family worldwide are vaccinated and my love for them is unconditional and you naturally worry about them and their futures. With my own daughter, who is unvaccinated, the fear is not quite so bad; but it came at a great cost for her as Beauticians were in the front line of discrimination, and the owner of a beauty salon in Sandgate, Queensland should now hang her head in shame. My daughter's five years of loyal service to the salon counted for nothing; and she was retrenched by text message, possibly because she would never get vaccinated. If you were a doctor who truly held the mantra "Do No Harm" close to your heart, is it possible that the doctor was able to inject patients with a placebo, following a kind of Triage, especially if the patients were young or healthy?

That doctor would also have a big ace up their sleeves and that was the Temperature it had to be stored at and with Pfizer it was -70°C. Also consider that Australia Post delivered them, and it was a "Total Farce" and we are supposed to live in an educated country but this must give you all hope to any of you reading this who only had two vaccines, and I truly pray you really did dodge two bullets? like in the "Matrix" movie. Storage also was so very crucial with the Temperatures it had to be stored at with Pfizer and Moderna vaccines having very different storage requirements. The Pfizer vaccine must be kept at a frigid -70°C while the Moderna vaccine can be kept slightly warmer. Experts say that the Pfizer vaccine's difficult storage requirements could pose challenges during Distribution and in order to ensure the "Efficacy of the Vaccine," people will need to be vaccinated at "centralised locations with access to minus 80 degrees Celsius freezers or dry-ice containers". This equipment is high maintenance in and of itself and dry-ice containers need to be replenished regularly, and dry-ice supply may prove to be difficult to maintain," and she states that, "Doing that in high-income countries like the U.S. is one thing, "Trying to do that in low- and middle-income countries around the world, (with) even a normal 2 to 8 degrees Celsius, refrigerator-like temperature, can be difficult in many parts of the world. So, it's an implementation challenge." Sheila Keating PhD.

When reading that there is logically hope that so many fridges were not maintained correctly? and as this travesty unfolds. It surely has to give us all hope that some of our loved ones only got in essence a Placebo you must feel for the younger generations because of the fear and the stresses that accumulate, and a healthy mind does literally mean a healthy body. What a terrible time for the young today growing up surrounded by so much fear, with parents and grandparents wearing face nappies. What examples are you showing them be very ashamed of your own stupidity as face masks do not and never will work and all you are doing is ending your own demise early as this is why you're encouraged to wear them. These parents are supposed to set good examples and not buy into fear and spread that fear like washing your hands constantly, and anyone and I do repeat myself a lot, who have vaccinated their children and have encouraged their children to do so to protect them or their grandparents over a cold and must truly hold their heads in shame, and you will go to your graves early, having destroyed the total innate immune systems of your loved ones forever after only 3 of these vaccines. Why do educated people who send their children to private schools as they have the means to do so are yet too lazy to have not studied that C19 basically was never a threat to their children and is just an mRNA experiment for a cold but still did the unthinkable and vaccinated them it truly beggar's belief.

We all have seen footage of children who are spiritually aware screaming that they did not want it, and I truly hope any of you reading this who are really are upset by my word's because you should never have ever been a parent if you injected your children with this poison. The peer pressure on unvaccinated children in school classes also really bothers me, and them noticing the behavioural changes in their vaccinated school mates. Home-schooling looms for them as a better option to protect their sanity.

Increasingly unvaccinated single women are avoiding single men who got "vaccinated" for the Wuhan coronavirus Covid-19) as they are concerned about the "shedding" of vaccine spike proteins through physical contact, unvaccinated single women are, in some cases, calling it quits as far as the modern dating scene goes. This is also causing severe relationship problems in marriages, and it is very common for me to have a lady who confides in me, and I have never ever seen such a breakdown in marriages that are often 20 years and more in standing and the issue mostly concerns sex with "Fully Vaccinated Men" something that is no longer an option for many unvaccinated women who are trying to protect their bodies against the Fauci Flu shot. It naturally causes hostility in some men like "most disgruntled, hostile men," who would seem to be those who "succumbed to the vaccine by force" meaning men who did not necessarily want to get jabbed but were forced to in order to maintain employment, for instance. Feeling penalised twice over for a vaccine they never wanted to begin with, many of these men don't handle these women's rejection very well. Guilt, annoyance, and just plain rudeness are known to occur in relation to these women's decision to stay committed to their stance."

To be fair, Unvaccinated men face the very same thing with "Fully Vaccinated" Women, many of whom militantly support the jabs and look down on men who just said no to experimental drugs from the government and Big Pharma. It is an act of self-preservation by both men and women who skipped the jabs to avoid other men and women who opted to take the shots and who are now shedding spike proteins and who knows what else. In many ways, it is better to just remain single than to couple up with someone who allowed his or her immune system to be destroyed by this and the reason I am and will remain celibate, as I walk the talk and the only leg over I get is when I throw my leg over my push bike. The more this disaster unfolds the more daunting it seems to get we all heard of lady's well out menopause and that it was restarted due to shedding, or because of the potency of the male sperm, because troubling now is female cervical cancer and is there a direct linkage due to the contaminated sperm. Men will also show up with cancer of the tongue and throat as "Dining at the Y" and enjoying the nectar of the gods does pose many risks with vaccinated females. But marriages are worth fighting for when the person you married did it to keep food on the table for you and their loved ones so, please "Do Not Give Up on Them and try to reverse some of the damage it has caused. It also should be noted not everyone who had 3 vaccines will be the same. It is possible that you could have dodged "3 bullet's" especially if you got powerful spiritual guides because I met some who seem very normal even though they had 3 stabs, there is always hope.

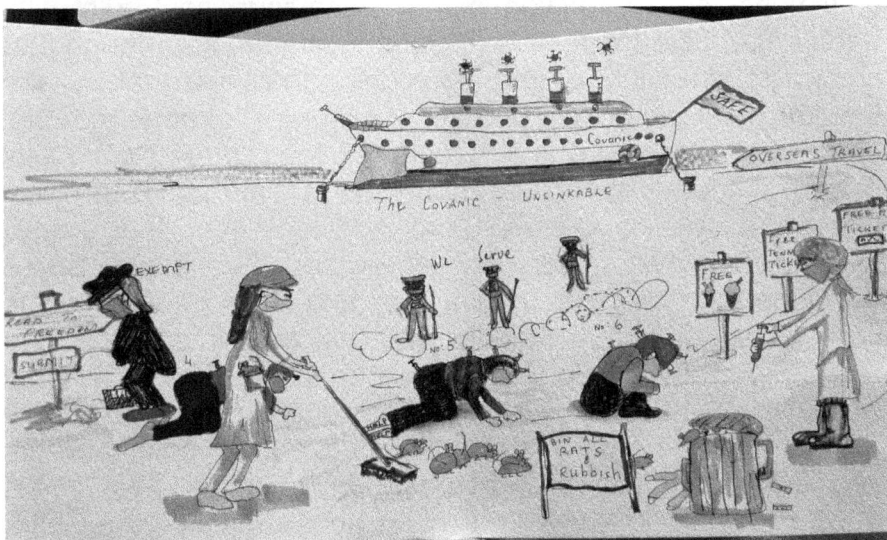

We Sink The Covanic © Harmonica Man

Chapter 4

Cognitive Dissonance

This is such an important part played out in this total hogwash for a lot of you will be aware of "Operation Paperclip." Operation Paperclip was a secret United States intelligence program in which more than 1,600 German scientists, engineers, and technicians were taken from the former Nazi Germany to the U.S. for government employment after the end of World War II in Europe, between 1945 and 1959. There would have been people very specialised in MIND CONTROL who would have helped in creating Cognitive Dissonance and we all have to be confused how easy people were sheep-controlled in such a short time frame worldwide over basically a cold, it is abundantly clear the brainwashing has worked and that is why on the book cover I feature the main reason that the TV (Idiot Box) caused C19.

Cognitive Dissonance was first coined by Leon Festinger in the 1950s, describing the discomfort people feel when two cognitions, or a cognition and a behaviour, contradict with each other. Like I smoke is dissonant with the knowledge that smoking can kill me and to reduce that dissonance, the smoker must either quit or justify smoking ("It keeps me thin, and being overweight is a health risk too, you know"). At its core, Festinger's theory is about how people strive to make sense out of contradictory ideas and lead lives that are, at least in their own minds, consistent and meaningful. So as with Con-Vid: I recently met a lady and often people can be very intelligent (but she sadly was not) I commented on the Spanish Flu and straight away in a nanosecond she stated it was started by "rats." She still passionately believed in this plandemic and how much she believed in this whole charade, and if I spent a year trying to debate it with her, I would get nowhere because 'down the rabbit hole she has gone' a bit like in Alice in Wonderland and never to return.

World-wide you will believe what you believe and sadly if you still watch the TV and if you disagree with these words, I can guarantee you do watch the TV news religiously and buy into the facade. I will also guarantee you will buy newspapers and use fact checkers often because a 'Lie to us is the Truth to Them' and that what they do watch on TV and they will never admit the truth that they could die or be disabled from this toxic poison? I sadly see this a lot, and they still believe it was never those vaccines that did it and even if they do admit it they make an absurd comment like "I am on this Train" which for you is actually "The Auschwitz Train Mark 11" and even after some of you would have had your cancers return or family members die from the vaccines you still line up for the next clot shot so what is wrong with you? and how many of you will be honest and true to yourself and would really admit there is a linkage, and it was properly the vaccine that has ignited its return and here is the linkage SV-40 vector is a chimeric Bio Weapon found in the J&J patent. It's known to cause rapid cancer growth. The SV-40 vector is provided to J&J by Thermo Fisher. SV-40 contains Human cells, Bovine Growth Hormone (Mad Cow Disease), E. coli, and Herpes. This would explain the Herpes outbreaks after "vaccination". The Pfizer patent also mentions gene 144 deletion which causes rapid cancer growth""

Until you accept responsibility for your own actions, we properly cannot help you, because you will not want us to, so you will continue to walk towards your own very sad demise "into your own Gas Chamber as history repeats." Please wake up and if you still believe in Covid19 I would bet you believe that men 'Walked on the Moon' and in that Lego craft seriously, and yet they have not managed to ever return funny all these years on because it never ever happened in the first place. It would test your belief systems and the power of that TV (Gogglebox) and a bit like you believing in Google, it is often a false reality and that two planes could crash into the Twin Towers in NY, flown by Saudi Arabian pilots who have only been trained on single engines and just like that, two structures fall down.

That also never happened, it is a bit like the illusionist who can create an illusion in his world of Magic, and I would suggest that 75% of people that believed they truly happened, would still even today, after three years of being scammed by this, Pandemic still will line up for the next Pandemic. Which is already planned and sadly coming, there is no method in their total madness is there? Even writing about this total genocide they will always believe it was for the greater good of mankind? So, if you believe in holding the hands of evil and by doing this you're playing into the hands of Lucifer, The Freemason's, The Jesuits, and all the cults who have beliefs in paedophilia, which we are all aware is a very sick psychiatric disorder, in which an adult or older adolescents experience a primary or exclusive sexual attraction to prepubescent children.

Please note there are some who are Freemasons who might just be naive and not truly aware as we the pure bloods are and for that they should be given the benefit of the doubt. This Agenda is trying to normalise these sick acts and the catholic church and some of their priests love to wear red shoes, a kind of advertising their sexual perversions. In the media of course, paid by satanic people they are really trying hard to make this the new normal, so be aware in every street there could be one lurking so be very aware and protect your children because with grooming and the internet they will do anything they can to satisfy their sickness. I would think it would be very hard to cure this evil and they need de-sexing like we do animals? These vaccines are the Mark of the Beast when you understand the Bible and the book of Revelation, and this very sad topic is also the sickness of this satanic New World Order they hold no bounds to what they want you to accept.

If you do not wake up soon, you will be living in their smart cities travelling the small distances under the guise of climate lock down, eating their bugs and their modified foods enhanced with mind altering ingredients like (GO), accepting the new norm with all its evilness.

You are living in their Matrix, all controlled for a reason, and it has all been well planned for many decades and it has sadly got you to where we all are today, having so much: an expensive car, house, family and all the luxuries that should be making you happy? But how many are truly happy but in reality, you have nothing, you're losing your Freedoms, your Minds and ultimately your Souls and you will truly "Own Nothing and Be Happy" is the mantra cry of the NWO and their programming for the reality that will be happening real soon. I am seeing that when riding around the Moreton Bay region of Queensland, on my push bike with my coloured hair living in my own high vibration, attracting like-minded souls through the power of synchronicity. But I also see written all over so many faces of total unhappiness, from those of you who complied and got vaccinated with these toxic poisons and are not very well physically, mentally and emotionally and what will make you happy? as you look very dubbed down. I believe eventually they will bring in new laws making it a new norm as in Thailand that Marijuana use is legal? that might cheer you up for a while? to comply more.

Then you will take more of these mind-altering poisons that never were a vaccine. Cognitive Dissonance is alive and well here in prison Australia with a high compliance rate. I was very proud to have to migrated here from Northamptonshire, UK, but I have to be brutally honest: I am ashamed that the Anzac spirit we all saw at Gallipoli is long gone and we are the laughing stock of the Western world due to our Vaccination compliance similar to Thailand where I having lived a lot where the vaccination rates are also very high, a friend of mine his wife works in 1400 people company and she is the only one not vaccinated, but they are used to complying, where as we Aussies with are "she be alright mate" attitude have meekly let all those freedoms that the Anzacs fought and died for, erode away basically over a cold.

The road back to regain that freedom is going to be a long one and me writing this book even under my pen name could end in my demise.

But am I truly scared Hell no; but if it was announced that I died because of C19 that did not happen or committed suicide by hanging by the door handle that also will not have happened but bring it on bang gong because I am ready. My own destiny has been decided spiritually to continue to walk in my own shoes, holding my head up and being able to look in the faces of my loved ones and say I really tried. There are so many freedom fighters around the world, pure blood warriors you will see them at all the rally's, many are of the spectrum with dreadlocks and coloured hair and they stand out with their individuality, they are passionate about one word Freedom. We stand up as one and protest peacefully, and the police in Qld have been very kind? but in another chapter I talk about paid opposition, which is another illusion, so was that the real reason and why did the police leave us alone? At protest rallies nothing ever is what it seems and the reason I often supported these events but maintained a low profile but not anymore .

Do you really understand how far you've been dehumanised when I see you while riding my bike, running and sitting in your cars wearing your face nappies? Humans have been wearing face masks for thousands of years as part of rituals, and cultural practices and celebrations. During the plague, the doctors began using beak-like face masks as a form of protection and in the early 20th century the early forms of surgical face masks became popular in surgical settings. Today, we are encouraged to use face masks to protect ourselves from infectious diseases and in some parts of the world, from pollution.

Even though face masks are 'in' and may even turn into a new 'fashion accessory.' God forbid. You may wonder about their effectiveness against germs and illness. This is what I am going to try and discuss here, by going over some scientific facts related to face masks, infectious diseases, and your immune system. Face masks do not work and never did work but the fear installed in you? must affect you mentally? and the need to wear them to feel safe.

Would you have worn them for a common cold? which is C19. There have been extensive randomised controlled trial (RCT) studies, and meta-analysis reviews of RCT studies, which all show that masks and respirators do not work to prevent respiratory influenza like illnesses, or respiratory illnesses believed to be transmitted by droplets and aerosol particles. What we know about viral respiratory diseases, as the main transmission path is long-residence-time aerosol particles (< 2.5 µm), which are too fine to be blocked, and the minimum infective dose is smaller than one aerosol particulate respirators that do not work to prevent respiratory influenza like illnesses, or respiratory illnesses believed to be transmitted by droplets and aerosol particles. How did we get here? The fear and the compliance of so very many to live their privileged lives and do as they're dictated to, when so many others I know had to leave the jobs they dearly loved, and some of them had very large pay salaries like surgeons and doctors but who took the "Oath: do no harm," and because they had a conscience, they have left the medical system. Let's be so proud we have them to give us faith in humanity, that not all in the medical profession are tarred with the same brush. A lot of you reading this would have your own tragic stories of losing jobs in professions that you loved dearly, and they are gone for now but surely sanity must return at some point. But I am also aware some of you will never ever go back and what a brain drain and a loss to society over what was always a cold.

The Australian government and the mongrels running it federal and the states here in Queensland such as the premier 'Pile a Chook' must hold their heads in shame, but the rats are leaving this "Titanic." Only recently New Zealand's Evil PM resigned, but she is only a puppet that they have thankfully cut the cord off and let her hang out to dry? And what evil she has done to New Zealand is sadly going to create its own challenges. We are so fortunate in this part of Queensland, the Redcliffe Peninsula, where Spiritual warriors thrive and are so numerous and is that because of the high vibration and frequency that has drawn us here? Twenty-five years ago, I came for a visit with my ex-wife and we spotted our surname Warren name on the Redcliffe wall, of the ship "Amity" monument that had settled and named Redcliffe, so I personally felt a pull to move here as my name from the UK is very rare, and in phone book in the UK there are not many of that surname. The aboriginal elder for Scarborough, Queensland, a man also named John, his father knew my namesake James Warren, who arrived as sailor on the Amity in 1824 with his wife also Mrs. Warren.

I have been fortunate to have met so many incredibly beautiful people in my life including people who I had lived with before in previous lives and one is Martina Batovska, who is in the book dedication; we were in life number five together I met Martina on December 5, 2021, at Scarborough bowls club, an event for charity. I had donated my book "John Warren "Our Soul Music Journeys' ' as a raffle prize. It was a very strange night, thunder and lighting, and I felt supercharged feeling this spiritually was going to be a very special evening, and how correct I was. I had bought only five raffle tickets and explained to my friends that I was going to win, and I did the 2nd prize, which was $300 which I did not take, and my friends said why? and I replied because I will win again. I did and won the 7th prize, a magnum of champagne. The man who won the 10th prize, which was my book, asked me to sign it. As I signed it this stunning lady Martina looked at me and I looked at her and within five minutes of talking we were in Egypt together, she was explaining she was a "King" and was very traumatised by that past life experience in her words, "I have killed lots of people." When the lights came on at midnight she came over and waved, then when she got to the door, she blew me a kiss and I returned with my own, so very bizarre. We met the next Monday at laughing yoga and for only five weeks before she accidently fell to her death on January 12, 2022. I met Martina a lot sometimes outside her unit in Sutton Street, Redcliffe and we would talk for up to three hours on the phone. She understood that in life number four we had together, she had drowned in 1790 in the UK and she was pregnant in that lifeline, and we had talked about this only four days before she fell to her death. The day before she died, she went to meet clients as Martina was a sales representative for an international property developer and doing very well. We met at lunchtime on the very last day together 11th, January 2021, and when we met, she was very distressed by what had just happened. She had just met two clients that she just sold a property to and was having a drink, when one of the managers of Mon Komo, Redcliffe, asked her to leave "You have not been checking in properly." She stood up and told him, "That is discrimination."" He then assaulted her by pushing her, she then left and took her clients elsewhere and was meeting me shortly after, she looked very distressed when she arrived, so I suggested doing a police report. She said, "Let's not let it spoil the day." We went to the beach, she swam, and then at 6pm I said goodbye never to see her again in this lifetime. I messaged her later that evening before I went to bed and she responded with, "I am still heavily traumatised by today's events."

In the morning I messaged her early before I rode to play my harmonica, and at around 10.30am, my sunglasses exploded on the beach at Sandgate Qld. I have never worn sunglasses again since that day and I never will. I was not aware 20k away she had just fallen to her death five floors down from her balcony in Sutton Street, Redcliffe. When she was in distress, she went into a past life to comfort herself, which she had done on December 24, 2021, when she successfully climbed over that same balcony. I had tried to encourage her to make it safe by putting a code lock on the door only the day before, but her words were always, "I know what I am doing". I rode my bike past her unit at 1.10pm on January 12th, 2022, on that fateful day the police were there, and the body was on the ground thankfully covered up on a stretcher and that told me everything and my heart broke and would she be alive today if it was not for silly check-in laws? I went to the police in Redcliffe Qld who are totally useless, they do not care but my messages from her I was told by the police would go to the coroner so that her death would be recorded as an accident due to sleepwalking. She had slept walked many times before and I often lay flowers on the wall at Sandgate where my sunglasses exploded and will continue to do so. I commissioned a local artist, Gabriel Buckley, a friend, to draw her for this book and to connect with her in-spirit which he did, and he did a great job thank you mate and it's included in the book dedication R.I.P Martina you were too good for this world but you left your mark. Not one person who met you would ever have forgotten your incredible "Aura" and the presence you had. You were a King when we met and died a Queen.

She is in a better place and will continue to be my spirit guide along with my daughter Ethan Elizabeth Warren. Some of you reading this will have your own tragic stories of what lockdowns and absurd checks did to change your lives forever. This is another reason why I am so passionate about standing up for Martina and all the other people who died through this total madness and by writing this book. She is also the spirit guide to another beautiful lady who I will call "The Vase" who was very kind to me and we will continue to help each other through the trauma Martina's passing has caused us both. True Spiritual people I find about 95% would never ever put a vaccine like this in their arms. They are so in touch with their "Inner Self" and really listen to their spirit guides. And if we truly listen, can we not change the destiny of destruction we might have chosen if it not was for them our spirit guides being there for us. Spiritualism, face and palm reading and transgression, are very influential in my current life as I keep evolving. When you are in that "high vibration" which I have already touched on, stay there; do not pick up people's rubbish Ignore them even though they may be judging you; "Just send them love and blessings" One of my friends Koota taught me that, and it has took me so very long to let that sink in because we are conditioned to react, and reaction creates reaction, and then we get into situations that often lead us down a very rocky path and then it takes quite a while to raise vibrations back up to where they were.

It takes a lot of practice, but the sheeple and the zombies want to trigger you and by doing so we become as mad as them. Just try to remember to be kind as they do not know what they do, and their paths are filled with uncertainty and often ill health unless they wake up. If they have not by now, they probably will never ever wake up. Be very thankful you were born not to comply and not to buy into this craziness, and when you find like minded friends nurture them. Appreciate how we can all evolve in this age of Aquarius and spiritual enlightenment.

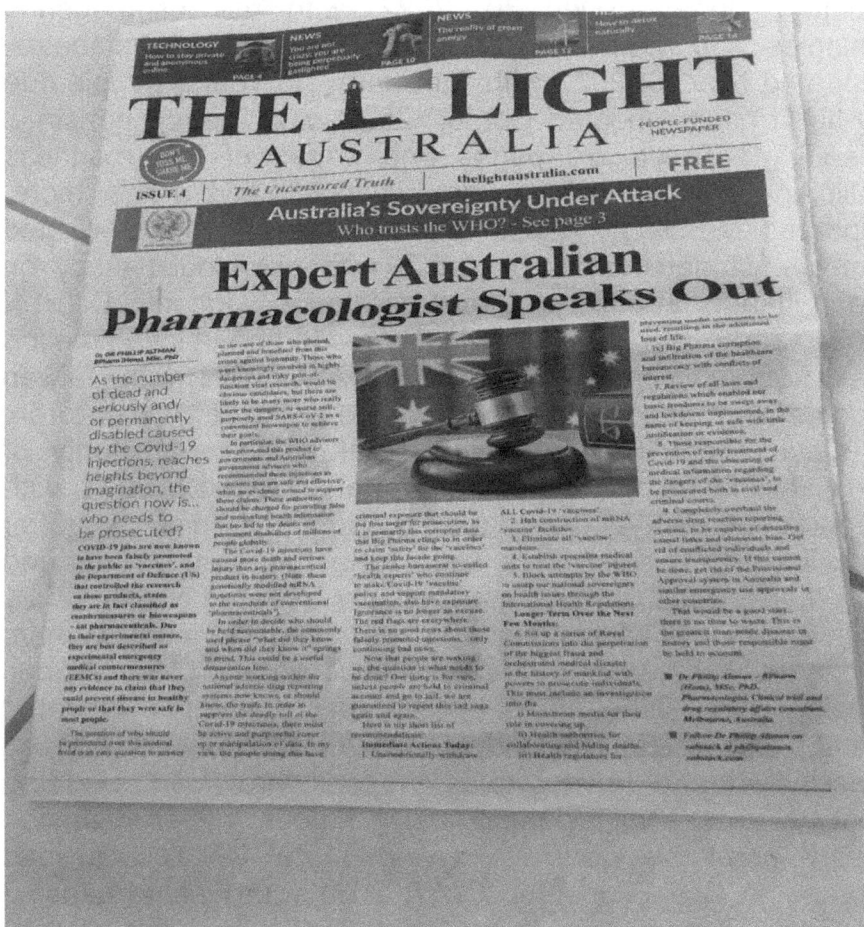

A real truthful paper here available in Qld and the truth will truly set you free.

Chapter 5

Vaccine Side Effects

These are the latest serious side effects from the vaccines up to January 2023. Updated Jan13, 2023 with CDC stroke data. Updated Jan13, 2023 with vaccine antibodies transmitted in breast milk. Updated Jan.12, 2023 with heart issues in young people. Updated Jan 1, 2023 with autopsy findings on heart deaths. Updated Dec 30, 2022, with risk of triggering shingles. Updated Dec 29, 2022, with links to diabetes. Updated Nov.10, 2022 with "net harm" to young people due to heart risks. Updated Oct 28, 2022, with "heavy menstrual bleeding". There are pages and pages of this madness inflicted on some of you so I just will add a few more. Updated March 12, 2022, with studies on vaccine-related tinnitus. Updated Feb 14, 2022, with pathologist study on heart deaths in children after vaccination. Updated Dec.14, 2021 with British study showing increased heart inflammation risk from vaccination. Updated Nov.14, 2021 with Taiwan suspending second dose of Covid vaccine for children. Updated Sept.10, 2021 with Israel study on majority of hospitalised being vaccinated. Updated July 12, 2021, with reports of Graves' disease autoimmune disorder after vaccination. This list of vaxxed injuries goes on and on and the media does not give it a mention! Updated Nov.10, 2021 with Germany limiting Moderna in young pregnant women. Updated Nov.7, 2021 with study showing 2 of 3 U.S. vaccines having under 50% effectiveness after 6 months. Updated Oct.30, 2021 with UK study showing no difference between vaccinated and unvaccinated in peak viral load. Updated Oct.10, 2021 with Iceland Pausing Moderna over increased heart problems people carrying more Delta viral load spreading Covid. Updated Oct.7, 2021 with Finland pausing Moderna vaccine for young males due to heart issues. Updated Oct.8, 2021 with Vietnam study about vaccinated people carrying more Delta viral load spreading Covid.

There are 1,246 other medical conditions following vaccination with just Pfizer. This is a bombshell," said Children's Health Defense (CHD) president and general counsel Mary Holland. So why is there no safety recall on these not safe vaccines? Well, the reasons for that are blatantly obvious and I personally often see people with some of these very distressing side effects and they are literally everywhere. You only must mention vaccine injury when you are in company, and you quickly get a story of a neighbour, friend or a loved one and words like 'They're Dropping like Flies" But then ask anybody, do they know of anyone who has died from Co-vid19? There is a big difference from dying "With Co-Vid 19." and this was part of the plan to report all the deaths as C19. Sadly, even when people die in a car accident and then they take a PCR test they will write it up as death due to C19.

Also, to compound this pandemic the PCR tests were flawed because of the amount of testing cycles they did. We now have Jab Injuries Australia, which is part of a global organisation, uniting 30 plus countries where vaccine injured people have a voice, and you can reach them on www.jabinjuriesglobal.com and they have over 300 published stories and many of them are very hard to read. The Mainstream media now reluctantly acknowledges that the PCR Tests are Flawed and after having sustained their propaganda campaign, the mainstream media as now tacitly acknowledged that the PCR tests are invalid, below is an excerpt from London's Daily Mail on something which has been known and documented by scientists and the independent media from the outset of the corona crisis in January 2020. The report is convoluted, and it is an obvious understatement: "Did flawed PCR tests convince us Covid was worse than it really was? It has been one of the most enduring C19 conspiracy theories: that the 'gold standard' PCR tests used to diagnose the virus were picking up people who weren't infected. Some even suggested the swabs, which have been carried out more than 200 million times in the UK alone may have mistaken the common colds and flu for corona." Logically for most of us it was clear as night is day that this trumped C19, was always a Pandemic fed on all the lies that we avoided basically by switching that TV Off. Life Insurance companies have noticed the rise in non-Covid deaths and disability claims since the rollout of this and they are very concerned about the working age groups and

Indiana Life Insurance CEO says that the deaths are up 40% in the working age bracket of 18-64. The linkage of what is causing this is very clear to me and the premiums are rising; accordingly, and technically, because you voluntarily took this poison you might find your policies in the future are null and void as it could be deemed voluntary euthanasia. Sadly, I feel this is going to be a major problem for the future, and this report is very alarming as Dr. Charles Hoffe, a medical doctor of 28 years in British Columbia, now working at the Lytton Clinic, has done the unthinkable when it comes to inspecting the so-called "safety and efficacy" of the Fauci Flu jabs that the CDC calls "Vaccines." He ran PET/CT scans on cancer patients who had received the Pfizer mRNA booster shot just eight days prior, and found rapid progression of T-cell lymphoma, a dramatic increase of gastrointestinal lesions, and a turbo-effect of spreading of cells in the lymph nodes under the arms near the armpits.

This is called **Turbo Cancer** where the spike proteins from mRNA jabs serve as a carcinogen literally "food that feeds the cancer", propelling it to multiply exponentially to invade the rest of the body. This happens because the spike protein turns off genes that fight off cancer (P-53, a.k.a. 'guardian of the genome'), so by getting the Covid jab it's like disarming your own army during a critical battle. This pet scan shows how the cancer cells were exponentially invading the rest of the body. So, have you been feeling tired all the time since you got stabbed with the Fauci Flu injection of billions of spike proteins? When will your body stop creating them, now that the pandemic is over and done? These toxic spike proteins are recognized by your immune system as enemies, foreign particles, that resemble a deadly virus.

Your body is trying to attack those spike prions that have travelled throughout your body to cleansing reproductive organs, the heart, and the brain. Now any cancer cells in your body are also being fed, as your vascular system delivers less oxygen and less nutrients to fight them off all thanks to the spike protein injections. Spike Protein Injections prevent your own immune system from recognizing mutations of your cells when they divide, enabling cancer cells to develop and multiply uncontrollably and under the radar of your natural defence system.

This is because the Fauci Flu jabs turn off your P-53 gene and now your body can no longer fight against cancer, as Dr. Hoffe has described, and all of this while the spike proteins clog the vascular system, depriving the body of oxygen and nutrients. Most natural health advocates already know that the clot shot effect is real and dangerous, but this research by Dr. Hoffe confirms any doubts or second guessing about it, so move forward with your organic lifestyle and natural remedies and detox to remove the spike proteins from your vaccinated bodies or unvaccinated bodies due to shedding. I am sadly meeting people who are being diagnosed with stage four cancer and reports are that since this gene therapy was introduced ⅔ cancers that are reported are Turbo Cancer. Some scientific evidence points to the fact that N-acetylcysteine can help in preventing some cancers and boosting cancer therapy.

Remdesivir an end-of-life protocol? An expert in medicine had warned that hospitals using remdesivir and the ventilators to treat COVID-19 patients are doing more harm than good, explaining "that these protocols are set up to kill." Speaking at the Truth for Health Foundation's latest virtual conference exposing human rights violations in American hospitals. Dr. Brian Ardis explained in detail the dangers associated with remdesivir, a drug that has been widely prescribed to patients with C19. In combination with mechanical ventilation, Ardis said remdesivir is responsible for expediting the deaths of "a lot of Americans [who are admitted to hospital] innocently looking for treatment." The medical expert explained that President Joe Biden's chief medical adviser Dr. Anthony Fauci originally pushed to have remdesivir administered to COVID-19 patients from May 1, 2020, at which point he attempted to discredit the effectiveness of the Food and Drug Administration (FDA) approved drug hydroxychloroquine, "saying it was ineffective and dangerous, and could kill C19 patients." Also "Fauci declared that there was one drug, and one drug only, that he was going to use in all hospitals throughout America to treat C19 hospitalised patients," Ardis said. That drug is Remdesivir and I myself am very wary of entering a hospital in Qld Australia, with their 'end-of-life protocols' and their vaccinated contaminated blood banks. Will there come a day when the unvaccinated can receive unvaccinated blood because we must work to make that become a reality.

Body Fluids Sharing body fluids with the vaccinated I would strongly avoid at all costs, if your partner is vaxxed then sadly he will infect you and then your health might very well deteriorate, I met so many who told me that has happened "It will be advisable for men and women to use contraceptives such as condoms after receiving any vaccination. This is because during sex the body fluids come in contact." They added, "Since we do not know how vaccines impact us, using a condom will be the best and most cost-effective prevention. We as social animals need touch and loving companionship, and that includes sex and sexuality, one option has been for people to refrain entirely from any kind of dating or sex. We learned that this is not a sustainable strategy in the last pandemic HIV/AIDS as initially, in response to a troubling wave of young gay men dying and soon followed by others, the official government response was to advise abstinence. There have been no Government directives this time because they want the vaccinated to infect us all and always was part of their Plan and a lot of us are so much smarter with so many unvaccinated dating sites, and we truly want to be around like minded people and not having to defend our actions, as why we are so dogmatic that we want to survive this pandemic. Having come this far, and for some sex is a lot of effort for a little result. So, the "Grim Reaper" is back and when anyone has had 3 vaccines or more and the Armed Forces of the United States has recorded a five hundred percent (500%) increase in AIDS .After administering the C19 Vaccine to US Troops, and the C19 Vaccine is implicated because White Blood Cells fight-off infection in the human body and normally the level of white cells in blood is usually about 5,000 cells per millilitre. During an infection, that level jumps to perhaps as high as twenty thousand (20,000) until the body kills the invading bacteria or virus so once the invader is dead, Doctors began seeing patients with 4,000, or 3,000, and some as low as 2,000 WBC and at those levels, the human body does not have enough of its front-line troops to fight-off infection very well so when the level drops below 1,000, a person gets sick from their own natural gut bacteria, which gets out into the bloodstream, and they become Septic. This leads to death and now the US military doctors are seeing AIDS-like levels of WBC in their troops because they cannot fight off infections. Doctors are calling this "Vaccine Acquired Immune Deficiency Syndrome. It turns out that the C19 "vaccine" contains three proteins found in the HIV virus and it now appears that some of those who got the C19 "vaccines" gave themselves AIDS and could die from it. Will that be the same for the military here in Australia? And around the world, you would have to assume if they got the mRNA vaccines then the results would have to be tragically the same and just when we need a strong military especially with China flexing its muscles. It really beggars belief yet the Labour Government Under Anal Albanese continues to waste taxpayers money on submarines and sending cash to Ukraine, the World is truly mad.

Efficacy of Nicotine in preventing C19 Infection as daily active smokers are infrequent among outpatients or hospitalised patients with C19 as several arguments suggest that nicotine is responsible for this protective effect because Nicotine may inhibit the penetration and spread of the virus and have a prophylactic effect in C19 infection.

Nicotine effectively stops the virus from propagating, acting as a type of brake that keeps disease from forming. As disturbing as this hypothesis might be, seeing as how tobacco and nicotine are largely vilified, it does have some merit. It could explain why smokers are faring generally well amid this pandemic.

26 March 2023. TGA Document Revelations. Dr. John Campbell Page 4 "Almost similar microscopic lung inflammation was observed in both challenged control and immunised animals (macaques) after the peak of infection (Days 7/8). Challenged with infection, immunised (vaccinated) animals also showed almost similar microscopic lung inflammation. We know from page 4/5 that 5 the lipid nanoparticles are systematically distributed, but the distribution of the spike protein that the RNA produces has not been tested. No data is available on how long the spike protein persists Page 5 "Antibodies and T cells in monkeys declined quickly over 5 weeks after the second dose of BNT162b2 (V9), raising concerns over long-term immunity." Page 6 Unknowns continue "Long-term immunity and vaccine-induced autoimmune diseases were not studied in the nonclinical program".Nonclinical Evaluation Report BNT162b2 [mRNA] COVID-19 vaccine Pfizer Australia Pty Ltd Freedom of Information Request. Yes, Pfizer the truth always comes out at some point and Governments would be very aware that these vaccines that are bioweapons should never ever be approved and they have blood on their hands bringing them out and at some point, the media can't hide this for much longer. We long for that day for all people who are vaccine injured and have died. Vaccinating Children with mRNA as I have already mentioned is a 'Crime against Humanity' and most of you with any normal brains who understand basic innate natural immunity would agree. There are also some brave medical receptionists here in Australia who are advising mothers of newborns that all vaccines are not safe and with the understanding that all will have mRNA in them at some point real soon they are 100% correct.

It must be realised they are poisons, and it has been quoted that a child has more chance of being struck by lightning than dying due to Covid, yet parents continue to inflict this on their so-called loved ones. 'Pfizer sales before child safety.' Information is coming out of how Pfizer will be held to account for misleading parents about Covid vaccine safety. Bill Gates was interviewed here in Australia in January 2023. "He really nails it on the issues that we're having: the short duration of protection, not a significant discernible impact on the transmission of cases, not a massive benefit for a lot of otherwise healthy young people.

Bill Gates, we were aware of all the above for 3 years as they never worked and you were always aware of this, and he had a conflict of interest whereby he invested $55 million in BioNTech back in 2019 and it's now worth north of $550 million. He sold some stock at the end of last year, I believe it was, with the share price over $300, which represented a huge gain for him. So, translating that interview, you come up with the admission from Gates that the shots are impossible to align with rapidly developing variants, they expire at lighting speed, and they don't stop transmission and they don't work for the only at-risk portion of the population. Also, Bill but were they not supposed to be "Magic". In 2021, Gates described the mRNA vaccines as "Magic," saying they would be a "Game Changer" in the next five years, and he stated: "everyone who takes the vaccine is not just protecting themselves but reducing their transmission to other people and allowing society to get back to normal."

We did warn you but why did you not listen? It always was an agenda how many of your loved ones will be infertile because of your actions. It makes me physically sick that the health officers around the world know we need to bring back the death penalty for when Nuremberg 2.0 is a reality. We all have waited several years for those of us who were deemed conspiracy theorists, to be vindicated in the media and what we were saying has sadly come to pass. So we got a new name "Truth Seeker's".

It will only escalate as the cat is now out of the bag; and it's inspiring when media like the 'Wall Street Journal' on January 22, 2023, published a highly critical editorial regarding the FDA's non-disclosure of data pertaining to the efficacy of the COVID-19 bivalent boosters. Alysia Finley, a member of the newspaper's editorial board, wrote: "Federal agencies took the unprecedented step of ordering vaccine makers to produce them and recommending them without data supporting their safety or efficacy. She also accuses the vaccine makers of "deceptive advertising." But are not some in the media leaving the sinking ship now that the damage has been done? and worldwide you have been very complicit in this Pandemic Agenda and we would not be where we are today with high levels of dangerous life-threatening toxins in people if you had not pushed it on the world as safe, so you must be held to account.

That is why the drawings I have in this book depict the Covanic, a play of words on the fated Titanic and with that the "Rats Drowned" and with pandemic there are a lot of Rats. Back to Pfizer, yet again and let's do a recap the patent of this emergency approved vaccine was in August 31st 2021, it really seems like a lifetime away and the devastation of this patent the first to show up in over 18500 patents for the very simple purpose of "Remote Controlling" which is the contract tracing of all humans Worldwide who will be or are connected to the internet of things by a quantum by a pulsating microwave of frequencies of 2.4 gHz or higher from cell towers and satellites directory to the Graphene Oxide in their fatty tissue of all the persons who had the "Death Shots", so maybe now you see why I intentionally concentrated on a few subjects like (GO) and Detoxing, Frequencies, 5G and Shungite. This pandemic agenda will just roll on if you let it and there is no stopping their intent such madness as recently JP Morgan Chase has announced plans to pilot a new payment technology that would allow customers to pay with their palm or face instead of a traditional credit or debit card.

Following similar technological implementations in China, if the pilot program goes well, the bank intends to roll out the service to its broader base of US merchant clients and usher in a new wave of biometric payments that privacy enthusiasts have been concerned about. The rise of biometric technology, which uses unique body measurements to authenticate a person's identity, is being pushed by many corporations to make this the default payment method across the world. After reading that and if you are not shaking your head, you are probably past saving and boy did we try to save you as your heading for transhumanism and the level of zombification which will reach extreme levels soon.

This madness just keeps on giving back to the present day April 2023 and this no letting up over vaccines mRNA Poison's the Biotechnology company Moderna is preparing to begin human trials on HIV vaccines as early as Wednesday, using the same mRNA platform as the firm's COVID-19 vaccine. An entry posted Wednesday to the National Institutes of Health's registry of clinical trials shows that the trials are estimated to start on August 19, 2023, and should be completed by spring 2024. Moderna has two HIV vaccine candidates, mRNA-1644 and mRNA-1644v2-Core, both of which have cleared initial safety testing before being used on humans for the first time. The randomised trials will include 56 HIV-negative participants aged 18 to 56. So, with the vaccines after 3 clot shots that have affected your natural immunity so much that you are compromised and then you will be asked to take another mRNA vaccine so you cannot see their Agenda 2030. You are probably past saving and boy did we try to save you as your heading for transhumanism and the level of zombification which will reach extreme levels very soon when they turn that frequency up the term dropping like flies will be on everyone's lips.

Thailand "On December 15, 2022, about three weeks after her third Pfizer booster shot, Princess Bajrakitiyabha Narendira Debyavati collapsed with heart issues and went into a coma "The 44-year old eldest daughter of the King in

Thailand, and likely heir to the throne, had reported to be in excellent health prior to the vaccination and collapse while training her dogs. The media seemed to generally lose interest after a January 9, 2023, update in which it was reported the princess remained in a coma and, according to the palace, has now been diagnosed with "severe heart arrhythmia resulting from inflammation following a mycoplasma infection and one authority recently suggested that Thailand was going to declare its contracts for Pfizer vaccine "null and void" and go after the vaccine maker for damages. It was Thailand which proved that the Covid vaccines cause heart injury in nearly 30% of young adults and in a later chapter there is more information that has devastated this great Country. My mate in Thailand has covered this country in more detail in his own chapter.

Aviation Industry One of the reasons I will not travel is because of this one, Pilot Josh Yoder reported that as many as 80% of pilots have taken COVID jabs, as many airlines mandated it. He said it is no longer safe to fly as there have been many incidents of pilots becoming incapacitated, but there is a massive coverup underway. A captain on a Southwest flight departing Las Vegas became incapacitated soon after take-off on March 22, 2023. He was removed from the flight deck and replaced by a non Southwest pilot who was commuting on that flight. On March 13, Emirates Flight #EK205 made a U-turn over the Atlantic and returned to Milan an hour and a half after take-off due to pilot illness. On March 3, a Virgin Australia flight from Adelaide to Perth was forced to make an emergency landing after the First Officer suffered a heart attack 30 minutes after departure. At some point this will have to be in the mainstream media there underwater with all the stories they're trying to hide. In the future getting on an aeroplane will be problematic as most pilots will not pass their health checks and all will be exposed to the reasons why.

Chapter Six

Graphene Oxide and Spike Protein

After the doom and gloom of the last chapter which would drop anyone's vibration, the good news is that with most of this gene therapy you can reverse the harm it is actually doing to you; but you need to set the spiritual intention for that to happen, which will be explained in the next chapter, combined with some of the Detoxes Protocols that I personally use and found to be very beneficial for myself and many others using them. It is important to notice your body weight and not take in too much of these. I will also list other detox protocols that might be more suitable to you.

Graphene Oxide (GO) I tend to bang on about this like a stuck record, but (GO) is the conductor for the 4G & 5G to work. It is so IMPORTANT to eliminate this Toxin out of your body if you're vaccinated or unvaccinated, otherwise this is going to really impact your health on a long-term basis due to the aid of your "Weapons your Mobile Phones, you are totally Microwaving your Brains." And do you want to be a Zombie? We all see so many of you, especially young teenagers with those brain damaging ear buds, being microwaved daily basis through the send-and-receive of the 5G towers, which are zapping you constantly via signals conducted by the (GO) and your mobile phones, especially the 5G Smartphones which are giving me very high readings on my EMF reader. And it's so very ironic that most seem to wear earbuds when exercising to get fit and destroy their brain in the process.

So, I will next explain how to help remove Graphene Oxide. **N-acetylcysteine** ("NAC") is a supplement that causes the body to produce glutathione. It is known as the precursor to glutathione and causes the body to secrete glutathione endogenously, just as it does when you do sports intensely and this is such a great way of getting the (GO) out to produce glutathione.

N-acetyl cysteine (NAC) is used as a powerful antioxidant to remove toxins from the body and boost immunity and many hospitals use N-Acetyl Cysteine because it can quickly treat acute liver failure in the event of an acetaminophen overdose. A study published in 2017 found that N-acetyl-L-cysteine can help to prevent bacterial infections in the lungs associated with chronic obstructive pulmonary disease (COPD). NAC supplementation is certainly good for your lungs because it helps to kill off bacterial pathogens in the lungs and reduce inflammation and other research points to the fact that nac helps to break up mucus in the lungs and I have already mentioned that I have lung disease and is another reason why I take this because taking nac supplements regularly can also protect against respiratory infections caused by the flu virus so nac is so very important in reversing the damage done by this Bio-Weapon that charade's as a vaccine. The antioxidant effect of nac can stop this flu virus from replicating itself and there was a study carried out in 2010 that found that nac can help prevent you catching the H5N1 influenza A virus and for example, pollution has led to more heavy metals like mercury, arsenic, lead, and cadmium being in the air and water. So, when examining the detoxifying effect of cysteine, scientists found that nac can help to avert the effects of metal toxicity, so regular nac supplementation can help to protect your brain against the negative impact of heavy-metal poisoning. Also, if you are struggling with weight issues this supplement might help you and in fact, the results of other studies have concluded that you could use N-acetylcysteine as an anti-obesity drug. Take ⅓ teaspoons in organic powder form with Vitamin C and Zinc and NAC supplementation is gaining wider acceptance in the medical community.In fact, the journal American Family Physician lists some of the many beneficial reasons to take NAC, including improving infertility, preventing kidney damage, reducing the severity of a flu infection, and improving lung health. I strongly suggest taking it in the morning on an empty stomach so finally taking NAC is the thing I recommend taking the most because eliminating the Graphene Oxide is crucial for everybody's well being, vaccinated or unvaccinated.

Blood clots You are all aware of this enemy and one of the side effects of these toxic vaccines is "Blood Clots" I have just spoken to an amputee nurse, and she is horrified by the number of amputations of vaccine patients, some very young. So, the ability of NAC to boost levels of antioxidants in the body is well documented by killing off free radicals helps to protect the heart and major arteries also NAC Boosts Brain Health, and Helps Treat conditions. Like Parkinson's and Alzheimer's. We move on to another detox that helps eliminate most of the metals out of your body and that is **Bentonite Clay** Cloud seeding is happening very high up and cloud seeding trials were carried out in Sydney, Australia, in 1947 and why do we have a weatherman when in 2023, they get it so wrong? it is obvious they do not have a "Crystal Ball. "When there is a protest rally or a major protest you can guarantee the powers-that-be will or sure it's a challenging day weather wise. Bentonite Clay (BC) also called calcium bentonite clay or Montmorillonite clay. (BC) is now taking off as a wellness trend among people who are looking to help naturally improve their skin's health, detoxify their bodies and improve digestion. It's possible to enjoy (BC) benefits by taking it internally (in other words, drinking and eating it), on top of using it externally on your skin and hair. (BC) is a product composed of ash taken from volcanoes as the clay is dried in the sun, filtered and then sold commercially in several forms, including as facial clay masks, ointments, pastes, and hair treatments, aiding in detoxification processes, protecting against bacterial infections, supporting digestive and so many respiratory processes and also aiding in dental health. (BC) is something I personally have been using for several years but I do not take it with NAC. Heavy metals are an issue for all of us due to their agenda to poison us any way they can, and do you really think those of you who are living here in Queensland that the weather has been normal for the last 18 months. So, the other benefits of Bentonite Clay removes the chemicals caused by the ''cloud seeding' and that it helps to expel toxins and heavy metals and it has antibacterial properties and fights off various pathogens responsible for disease, such as E.coli and the virus that causes staph infections and it contains a range of nutrients. (BC) is known to have an abundance of minerals, including calcium, magnesium, silica, sodium, copper, iron and potassium and it nourishes skin-hair balancing oil production, removing dead skin cells, clearing clogged pores, and fighting bacteria. I strongly suggest you add this to your detox protocol because apart from all the above, (BC) can help to reduce the negative effects of toxins that we encounter every day, such as those given off from paint, cleaning supplies, substances used in building homes, unpurified water, and even pesticides. The way it works, (BC) essentially seeks toxins in the body to bind with due to its chemical composition and then it acts like a magnet and sponge, absorbing harmful substances so they can be removed from the body.

The" Heavy Metal Toxins" usually refer to substances like mercury, cadmium, lead and benzene so upon binding, Bentonite Clay can help remove meats, toxins, chemicals and impurities from the gut, skin and mouth. Additionally, it's used to reduce the presence of toxins in the food supply and so when it's ingested into the body, either in a drink form or by eating the clay, its vitamins and minerals are similarly to how a supplement would be when combined with water and left to dry on the skin as a clay mask, (BC) is able to bind to bacteria and toxins of the skin and within pores, helping to reduce breakouts and thanks to the clay's special ability to act as an antibiotic treatment when applied topically, (BC) can also help to calm skin infections and contact dermatitis.It also removes fluoride from drinking water as BC has been researched as an effective way to remove some of the dangerous fluoride often found in drinking water, which is linked to serious diseases such as diabetes, thyroid dysfunction and brain damage. Dosage. Internally, you can take 1/2 to 1 teaspoon once per day, as many days of the week as you'd like, and most experts recommend that you don't consume (BC) internally for more than four weeks in a row. For the best results, do not take bentonite within an hour of food and avoid taking it within two hours of medications since it can interact with other substances.

Side Effects. Stop using it if you experience any side effects, such as skin rashes or digestive issues. Although both Bentonite and Zeolite are used to cleanse the body, the two purported healing agents come from different sources. Bentonite is a clay whereas Zeolite is a crystallised mineral created by lava and water. Drink lots of water when using both these detoxes.

Zeolite This is also another great detox, and I would suspect many reading this either use Bentonite Clay or Zeolite, but I suggest you alternate both, especially with (ZO) ability to detox Mould. Where I live in tropical Queensland, mould is a MAJOR issue, with the humidity and the amount of rain we've been subjected to through their agenda of persistent "Cloud Seeding"."(ZO) is also very beneficial at removing leftover radiation from your body from scans so (ZO) is one of the most fascinating and powerful supplements on the market today and I truly believe in the healing potential of this amazing substance when used properly. Zeolite is a silica-based volcanic ash (sand-like mineral) that forms over time when ash and lava from volcanoes chemically react with seawater, and this results in a compound with a very strong "cage-like" structure and negative charge. (ZO) is an alkaline mineral that is very porous and is one of the very few minerals that is negatively charged by nature and since most toxins, such as heavy metals, radiation, and pesticides are positively charged, zeolite is pulled to the toxins, like a magnet, and sucks them up into its structures. Since most toxins, such as heavy metals, radiation, and pesticides, are positively charged, (ZO) is recognized as a player in several serious chronic conditions. Even if you are not currently exposed to mould in your home or workplace, is it possible that mould from a previous exposure is multiplying in your body as mould spores can linger and continue replicating in your body for years even in the absence of external mould exposure. Zeolite is an incredible **detoxifier of mould** and is a must have in any mould detox protocol and after being exposed to ionising radiation, radioactive materials are left in your body will stick around for years if you don't take action to remove them, so the chances are you've got a fair amount of radioactive radiation over the years from CT scans, mammograms, X-Rays, naturally occurring radiation like radon, etc. In the 21st century we face an unprecedented number of toxic stressors in our daily lives, from the air you breathe, to the food you eat, toxins are everywhere and over time these toxins accumulate in your body wreaking havoc on your health and fatigue, brain fog, weight gain, a weakened immune system, and countless health issues are common side effects where these toxins build up. So, in conclusion, I suggest alternating both Zeolite and Bentonite Clay, as both are great at mopping up toxins in the gut and even in the bloodstream. Side effects of (ZO). It does not absorb in your body; it simply passes through your bloodstream, collecting positively charged toxic elements and then is excreted. Therefore, you cannot overdose on zeolite but you need to drink plenty of water, suggested dosage for basic detox 1 teaspoon of powder with water or juice daily. The approach which I would highly recommend with most supplements, is to start with a very low dose and work your way up.

Activated Charcoal This is another important detox because it is made from a variety of materials such as wood, peat, bamboo, and coconut and most activated charcoal that is sold for ingesting is produced from coconut and the charcoal is activated by heating it to very high temperatures of over 1,400°F and treating it with oxygen. This process causes pores to form in the charcoal giving it a large surface area and it is this porous surface which makes it a powerful substance to rid the body of certain toxins. Activated charcoal has been used for centuries to treat cases of poisoning and it is still used for this reason in many hospital departments and one of the most common is activated charcoal for treating certain cases of drug overdoses. Some of the drugs that activated charcoal is effective on are aspirin, paracetamol, tricyclic antidepressants, and barbiturates. Activated charcoal is also good at helping to rid the body of toxins as you can use activated charcoal as part of a detox regime, by taking it as a supplement to the suggested dosage you should take 10 grams of activated charcoal about 90 minutes before each meal and do this for 2 days. It also removes harmful toxins from drinking water, and it is the main component in water filters. It can be also used to treat food poisoning as well as alcohol poisoning.

Colloidal Silver I personally use this daily and spray it in my face before I go out and use it through a vaporizer. I have mentioned in an earlier chapter that I have a condition called Aspergilloma (fungus ball) and this helps keep my lungs clean. A lot of you will have heard of this 'miracle' product known as Colloidal Silver and the basic reason for any colloidal silver efficacy and safety controversy is that the medical establishment (medical mafia) and the pharmaceutical industry (Big Pharma) see colloidal silver as a financial threat. Any useful and beneficial thing is tarred and feathered this way, maybe because it is very cheap. You can buy a one litre bottle online for $40 and many consider colloidal silver an antiseptic because it kills more than bacteria; as it destroys viruses and eliminates fungal infections and so far, bacteria that are resistant to silver haven't developed. The approach which I would highly recommend that with most supplements, is to start with a very low dose and work your way up. Colloidal silver can destroy antibiotic-resistant pathogens, even the dreaded MRSA. As a matter of fact, we hear the medical mafia has been covertly adding colloidal silver into antibiotics to conquer the superbug strains that have developed immunity to those antibiotics and I say covertly because they aren't talking too much about it. Keep in mind that while antibiotics don't touch viruses and fungus and my lung condition is Aspergilloma (fungus Ball), colloidal silver helps eliminate them, making colloidal silver benefits incredibly useful. Silver has been used for its antimicrobial and other health benefits in folk medicine for centuries to treat wounds, colds, and infections but with the invention of antibiotics, the use of silver for bacterial infections has decreased. However, with rising antibiotic resistance and the growing renewed interest in natural treatment options, colloidal silver is an alternative option for all of us? and back in the day when people didn't have refrigerators, they commonly put silver coins in their milk containers as a preservative to prevent bacteria and algae growth so there was no spoiled milk, thanks to silver. Research has been done on it in treating colds and viruses, you may be excited to hear that colloidal silver seems to be effective against the common cold and the flu as research has found that nanoparticles can prevent viral replication in these viral infections. Also, thanks to its antimicrobial and anti-inflammatory properties, colloidal silver can be effective in treating cuts, burns, and other wounds of the skin so colloidal silver may also be effective in treating wounds infected by drug-resistant strains of bacteria. Colloidal silver may also be beneficial for people with eczema, psoriasis, acne and other similar skin conditions as colloidal silver-based nanogels are both an antibacterial and antiviral supplement; it can soothe scrapes, repair tissue damage, and be a helpful dressing for various skin wounds. Colloidal silver is also a powerful antiviral and antibacterial substance that may be helpful against pink eye and other eye infections. Met a man who could not get rid of prickly heat and had this condition for months until he got lucky using this amazing miracle cure. When inhaled into the lungs, colloidal silver can directly contact the invaders and clear up the lungs effectively. A word of warning: be very careful how much you ingest because a condition called Argyria is a condition that makes your mucous membranes and skin look greyish blue and taking colloidal silver by mouth can result in a build-up in the tissues leading to agyria.

Beetroot Powder This is another supplement that I use regularly, and I buy it in powder form, 250g for around $15. Have you ever stopped to think about why beetroot powder is so popular or about its health benefits? Why were you forced to eat beets as a kid? And why is beetroot so good for you? Well, it turns out that beets are a superfood full of antioxidants, vitamins, minerals, you name it, and beets will have it and is full of nitrates and that is why beetroot powder, a neutral tasting version of beetroot, is a popular dietary supplement. The benefits of beetroot powder are very immense including the heart because the antioxidants present in beetroot are of utmost value to the circulatory system, especially the heart and for example, betaine is an antioxidant present in beets also as an antioxidant, one of its responsibility is to save cells from environmental stress that can potentially cause damage. But aside from this, it is also partly responsible for proper heart function and some studies suggest that eating beetroot may help to relieve high blood pressure which is a condition common in patients with type 2 diabetes. The nitrates present in beets are one of the vital nutrients that helps ensure that blood pumps efficiently through the blood vessels, resulting in better blood circulation and healthier blood pressure. Studies have shown that drinking beetroot juice prior to a workout may help enhance performance so if you are a fitness enthusiast, like me you may be able to have a more successful and efficient workout with better results. That's because the nitrates present in the beetroot may provide better blood and oxygen flow so theoretically, if the respiratory system is able to supply these nutrients throughout the body, you may have an easier time performing during workouts and may even have a faster recovery time.

We talk a lot about Cancer, because these gene therapy vaccines have a lot to answer regarding cancers and especially turbo cancers. Beetroot also contains betalains that have been found to have anti-cancer effects in cellular models in the laboratory as clinical trials are now needed to assess if there are potential anti-inflammatory and anti-cancer effects and the nature of these effects. Also, more benefits are that beets also contain the minerals iron, manganese, and potassium and Iron has a vital role in the transportation of oxygen by healthy red blood cells. Eating beetroot can help to increase your fibre intake and support a healthy gut community and it's very clear that for relatively few calories, beetroot contains a variety of vitamins, minerals, nitrates, and antioxidants. Beetroot is the one vegetable that can have an immense impact on your sexual life, especially for men.

That is not to say that women won't benefit from the root' vegetable to beat sexual inactivity as when you eat beetroot, the nitrates present in the vegetable are converted into nitrite in the mouth by the bacteria present in the oral cavity. When the vegetable is chewed and swallowed the bacteria in the stomach converts it into nitric oxide, a gas that helps blood vessels to dilate and boost circulation. Regular consumption of beetroot helps blood vessels in the genitals to open and improve circulation. This helps in better erection in men during sexual intercourse and helps last longer in the bed, too. In fact, nitrate supplementation from beetroot juice is seen to give best results for improving sexual health and stamina. I personally alternate this amazing health enhancer; and apart from adding in my meals, I also supplement it with organic beetroot powder, and I will say it will make you feel very "horny" and men should never ever waste an Erection.

Carbon 60 This is a microscopic molecule with 60 carbon atoms, which looks like a buckyball and C60 works as an antioxidant in the body, removing harmful antioxidants and because they're so small C60 molecules can reach individual components of your body's cells.That's one reason why this compound is being researched for the fields of nanotechnology and nanomedicine as in very basic terms, carbon 60 is a collection of 60 carbon atoms. During a study, the research team bought C60 to see its effects on Wistar rats when they separated the rats into several groups and some groups were given 1 ml of water, some were given 1 ml of olive oil, and the rats urine, blood, and brain samples, they discovered something amazing which was that the rats that were given olive oil had increased their lifespan by 30%. But the rats that were given the olive oil with C60 increased their lifespan by almost 90%. I am currently using C60 olive oil for my own detox regime because it Fights Bacteria and Viruses: C60 eliminates bacteria and certain viruses. It also boosts white blood cell count, so the body is more effective at fighting off infections and protects against the effects of ageing: C60 is an antioxidant, which means it reduces oxidative stress caused by free radicals so free radicals are largely responsible for symptoms of ageing, so consuming C60 may slow down the ageing process. Minimises Inflammation: According to clinical research that has anti-inflammatory properties and also energy, many C60 users report increased levels of energy after consuming the supplement regularly for some time. It provides better enhanced sleep, which most of us need, and a well-reported benefit of C60 is that it improves motivation and strength: Athletes report that C60 supplementation helps to improve sports performance and motivation. Enhances brain functions: as a nootropic, C60 improves learning and memory also since C60 olive oil acts as an antioxidant, it can help your body look, feel, and function better. By using olive oil with C60, you may be able to avoid diseases and illnesses and I hope that this will interest most reading this as one of the biggest questions bouncing around scientific circles right now regarding C60 that in theory, carbon 60 has qualities that look like they should improve cell health and help people live longer. For optimal results, it's best to take a C60 product that's at least 99.5% purity and you may only need a very small amount of a product of this purity.

It is recommended to have about 5 ml per day which equates to approximately 1 teaspoon and you can squirt the product directly into your mouth and wash it down with a sip or two of water. If you dislike the taste of olive oil, you may want to mask the flavour of the Cod. There is also a very expensive Supercharged C60, a specialised form of multi-layered fullerene nano-carbon structures that act as a powerful antioxidant. It's at least ten times more potent than standard C60. **Detoxing the spike proteins** out of your body especially if you have been vaccinated will come with its challenges but it's very doable and according to studies published by The Lancet, people who've recently been vaccinated carry a viral load that is 251 times higher than those who are unvaccinated, endangering them and their co-workers. If you had Covid-19 or received a Covid-19 injection, you may have dangerous spike proteins circulating in your body.

Spike proteins can circulate in your body after infection or injection, causing damage to cells, tissues and organs. **Spike protein inhibitors** and neutralizers include Pine needles, Ivermectin, Neem, Ivermectin, Neem, N-acetylcysteine (NAC). Research into this naturally is ongoing as this "Nightmare Unfolds" some of the other spike protein detoxes include Vitamin D, Vitamin C, Quercetin, Zinc, Curcumin, Milk-thistle extract, Magnesium while the spike protein is naturally found in SARS-CoV-2, no matter the variant, it's also produced in your body when you receive a C19 shot. In its native form in SARS-CoV-2, the spike protein is responsible for the pathologies of the viral infection but in its wild form it's known to open the blood-brain barrier causing cell damage (cytotoxicity) and, as Dr. Robert Malone, the inventor of the mRNA and DNA vaccine core platform technology, said in a commentary on News Voice, "is active in manipulating the biology of the cells that coat the inside of your blood vessels, the vascular endothelial cells, in part through its interaction with ACE2, which controls contraction in the blood vessels, blood pressure and other things. It has been revealed that the spike protein on its own is enough to cause inflammation and damage to the vascular system, even independent of a virus and please remember the spike protein is a "Deadly Protein". It will cause inflammation and clotting in any tissue in which it accumulates as Pfizer's biodistribution study, which was used to determine where the injected substances end up in the body, showed the Covid spike protein from the shots accumulated in "quite high concentrations" concentrations" in the ovaries. A Japanese biodistribution study for Pfizer's jab found that vaccine particles move from the injection site to the blood, after which circulating spike proteins. Which are free to travel throughout the body, including to the ovaries, liver, neurological tissues and other organs. You might be aware of this, because this could be life or death for you or one of your loved ones as the virus spike protein has been linked to adverse effects, such as: blood clots, brain fog, organising pneumonia, and myocarditis, it is very probably responsible for many of the C19 injection side effects.

Even if you have not had any symptoms, tested positive for Covid-19, or experienced adverse side effects after a jab, there will still be lingering spike proteins inside your body, and it is essential to remove them.

This is such a beneficial detox. **Intermittent Fasting** I intermittently fast most days from 8am till 5pm to help remove the spike proteins even though I am unvaccinated, but with being around so many vaccinated people daily, I feel it important to take this seriously and treat it accordingly. but for the vaccinated it is far more serious, and some people still had the spike proteins after two months post-vaccination and is it possible that fasting could help clear out lingering spike protein, or cells that contain spike protein. A study found that for a given amount of mRNA, more protein was produced from it in fed men, compared to fasted men. I hope you're starting to see the connection with mRNA vaccines and if someone were given one of these vaccines, and they wanted to make sure they didn't produce too much spike protein, isn't it plausible that fasting would lower the overall protein synthesis rate, including protein synthesis from the vaccine mRNA, all other things being equal? Remember also that the mRNA vaccines are supposed to be given intramuscularly and it's supposed to get taken up by muscle cells. Under fasting conditions we'd expect that the muscle cells would lower the rate of protein.

Colloidal Gold This is very exciting news about Colloidal Gold and recent studies worldwide and even here in Queensland Australia, and the hope we are getting in treating this Toxin, the news for vaccinated people is immense and gives you all reading this so much **'HOPE'**. That you can take the control of your loved ones back and I am quoting from a recent report. This book is all about hope for everyone and a recent case study of a patient called Bill in Brisbane showed blood slides showing 'Micro Clots' and what looks like Graphene Oxide on the slides. These bloods were from vaccinated people including Bill's own blood and unvaccinated blood showed a smaller amount of Graphene unvaccinated blood showed a smaller amount of Graphene Oxide but 'NO CLOTS'. We also looked at "Three Drops of the Pfizer vaccine on the slide" and please remember that three drops is a fraction of the dose you get with each jab and he watched in a sped-up video the vaccine material moves and manages to self-assemble on the slide and the material formed lots of squares and unusual shapes and structures and this seems to occur when exposed to frequency or EMF, and when not exposed breaks back down but will reform when exposed again.

Now the interesting part is when Bill dropped One drop of a liquid next to (not touching) the three drops of the vaccine and what happened next was amazing: The structures just kind of melted away and the drop of this amazing liquid was Colloidal Gold. Next David discussed some success he had with a person named Pete, who is 26, a professional fisherman, a very fit healthy man, married with one child and one more on the way. Following his 2nd jab he had many negative side effects, so Bill then advised Pete he had treated himself with colloidal gold, high doses of Vitamin D and Ivermectin. Bill reported that within an hour Pete had done a complete 180 degree turn around and was doing great so fast forward to a Saturday and he was driving to Boondall Queensland, where he was introduced to Pete and his friends and family who were there meeting with Bill discussing the changes in Pete since he had tried the above. Bill had brought along his microscope and had it hooked up to the laptop and anyone who was interested could sit with Bill and he would take a drop of their own blood and we could watch as he scanned through the blood while having a look. The process only took about 15 minutes per person and was great to see in real time what's showing up in the blood as we looked at many 'vaccinated and unvaccinated bloods.' It is as clear as day, even to the untrained eye the difference between the jabbed and un-jabbed blood. Vaccinated blood showed micro clotting and lots of what looks like (GO) as the Graphene Oxide structures seemed larger and more complex in the vaccinated blood.

The Unvaccinated blood also showed (GO), and why must you all remove it with NAC. Why and how is Graphene Oxide getting in 'Everyone's blood'? The answer to that is also as plain as day: the food we consume and the water that we drink? Also, all the vaccinated around us unfortunately do infect us but there is HOPE to help the people injured by these toxic vaccines. So, what is Colloidal Gold as some health-conscious individuals are familiar with Colloidal Silver, and the scientific research into antibacterial and germicidal properties speaks for itself. Less popular and understood, however, is Colloidal Gold which is a tasteless colloid made from minute gold particles mixed with water, and its health benefits are altogether different from those of Colloidal Silver. The health benefits are Anti-inflammatory properties and research has shown that colloidal gold can ease the swelling associated with inflammatory conditions like arthritis, bursitis, rheumatism, and tendinitis and it can enhance moods.

Pine Needle Tea Word spread that pine needle tea may offer a solution against covid vaccine "shedding" or transmission where vaccinated people are spreading harmful particles or substances to others around them. It is rich in vitamin C and 5 times the concentration of vitamin C found in lemons. **Quercetin** you can treat the spike protein damage from Covid vaccines with Quercetin, a flavonoid with multiple proven health benefits to both man and animals, displaying a plethora of biological activities as Quercetin-treated neutrophils exhibited a remarkable suppression in mRNA expression of various proinflammatory genes. One of the lesser-known and recently discovered roles of quercetin, is modulation of microRNA (miRNA) expression, which plays a vital role in health and disease bring relief to conditions such as heart disease, varicose veins, skin complaints and fatigue and it can be used as an expectorant for coughs and to help relieve chest congestion. It is also good for a sore throat, and it brings you mental clarity and you can treat the spike protein damage from Covid vaccines with Quercetin, a flavonoid with multiple proven health benefits to both man and animals.

Zinc This would be on most people's health regimen, for it also neutralises spike protein damage from Covid vaccines with Zinc, it contributes to wound healing, and plays a role in childhood growth and development and it also has antioxidant properties and plays an important role in cell mediated immune function and modulates mRNA levels of cytokines also Zinc has been shown to regulate gene transcription in cancer cells, proteins necessary for microRNA maturation and stability and lastly Zinc-finger protein serrate is among the plant compounds that may silence mRNA.

Our Diet Which is very important and there are many anti-inflammatory diet protocols that will help; coffee also promotes autophagy. We already talked about fasting; this is extreme, but you could also start with a 3-day fast with only water or herbal tea if you can handle it? Hereafter institute intermittent fasting: Eat all the day's calories within a 6-8-hour window and no snacking between main meals as this helps eliminate the spike protein from within the cells. Sauna and hot-steam shower also help boost autophagy, the cell's way of getting rid of toxic substances, the natural elimination of abnormal cells and damaged proteins. Alter your diet so to reduce consumption of pro-inflammatory food items and a low histamine diet is recommended, avoid processed foods and GMOs and broccoli and especially broccoli sprouts have been shown to repair spike protein damage throughout the body. Hesperidin sources to help disable spike protein Citrus fruit (especially blood oranges, due to their high hesperidin content hesperidin is a chalcone like quercetin that deactivates the spike protein. Peppermint (is also very high in hesperidin). Carrots, Carrot Juice is (rich in Shikimate), Dandelion Leaf the common dandelion efficiently blocks the interaction between ACE2 cell surface receptors and some spike proteins, Wheatgrass and Wheatgrass Juice, Shikimate neutralises the Spike Protein.

Urotherapy hopefully you have sorted your diet out before you read this? This is a 5,000-year-old practice, the rejuvenation method of Urotherapy uses your own perfect medicine to heal the body from the inside out as your body produces antibodies and antidotes to all invading organisms and poisons and those natural substances come out through your urine. Your body knows what it needs to heal itself and what your body needs is contained in the 'golden nectar of your urine and this is one of the most guarded secrets of the dark forces at work. Its proponents believe that drinking your own urine can eradicate any health condition you may have, over time. Directions for use: First morning urine. Wait 3 seconds after starting urine flow and then catch about 3-6 ounces mid-strength and drink it straight or you can mix in fruit juice and if this is too much for you to handle, start with putting 9-12 drops off your urine and hold it under the tongue for 1 minute and swallow. I bet that got your attention but never ever when it comes to your health dismiss anything that could make a big difference to improving your health.

Shungite Water I have talked a lot about shungite and its ability to reduce the dangers we have with EMF'S, but I encourage everyone very strongly to make their own shungite water. It's not that expensive to do so I suggest buying a water system like a 7/8 Stage Ceramic Carbon 10-32L Water Filter Bottle Bench Top Dispenser Purifier that is not expensive at around $50 on ebay and then buy your shungite stones. Shungite is widely applied as a natural filtering instrument to clean and mineralize water as it is proven that digesting shungite water provides a positive therapeutic effect and helps to cope with a great number of diseases including skin related problems, chronic respiratory issues, headaches, aches in joints and muscles as well as the problems with the digestive system. In order to make shungite water you need to carefully wash, by boiling, your shungite stones; this activates them before using them and rids them of any post-production dust and are widely applied. Regular shungite contains from 35 to 60 percent of organic carbon, while the percentage of Carbon in elite shungite is much higher and totals from 92 to 98 percent In order to make shungite water, infuse 150-200 grams of regular shungite stones or 50-70 grams of elite shungite stones per one litre of water for two or three days and drink it fresh. Shungite starts filtrating water within the first few hours, but the more you keep shungite in the water, the more effect you will receive and the stones are supposed to be cleaned and activated regularly so that it is easy to just leave them in the sun and shungite water is also designed for making shungite baths that are very popular since taking a bath with shungite water benefits your health, well-being, growth and recovery. In order to make a shungite bath, infuse 400-500 grams of shungite stones into the bath with the hot water and keep them there for about 15-20 minutes. Then take a healing bath and enjoy the positive changes shungite gives to your physical and spiritual health. Another major advantage of water filtration with shungite stones is that it helps to balance pH level.' Some will know, water we consume shouldn't be too acidic (pH level of less than 6.5) or overly alkaline (an 8 on the pH scale) and one of the well known facts about shungite water is that most animals really like how it tastes, and as a result drink much more than they normally would and because animals are especially vulnerable to pollution from the environment, lawn, garden and household chemicals, exposure to these harmful substances can increase the risk of many diseases so one way to mitigate dangerous effects of hazardous chemicals is to keep your pets very hydrated and shungite infused water is a simple but very effective solution.

According to Regina Martino, a French Bioenergetics researcher who has been conducting experiments on shungite since 2016, it will keep indefinitely. So, they are a great investment for you and your family, and your pets and some things are worth repeating. Shungite is a powerful antioxidant so it helps rid your body of toxins, too as shungites are effective for protection from radiation and can increase energy in your environment. Shungite necklaces have been used for centuries to protect the body from negative energy and shungite is often used in grids in the home or office for cleansing and purification purposes and a person can do so by placing them in each corner of an entrance way or carrying a piece in their pocket when going out. It has the ability to absorb negative energy which makes it an incredible stone for transmuting internal blockages, fears or other unsavoury feelings that you might have about yourself, and I actively do all of the above. Who needs shungite the most? I suggest everyone needs shungite, and if you fall into one of these categories, then 'you will need it now.' Shungite is a must-have for anyone working as a healer including doctors, nurses, holistic health practitioners and light workers and essentially anyone helping people who are not in top shape shungite is a must for anyone working in stressful environments. Where work and the people at work are stressing you out and this quote from a nurse "Another one of the main reasons that I started using shungite was because of the heavy energies, and sometimes entities that I was picking up on when I was working as a nurse in hospitals.

We are all empaths, designed to connect with one another on a physiological level and our brains were designed to connect with other brains, so that we may become relatable, and we're physically designed to feel what another is feeling in order to increase our degree of compassion. Some of us are not taught this and we move through life, taking on the energetic and the form of emotions and thoughts, not realising that we can experience these interactions without being grossly impacted by them. Shungite could help us to set healthy boundaries in this area of our lives and help us to connect with one another in a more empowering way. I talk a lot on the spiritual level and as a Meditation Tool because shungite's grounding properties restore balance to your auric field by dissipating overactivity of the higher chakras and stimulating the lower ones. Also meditating with shungite is an amazing way to boost your energy levels, dissolve stress and anxiety and relieve muscle ache and tension and in this way, it increases your personal power and raises your vibration. I talk a lot about vibration because life is all energy and vibration and for those of you already on a spiritually high vibration you do not need anything but synchronicity to meet your like-minded friends, shungite is still so beneficial as shungite 'grounds you to mother earth through the root and earth star chakras, thereby activating them both. The benefits of connecting those two chakras to one another provides a powerful surge of security and energy. The earth reminds us that we are taken care of and supported in this life and she gives us permission to explore as shungite clears and balances your aura and aligns all of your chakras. When you have a clear aura and aligned chakras, energy flows through you with ease so you're able to release the brain and move into flow with the heart and shungite enhances your metaphysical abilities. When you are clear, you become channels for connecting to your highest self and other realms and by being able to use your metaphysical abilities to align you in this way, is a fascinating reminder of just how powerful you truly are so shungite assists in your spiritual evolution.

Shungite evolved with the planet and within the codes of evolution may be found and maybe this explains my addiction to buying so much shungite and I like to give some away as the power of giving is all powerful. Spotting fake shungite the first distinguishing feature of authentic shungite is the intense black colour and often, it has infusions of golden, grey, or brown colours. These are traces of other minerals like pyrite and quartz, found in the same layer as shungite. When you touch it a black residue will come off a bit like coal dust so raw or regular shungite stone is a greyish-coloured mineral.

One of the latest detoxes for removing the Spike Proteins is combining **NAC with Bromelain.** In a study, bromelain was found to be effective in dissolving SARS-COV-2 spikes and envelope proteins. When combined with 20 mg/ml of acetylcysteine, the SARS-COV-2 spike, and envelope proteins are fully disintegrated. So, clearly this is very good news. If we can literally dissolve the Spike Protein before it interacts with our ACE2 (and clearly many other) receptors, then the Spike, in essence, becomes as the nonillions of other viruses on the planet that cannot enter our cells. Bromelain, the key component of pineapple fruit.

Nattokinase Dr. Peter McCullough, MD, MPH, has also recently dropped another bombshell revelation, this time about how Nattokinase, a natural enzyme found in fermented soybeans, is a powerful remedy against Wuhan coronavirus (Covid-19) spike proteins. McCullough says he is asked all the time by people who got "vaccinated" to covid what they can do to "get this out of my body." This inspired him to write a piece about nattokinase that calls the substance the "holy grail of covid-19 vaccine detoxification." The mRNA and adenoviral DNA products were rolled out with no idea on how or when the body would ever break down the genetic code," McCullough writes "The synthetic mRNA carried on lipid nanoparticles appears to be resistant to breakdown by human ribonucleases by design so the product would be long-lasting and produce the protein product of interest for a considerable time period "This would be an advantage for a normal human protein being replaced in a rare genetic deficiency state (However, it is a big problem when the protein is the pathogenic SARS-CoV-2 Spike.

Nattokinase, McCullough says, holds the greatest promise out of any other detoxification agent of which he is aware and the best part is that it is relatively inexpensive and is sold over the counter as a dietary supplement. "Nattokinase is an enzyme [that] is produced by fermenting soybeans with bacteria and has been available as an oral supplement," McCullough explains. "It degrades fibrinogen, factor VII, cytokines, and factor VIII and has been studied for its cardiovascular benefits. When studying this cheap product, you will find Natto is popular in Japan, where it has been a staple breakfast food for thousands of years. It gives off a nutty, salty flavour and is often paired with rice and researchers from the University of Chicago isolated a specific clot-busting enzyme within natto. This enzyme is called nattokinase so when nattokinase was applied to blood clots at body temperature, the clots dissolved within 18 hours as a person ages, their body produces less plasmin. Blood clots are a major issue with so many amputations happening now you start to see more people in society have had this happen to them the common theme will come up in conversation "I was vaccinated" and it's beyond tragic. If fibrin is not properly dissolved, it can become a dangerous clot that leads to heart attack or stroke and a single dose of clot-dissolving drugs is good for only a few minutes and can cost up to $1,500. On the other hand, a hospital emergency can be prevented altogether with a $20 weekly serving of natto, also natto is a healthy option for treating osteoporosis, the substance spurs the synthesis of vitamin K2 in the intestinal tract and this vitamin helps the body preserve its calcium stores in the bone. If this food was adopted into cultures outside of Japan, the quality of life would be improved for hundreds of millions of people around the world, Especially for adults transitioning into old age and doctors should be recommending natto supplements for anyone who received a C19 vaccine and survived thus far but because it's cheap call me cynical they probably will never if you're a proper doctor reading this prove me I am wrong but what would I know.

Hydrogen Peroxide 3% food grade hydrogen peroxide is sold in many chemists, supermarkets, and online as an over-the-counter antiseptic solution. Doctors warn that 3% H2O2 should never be ingested, and you shouldn't use the solution for longer than a week but hydrogen peroxide even at 3% concentration has an antibacterial effect, gargling with hydrogen peroxide can also help cure a sore throat. For this, you should mix 1 part of 3% food hydrogen peroxide (H2O2) and 2 parts of water. Gargle for up to 60 seconds, taking care not to swallow any of the solution. Another use is food grade hydrogen peroxide is very effective against mould and mildew. A word of warning: food grade hydrogen peroxide, even in concentrations as low as 3%, can cause some irritation to your skin, eyes, airways (if you breathe it in), or oesophagus (if you swallow it). There will be some protocols that I have left out because I am not a doctor or naturopath, and these are things that I have tried and currently use on a regular basis.

Herbalists who may use herbs and natural ingredients to make their own holistic preparations for clients and herbal products businesses must keep informed about FDA dietary supplement regulations surrounding the use and sale of herbs as dietary supplements. In 2019 this came in to review for obvious reasons: anything that might make you well will not want that so anything good will become deemed as very bad. So, herbalists and naturopaths be on your guard, things like NAC worldwide, Colloidal Gold, Pine Needle Tea, Bentonite Clay and Zeolite to name just a few will be banned. So many more like these also might be targeted and if you use herbs, essential oils, supplements (vitamin and 82 minerals), and/or compounds, or make or sell them, even from your garden, the FDA is currently undergoing hearings to determine the fate of 68 substances commonly used by herbalists, such as nettle leaf, Astragalus extract, and tea tree oil. B12 methylcobalamin, the best form that the body can utilise, could be eliminated which then will stop detoxification or make it more difficult and in addition, 242 additional substances were deemed unworthy these include alfalfa, Chinese rhubarb, dandelion, grapeseed oil, ginger root powder, Ginkgo biloba extract, cedarwood essential oil, Jamaican dogwood (Piscidia erythrina), mullein, myrrh tincture, parsley, passionflower extract, peppermint oil, pine tar, pipsissewa, psyllium, sage oil, saw palmetto. Going back to the so important NAC which I talked so much about, however, the U.S. The Food and Drug Administration suddenly cracked down on NAC in 2020, claiming it is excluded from the definition of a dietary supplement, as it was approved as a new drug in 1963, before it was marketed as a dietary supplement or as a food but on Amazon.au it's still available but be wary any products coming out of China or India.

Andrographis I recently added this to my detox regime to reduce fever, combat inflammation,reduce oxidative stress and relieve symptoms of the common cold and flu.

Chapter 7

mRNA & Poisons in Your Food

This will be a brief but very necessary chapter, as I have already given my views on these non-vaccines for a virus that everybody accepts that C19 is possibly just a cold or flu variant? but trumped by fear and money to exploit all those who did not have any critical thinking? But we must acknowledge that people and most of the purebloods (unvaccinated) would have family members and friends who did not want these vaccines? but were coerced by the evil governments, who are complicit in this Plandemic Agenda. They needed to feed their families and basically survive so there is no judgement from me, and we really should not judge as we are all born perfect-imperfect. Some may have been lucky to have gotten away with it when they have only had two stabs.

As of January 2023, the EU has given permission to add insects (house crickets) to baked goods, pasta and other semi-finished products "for the general public." Although there is too little published knowledge about allergies and possible anaphylactic reactions, the EU Commission is of the opinion that no specific labelling requirements about possible allergic reactions need to be listed. But those of you who have allergies to crustaceans, molluscs and house dust mites are highly likely to also suffer allergic reactions when consuming products with house crickets added. It can also lead to new allergic reactions to the substrate that is fed to the insects but, there is only a labelling requirement if the product contains powder "Acheta Domesticus." Commonly called the house cricket, it is a cricket most likely native to SouthWestern; but between 1950 and 2000 it became the standard feeder insect for the pet and research industries and spread worldwide. What this means is that people have to find out for themselves that "Acheta Domesticus" is ground into powder and added to food products and have to check for themselves whether they could be allergic to it so the admission into the foods began on January 24, 2023. In the EU as it is the aim now as I have already mentioned to get the vaccines into us all by stealth through the Food Chain. **The NSW Government** has 'already' made it compulsory for any livestock going through sale at stockyards to be Vaccinated with mRNA and Bio-Tagged, so although we who have worked so hard not to get vaccinated are having our food supply randomly injected with mRNA now which as happened for at least six months in NSW, and two out ten cows that are injected die. All dairy, cheese, milk, beef, chickens, eggs, pork now must be considered tainted and unsafe, and we cannot buy food from Supermarkets and no more take-away fast foods, no more restaurants unless proven they're organicIf you don't GROW it yourself, then treat it with suspicion and we must now confirm for ourselves (by speaking to our local butcher directly) that the meat is fully organic and not mRNA injected.

We must NOW in earnest start to form very close protective communities, also buy farmland and go bush and do the serious survival prepping. Where to buy meat that is not mRNA and vaccine free the good news though is if you are hunting around online and been to some local butchers ensure to see their stance on this topic. I am pleased to say there are few I contacted who have all confirmed they have no intention to vaccinate their cattle with any mRNA, so they are out there as freedom fighters in all walks of professions thankfully. Fake Meat Globalist and Microsoft co-founder Bill Gates has invested in and pushed for the consumption of fake meat, which can possibly cause cancer due to the ingredients used to make it. The technocrat expressed his desire for everyone to eat fake meat as a "climate-friendly" alternative to the real thing. "I do think all rich countries should move to 100 percent synthetic beef," Gates told the Review. But a new study published in the Journal of Agricultural and Food Chemistry reveals that plant-based meats are not as easily digested in the body, therefore way less nutritious because the body cannot properly absorb the patty's nutrients. Another study showed that when the infamous Impossible Meat patty was fed to rats, the rodents developed inflammation and kidney disease in weeks, and the potential for anaemia. All fast-food outlets and their food products should be treated with caution Brands (the parent company of KFC, Taco Bell, Pizza Hut, A&W, and Long John Silvers), made a deal with faux meat producer Beyond Meat to make plant-based chicken for KFC and faux sausage toppings for Pizza Hut. Their competitors, such as McDonalds, were also introducing their new McPlant Burger. More fast-food chains have gotten in on the action as well. This includes mega-brands such as Burger King adopting their own plant-based Whopper, and the international food and water giant Nestlé joining the market too and more joining in Beyond Meat and Pizza Hut are now teaming up once more because Pizza Hut will soon be debuting a new plant-based pepperoni.

This is a statement from Bill Gates "You can get used to the taste difference, and the claim is they're going to make it taste even better over time." Bill you a total and utter moron making statements that are truly "Moronic" and like cow's love to fart you blame it all on climate change on "Gas Emissions" so maybe at the Nuremberg 2.00. It will be the "Gas Chamber" for you laddie.

The problem is that the materials used to make the product 'immortalised cell lines' replicate forever, just like cancer and which means, in effect, that they are cancerous. Industry types are 'confident' that eating such products poses no risk and you're all despicable in your thoughts and your actions. But it's not difficult to see, even if the products were 'proven' safe, how people might be put off by the thought that they're eating a glorified tumour." Labelled a "flop" in a January 18, 2023, article by Bloomberg, the fake meat industry appears to be tumbling before our eyes. The food supply of every American is going to start being Intentionally Poisoned with mRNA genetic modifications being fraudulently called "vaccines." Lobbyists for the cattleman and pork associations in several states have confirmed they will be using mRNA vaccines in Pigs and Cows starting in April 2023. It will become "vaccine food" and sold to you without your Informed Consent and buying and eating this beef or this pork may adversely affect you and in some cases, it may Kill you. Back here in Australia a processing ingredient called GM soy leghemoglobin SLH is produced from a GM Pichia pastoris yeast strain. Pichia pastoris has no history of being used safely in food. Australian/New Zealand food authority FSANZ has already approved SLH for use in foods, and it is expected that Impossible Meat will soon be available here. By keeping the amount of the controversial substance to 0.8 percent, Impossible Foods can even avoid having it labelled on its items and you can see why I strongly suggest not buying at major supermarkets and labels will mean nothing.

Attacking the food chain and the reasons for that are very clear: they need to get to all of us through it, and they're attacking from all quarters. Much of the conversation surrounding mRNA (messenger) "vaccines" centres around their impact on humans, but how about all the animals that are being injected with it? Believe it or not, cattle are now getting jabbed with the poison, which in a recent mass "Vaccination" campaign of an Australian herd resulted in 35 of the 200 animals dying immediately. We are told that dairy farmers and others are now being forced to inject their animals for the Fauci Flu in order to remain in business, and that the animals are not responding well to it. Just like in humans, these shots are causing such profound damage that many of the animals are succumbing to instant death, while the others are getting sick and dying over a period of time. (mRNA spike proteins linger in the heart and brain long after injection.) For the animals that do survive, one wonders what is becoming of their milk, which gets passed on as food for other animals as well as humans. Is it safe to consume mRNA-tainted milk and cheese from a "fully vaccinated" dairy cow?

The answer to that should be very clear. I have repeated myself on purpose because it is "Food for Thought" If "Milk is altered, and you consume it and then Butter constitution, yoghurt, cheese and be next? The answer to that is also blatantly obvious.So why would they do this madness when it is mysteriously absent from the "science" behind forced mRNA injections for animals is any actual evidence that animals are getting sick from Covid. A deal was forged with a United States-based biotechnology company called Tiba BioTech that, just like Pfizer, BioNTech, and Moderna, is now raking in the dough. There's soon going to be another reason to either choose vegetarian food options or get your meat from local, trusted sources: the mRNA vaccines are about to be heavily implemented across the meat industry, with cattle, chickens, pigs, goats and other livestock targeted for regular mRNA injections. As we've seen with human beings, mRNA injections can and do circulate throughout the entire body and end up in blood and organs. The body produces toxic proteins which can cause toxic effects and clog arteries that end up killing or harming people from strokes or heart attacks, when you alter chromosomes and cause permanent genetic changes to the organism. Merely handling raw meat contaminated with mRNA products is likely the equivalent to being exposed to "shedding" from vaccine recipients. And even though stomach acid likely destroys mRNA sequences, there is absorption that takes place in the mouth, under the tongue, which is why many medications and supplements, including Cbd Oils and Zinc, are often best absorbed under the **tongue rather than being swallowed.** So, merely introducing mRNA-vaccinated animal meat products into your mouth, if not fully cooked, may expose you to a kind of "food shedding" of mRNA products that can be absorbed into your blood and circulated throughout your body. This can include proteins which are alien to the human body, most of you will not know whether to eat anything that has mRNA in it, cooked or not but logically don't. It seems obvious that globalists are trying to both contaminate the meat supply and wipe it out over time, replacing animal meats with grubs, mealworms, crickets and black soldier-fly larvae, among other creatures.

Meanwhile, no doubt, the globalists will enjoy prime rib on their private jets while they nibble on non-GMO organic salads, because they know clean food promotes longevity. The UK government is actively considering vaccinating the country's poultry flock against bird flu in a bid to curb the worst-ever global outbreak of the virus and prevent it turning into a new pandemic in humans. In what would be a major change of UK policy, government officials and scientists are looking at overturning a ban on vaccinating tens of millions of birds as the H5N1 virus shows no sign of abating.

Wildlife Nothing is sacred and vaccinating wildlife is not a new idea, in fact, it was first conceived in the 1960s. Following trials and research, oral rabies vaccines were administered throughout Western Europe 188 from the 1980s onwards focusing on red foxes and leading to the virtual elimination of the virus in the region. In 2022, the UK government reduced the paperwork necessary to vaccinate badgers against tuberculosis.

Honeybees Meanwhile, the US Department of Agriculture, has conditionally approved an accelerated track to market for a vaccine that will protect honeybees against American foulbrood, a disease that has run rampant through bee colonies since the 1800s. The honeybee vaccine is administered to queen bees in a jelly that contains dead versions of Paenibacillus larvae, the bacterium that causes the disease. This then means that the queen bee's offspring have resilience against the disease. Now, let's once again, get back to our food chain, as it relates to Agenda 30. This has never been more important, especially if you're buying from the big food chains, because insects in our food or edible, insects and insect species used for human consumption; they are not as safe as you may believe. More than 2,000 insect species worldwide are considered edible, and can you really believe that, and how many are not safe. I was brought up in the UK eating offal which might grouse some of you out and still enjoy "Lambs Fry" sheep's livers and also sheep's kidneys.

But insects are not for me and in a country abundant with food like Australia why would we want to. Many countries like Thailand, Indonesia, Mexico, India, Japan and Cambodia have eaten insects for a long time, but I never ever tried them and never will, but we are not talking about these insects. But ones created in factories in Vietnam, Canada and anything the EMF have planned and this part tie Agenda 2030. I spoke to some of the vaccinated. They go "Yum, it's Protein" because they are programmed and after 3 vaccinations their natural immunity is already at zero this might be the final death knell for them.

Brussels, Belgium the most recent approval was on January 5 2023 and from now on, mealworms, grasshoppers and crickets, the grain mould beetle can also be used as an ingredient in foods such as bread, soups, pasta, snacks, peanut butter and chocolate products. Avoid processed foods as much as possible from today because if you do not your health will suffer from this Plandamic Agenda, as permission has already been issued for manufacturers to add insects to all food products. Now all of you reading this are required to read the ingredients of the products and they obliged the producers to write what was added there, but unfortunately it will be in Latin. Remember when looking at the product composition you will find so welcome to the New World Order of 2023. The evil multinational corporations are using one excuse or another to inflate their profits and continue this 2030 Agenda and if people get sick or die, it is not their problem as they will still make money from the sick and also be aware they will always fool consumers by mentioning just the numbers or codes of the ingredients they put into your food. Insects in flour which are already in Woolworths Macro brand Cricket flour from February 2023, snacks, peanut butter and chocolate products avoid processed foods as much as possible from today because if you do not your health will suffer this Plandamic Agenda, as permission has already given to manufacturers add so many insects, beetles, cockroaches, crickets and domestic grasshoppers.

Carmine used for food colouring is extracted from insects and these insects will give us a lot of parasitic flora. Over 4,000 species of parasitic plants exist and most of them are flowering plants. Successful, ongoing parasitism is an easy way to make a living, since the parasite doesn't have to expend or absorb as much energy as would be expected in order to fulfil its needs. The parasites may be either holoparasites or hemiparasites and the symptoms of **Body Parasites in Humans**, are many including constipation, diarrhoea, gas and bloating, ibs, muscle aches, anaemia, skin conditions, sleep disorders, anxiety, chronic fatigue, and tumours. The list is endless so if you want your body and life to turn to crap just eat these insects.

Chityna is a hard outer cover for insects that destroy internal organs and cause diseases, such as things like Cancer and insects are a reservoir of parasitic and pathogenic flora that cripples human organs, and you cannot get these parasites out of your body. If you look at the product compositions, you need to look at these numbers for **E 120 Carmine** (Red Dye) is a mixture of cochineal beetles and for **E 904** refers to shellac, a natural product and shellac consists of excrements of the female varnish scale insect. Shellac is a food additive approved in the EU and can be used (without maximum quantity restriction) as a coating agent for the treatment of foodstuffs. I wish I was making all this up as It is total madness and everything that is done like the small print is well thought out and insects are now being added to confectionery. Not surprising they target this as people are depressed and chocolate for many is an outlet to cheer you all up. It is also in baking products, pasta, pastry products and drinks. This is well thought out by the NWO and eating crickets could be the fuel for the next "Pandemic" and wipe out several million people, if not a few billion. There is a method in their total madness and do the globalists and their insidious scientists know this? Is this new push for the populace to consume insects all part of the depopulation plan? This requires careful consideration when you are eating your locusts, crickets, ants, beetles and worms.

There is a method in their total madness and do the globalists and their insidious scientists know this? **Is chitin the kill switch?** Ironically Ivermectin is an anti-parasitic medicine that has an amazingly high percentage of success beating Covid infection at all stages So, could it be that chitin consumption will be the parasites and virus mutations of the next pandemic in such a way that ivermectin won't work anymore?

The Green Lizard King Charles 111, King of England we all aware he a reptile and here is further proof and one of the more shocking hypocrisies of this year century so far, Charles 111, King of England considered to be a strong supporter of organic farming and environmental causes has given his Royal Assent to a biotechnology 'innovation' which will provide an open book for UK firms to alter the genome of animals and plants, so as to create "novel engineered species and biotech 'foods'. In taking this step Charles has committed an open act of betrayal of all bona fide farmers, and particularly of organic farmers.

The Genetic Technology Precision Breeding Act 2023 was given the royal go ahead on 23rd March 2023 and this piece of legislation will, for the time being, be unique to the UK, as such animal and plant biotech deformations are not allowed in the EU and many other countries, and another deception relates to the marketing of such novel recombinant DNA experiments. But the EU and the rest of the world will follow the evil King's lead as soon as he gives it the "Royal Seal of Approval'. The UK government has stated that no separate definition will be given to gene technology engineered products, so therefore no special labelling will be required because they're going to poison you as planned and all Agenda 2030 which just keeps on rolling on to achieve its aim. The conclusion and the dark irony of King of England launching unlabelled biotech foods, animals and plants on citizens of his own country, is not hard to understand when Charles is already in conflict with the constitution of his country by standing shoulder to shoulder with Klaus Schwab promoting the World Economic Forum's 'Great Reset'. The UK government has stated that no separate definition will be given to gene technology engineered products, so therefore no special labelling will be required because they're going to poison you as planned and all Agenda 2030 which just keeps on rolling on to achieve its aims. One of the main objectives of which is to render nation states obsolete and to centralise all power within the control of a small despotic elite, whose sole stated intention is to make all private property illegal and to re-engineer human beings into "Transhuman Cyborgs".

On May 6, 2023, at his coronation in London, Charles will be officially crowned monarch of the United Kingdom and its Commonwealth, and it is a large empire and the centrepiece of the coronation ceremony, Charles will swear 'The Coronation Oath', essentially pledging his allegiance to the people of Great Britain and to protect the sovereignty of the country and its traditions. If Charles does not break his relationship with the World Economic Forum before this point, he will be performing an act of "Treason" and the implications of this are very profound. Yet, the British people have not woken-up to their fate and most never will, but should the truth emerge from this singularly blatant hypocrisy, the future of the British monarchy that already has a dark past when you understand the ties they had with Germany in the second World War and time to end this monarchy for good and as the UK is officially recognised as a 'constitutional monarchy'.

With an unrevoked Common Law constitution stretching back to the Magna Carta of 1215, the true political power lies with the people and not with parliament and something which has been largely hidden from public knowledge as the sheeple don't really care as long as their mobile phones are still switched on and will do as they are told. We all have heard of the "Stolen Generation" in Australia. Sadly, I must be very unkind that most of the youth of the UK and the World will be known in the future as "The Lost Generation" if they don't "Wake Up Today" and fight for their freedoms.

If there is to be a future king or queen, the country needs that person to exercise his or her power to stand-up against the continual parliamentary usurpation of the people's power. The people need a monarch with some guts, some wisdom and a genuine respect for truth, and you would wish someone who will use his very time-honoured constitutional powers to block anti-life legislation like The Genetic Technology Precision Breeding Act 2023; thus, setting a proper precedent for Great Britain's 'first among equals' to act like a real King.

But he was never going to be a real king and you only got to look at his past history of being best friends with Jimmy Saville and he would have known all about what that evil man was doing to disabled children and his own Brother Prince Andrew and his connections with Jeffrey Epstein and do not tell me he did not know. For any you really switched on you be aware of what truly happens behind the doors of the royal families of the drinking of children's blood and the eating of the flesh. Its logical they had insects added in to the "Royal Feast" Sadly he live to be nearly 100 and the reasons for that also very clear, so let's just hang Him "For Treason" alongside Klaus Schwab, Biden, Scomo, Anal, Gates, Fauci and all who will be proven in on this Genocide.

No Farms No Food™

We are literally witnessing a worldwide coordinated plan to shut down farming. This is all about controlling the food chain. When they control the food... they control us.

Chapter Eight

The Freedom Movement

We have all seen the inspiration of Truck conveys in Canada and all the other Worldwide protests for our freedoms and basic human rights, and how inspiring was the Canberra protest that lasted many weeks in 2022. Ordinary people have just had enough of this evil tyranny yet the media, as they have done all along just played us down as Conspiracy Theorists, and in some cases the use of weaponry by the police in Melbourne and Canberra was deemed acts of War by all of us and even when we protest peacefully, they resort in this manner which is totally Un-Australian and not acceptable. We have all seen footage of the protests during the Vietnam War, but then there is no war bigger than this Spiritual one which we must Win for the sake of mankind. I personally have had reservations for a long time regarding the freedom movement, and I truly believe it is not what it seems? and who is the enemy. Sadly, some amongst us would have to be treated with suspicion and are 'Paid Opposition' and will be exposed at some point and they will need to really fear that. One of the true heroes though is Dr William Bay, who worked at my local medical centre here in Woody Point, Queensland before having his licence revoked, he stated ''People and Doctors should be allowed the Legal and Moral right to question Government directives and Public Health messages. The Government should not get in the way of the doctor-patient relationship and doctors must be allowed to exercise their thoughts on issues affecting their patients or otherwise the public will NOT have confidence that doctors are doing the right thing by them. I have personally watched lots of public speakers in the freedom movement and Dr William Bay is not in my humble opinion paid opposition and an incredibly passionate speaker from the heart with God on his shoulder. Please show him your support by attending a QPP rally or donating for his fight to take this matter to the

High Court of Australia, Dr Bay urges you to stand with him to make it possible again for doctors to speak freely in the interests of you the patient, lest we lose our ethical medical system forever. There are so many Worldwide in the medical profession who are standing up like Dr William Bay and we all owe them a great debt; they are doing God's work and fighting the great fight for all of us. In a later chapter I will highlight some of the brave businesses that in my local area that did not comply with the bullshit of checking in, and mask wearing and treated us all equally. All of you reading this will have many experiences of the discrimination we had to endure and in front of our own family members.

I remember one such incident vividly which happened on Boxing Day 2021, when going out with my vaccinated family members and not being able to enter a fish and chip shop here in Scarborough, Queensland as I had to show vaccination proof and check in to enter. It was a total madness that divided all of us, and the divisions in some of our families are now etched deep. So to all those businesses Worldwide that did not treat us like 'Vermin' thank you, and I will bet you are like the ones here in Queensland that your businesses are thriving and the others who were a disgrace like one certain chip shop here in beautiful Scarborough, Qld, this owner had a sign on his window "you know the drill regarding checking in"; I have since noticed his business is suffering, and it's currently selling coffees as well as fish and chips now to survive.

Never forget how badly they treated us, the Unclean and "Karma is a real Bitch" They truly need to be treated with disdain, and no longer will we accept their compliance and dictation to us, because we are truly free, happy and healthy. We are the true survivors, and they are not and feel how truly lucky you are to be alive and if you listen to your heart and not some of the paid opposition you can and will Survive Agenda 2030. We have all seen all the court cases being squashed; well, legally they never were going to stand up in court.

Controlled Opposition This topic really bothers me and being spiritual sometimes does give you an edge on reading people and their Agendas? and all of us in the freedom movement I feel we are our own worst enemies. We were so divided in the last Federal election here in 2022 in Australia, and so many of us across Australia worked so very hard for our freedom parties for a change to happen. I had met Kelly Guenoun when she was speaking as a representative for the United Australia Party event at Redcliffe, when we got to meet all the candidates.A true honest politician that means what they say, does truly stand out. It was a very interesting night and I got to meet Mrs. Death and her energy truly bothered me and, on the way home at 10pm a bat attacked me on my face and body. After that I was ill for twelve days, since then I have given Mrs. Death a very wide berth and was that a coincidence the bat attacked me? She has been very instrumental in what has happened here in Queensland, and her actions have been very disappointing, and everyone is accountable at some point in time. When you put her name into "Word" it converts to death and is very apt. I really do not have time for most politicians usually, as they just kick the can down the road once they get into Parliament and are then often corrupted by "The System." But we are fortunate to have a few upstanding ones like Malcolm Roberts and some of the others I have already mentioned. We salute you all and Godspeed you help end this Australian and Worldwide Tyranny, as you call out all of them out that are complicit in the Genocidal Agenda. Let's be totally honest, all of the major parties are in bed together and they are all one party. So here was our big chance in the 2022 Federal election; and I don't think people could have worked any harder. Here in the Petrie Division, we had the Pauline Hanson candidate living in NSW and it is a total mockery of the system. If all the Freedom Parties, The United Australian Party, One Nation, Liberal Democrats and Australia One, had all treated this like a war against one common enemy, we would have done so much better.

The Australian Election of 2022, as with a lot of elections Worldwide, was rigged and we all are aware of that and they are rightly so fearful of us and will do anything to keep this total charade going, and protect themselves and the 'NWO' and all the evil that pervades this planet. Kelly Guenoun has kindly written a chapter and she has become a friend. Australia loses when honest politicians like Kelly do not get a seat to help "keep the bastards honest." As I already said, 'The Freedom Movement' really bothers me. We have all attended the rallies which have been uplifting being around so many "Normal People" with normal people that truly care about the future of this great nation Australia. The future of our Planet and our children's futures that are all being flushed down the toilet by some very weak "Specimens" who are holding on to power all based on greed, ego and pure evil. When we attend these rallies which are held in cities worldwide, we are all being microwaved by all the 5G towers that pervade the cities, and my EMF metre alarm is ringing all the hours while I am attending. I must be brutally honest, some of the speakers are not what they seem: they're maybe "Paid Opposition" and a lot of us are becoming increasingly aware of who they are, and they will have to be held to account.

Ego is also in the forefront; and they're mostly men, and nothing changes with some men. We all naturally have "Ego," and I am no different born imperfect- perfect but some have agenda's that run very deep and very concerning and we have all seen it. I am not going to name and shame as there is no point; but just remember there are people dying while you "big-note yourselves' with your trumped-up little bit of power. Hopefully soon we can unite as we are very splintered, and our enemy just loves that. I also saw that a lot in some of the Common Law groups and it really annoys me how just a few spoils it for the rest of us. One Group at Caboolture Qld I was allowed only to speak for 3 minutes which I thought rather strange when I worked as an entertainer and I was trying to save lives by not using 5G.

Those who are not so lucky and have family members treating you incredibly badly, and that seems to get worse when they have had the booster and seeing the emotional pain, you're going through cuts very deep. It is no coincidence when you understand the poison and its effects on the brains of those receiving these toxins; It is like your loved ones have been hijacked and in their place is someone you will never, ever understand or might never understand again, unless they eventually wake up.

Brainwashing runs so deep in this Agenda that those who should love you unconditionally as we love them, choose to ostracise you because they truly believe we are a danger to them, and mankind. If only they had listened and switched that damn TV off, but we will still be there to pick up the pieces and help those who need help with their self-inflicted health conditions, having destroyed their innate natural immunity for ever. Some will ask for help in detoxing, and I am starting to see that more and more, which is so encouraging when maybe some of you get to be able to 'switch the lights back on' in their brains after they were duped. While I attempt to write this book this Plandemic is evolving at a great pace. The division this Plandemic Agenda has on society has been immense, especially in families, and there may only be a few families not having problems between unvaccinated and vaccinated members? all over a COLD. It really beggars belief that we can be ostracised because of it. Luckily for me my family has found some common ground and we don't talk about 'The C (covid) Word' as it really is not worth falling out over. Those who are not so lucky and have family members treating you incredibly badly, and that seems to get worse when they have had the booster and seeing the emotional pain, you're going through cuts very deep.

Never have we lived in more uncertain times but there was more good news today which I have already touched on. It was not rocket science that would happen that all Doctors, Nurses, Medical Practices, Health Government Employees are liable for vaccinating patients without proper informed consent and warning patients the truth. I predict the insurance companies will be null and voiding the doctor's indemnity and the doctors and all be held accountable as they should because in reference to the Australian health department "It has now been confirmed by your department that health practitioners are not covered by a specific Covid-19 government medical indemnity scheme.

So, the Australian Government lied and what is new and will this latest bombshell ever be given media coverage? This has the appearance of the government throwing medical staff under the bus on liability and requirements for informed consent. I think most reading this have no sympathy for anybody who coerced people to make such an important decision without informed consent especially and the lawyers will love this, it was an experimental approved only vaccine which has since been found to be based on mistruths and that it was deemed Safe.

But we who did not buy into this Agenda always understood it could never be safe, but it was such a tragic day that so many brought into the scam. For all those who took these poisons and paid the ultimate price my heart goes out to their families. I predict a lot of the medical practices will fold and go into receivership. You notice most of them seem very quiet as most are charging everyone to see a doctor, so people are put in the position to go to the emergency departments of their local hospitals. **Warrior's** I would like to mention all the warriors who put their lives in danger by calling out this evil and they are very brave and courageous along with ethically minded senators and politicians from all over the world, like Senators Gerard Rennick, Alex Antic, Malcolm Roberts, Matt Canavan, Ralph Babet, Pauline Hanson, Craig Kelly (former MP), Senator Rand Paul, Rob Johnson (USA), and European parliamentarians who have continually voiced concerns over the manner in which the injections were rolled out across their respective countries. Also, lawyers from around the world have united, strongly driven by perceived injustices against humanity, such as Aaron Siri, Thomas Renz, and Reiner Fuellmich ect, and have launched actions and continue to do their duty to ensure the Rule of Law is followed internationally. To any who I have not included it was not intentional love and respect to all.

WHAT IF I TOLD YOU THAT ALL OF THIS:

@TRUTH.VIBRATIONS

WAS ENGINEERED TO CONDITION THE MASSES TO ACCEPT THIS:

DIGITAL IDS   DIGITAL CURRENCY   SOCIAL CREDIT

5G SMART CITIES   TRANSHUMANISM   WAR AGAINST DISSENT

Chapter 9

The Dangers of EMF Radiation

This is such a very important subject. You will probably have seen people exercising and so many of them are school children wearing these very dangerous '' Earbuds. Some of my friends had switched over to earbuds (wireless earphones), and then asked me if earbuds emit EMF radiation. It was obvious that I knew the answer, but I decided to do a bit more research on the issue. Most of my friends were unvaccinated, but they had family members, children and grandchildren who were following this agenda fashion accessory, and the results were extremely alarming that I made it a chapter title. Wireless earbuds, including Apple Air pods, emit high levels of EMF radiation, mainly in the form of microwaves. They rely on Bluetooth technology, among other things, and this is a potentially dangerous thing to have so close to your brain. Like me you properly are not surprised and when you consider the high levels of Graphene Oxide around the blood brain barrier it was easy to work out why. So, to all you exercise freaks in your sexy gear trying to look great, can you see why they seem like they're brain dead because they're basically heading that way. So please educate all your loved ones to ditch them and all of these devices rely on 'microwaves' and for Bluetooth, it's specifically between **2.4 and 2.8GHz** in frequency. It's what's known as non-ionizing radiation, although Bluetooth devices give off other forms of EMF radiation, such as heat energy. General EMF radiation safety guidelines for these appliances and devices are often to stand a large distance away for some Wi-Fi routers, it can be up to 20 ft. Similarly, for cell phones, it's recommended that you don't spend more than 20 minutes a day on calls, specifically with the device against your ear. When you do, your brain becomes Zombified over time and it is very scary and incredibly sad if it is a family member who becomes one.

What is at stake is that all freedoms are eroded one by one, a they have already for most of us in the last three years. The divide and conquer has only just started so what is next, so very much and not in any particular order this is their future all of those that have complied and are owned by the NWO who have become "Vaccine Addict's" and will basically do anything they're told as they truly believe they must and a lot lined up for clot shot number five that was available here in Australia on the 20th February, 2023. They will eat their bugs and the plant food and even enjoy it, or they think they will, as their mind is no longer their own. There is no limit to their compliance which should be a real warning to all of us as I already will mention the five levels of zombism in a later chapter. I already see quite a lot of them every day.

Are they very easy to spot? yes if you're truly in tune with their actions, which in some ways are bizarre especially if there is someone you thought you knew well. EMFS caused by 2G-4G & now 5G affects every living thing and we have seen a great reduction of 70% in fruit as there is a 60% decrease in insects that pollinate as a low dose of emf can be equally or more dangerous than a short high dose of EMF. It is already suspected of killing cattle and birds, Wi-Fi is a known weapons frequency and countries like Poland that have a lot of forests will sadly disappear at some point. People underestimate and do not understand how useful trees truly are because trees communicate with each other through their root systems and the soil and help each other and most do understand they take out a lot of carbon dioxide from the air and trees do not like it. Fish and especially around inland lakes are very dependent on trees and are up to 70% of a fish is tree matter that is acted on by microorganisms and other microorganisms start the fish web. So, if you destroy the tree and the ground soil you then destroy the Fish and it's interesting to note that in the last 20 years, we have lost 80% of our insects. With 5G, we're going to lose 100% of our insects so when the insects go, we go too. Both insects and 5G need antennas: insects use them, among other things, in their sense of smell, while 5G uses them to propagate waves.

Not surprisingly, insects are sensitive to 5G EMF waves which is very logical; there are recent studies showing that insects exposed to 5G radiation experienced an increase in their body temperature and this phenomenon was not observed with 4G or Wi-Fi. Bee's will also disappear due to microwaves and the fact there are plans to inject mRNA into the bees.

Mitochondrial Damage Due to Emf radiation. The MMW frequencies of 5G cause mitochondrial DNA damage which is then passed down through the generations as 5G is mutagenic and the mutations are inherited by the next generation. This is very grave for genetic purity and how many people are thinking about this when they can't stop looking at their phone screens? phone addiction is rife in all ages. You will see a beautiful lady out with their man and they're both "at it" looking at their phones. There are many studies showing the mitochondrial damage that occurs after exposure to EMF radiation and with mutagenesis usually comes carcinogenesis, in other words, once something is powerful and dangerous enough to cause DNA damage, chances are high it will lead to cancer. It has been reported that 5G is a class 1 carcinogen although the WHO, very classifies cell phone towers as a class 2b possible carcinogen.

It's important to note, however, that the WHO is an agency of the UN, which was set up by the Rockefellers, an illustrious NWO Illuminati family who plan to use the UN as a vehicle to usher in a One World Government which most of you are aware of but needs 5G it is being rushed out without the proper safety testing being done, so we don't have much data on how 5G specifically causes cancer, but there is an abundance of evidence showing how 2G, 3G and 4G EMFs are implicated in many kinds of cancer, including brain cancer. 5G is planned to be an inescapable grid with plans afoot to beam it down from space with "At least five companies are proposing to provide 5G from space from a combined 20,000 satellites in low and medium Earth orbit that will blanket the Earth with powerful, focused, steerable beam.

Each satellite will emit millimetre waves with an effective radiated power of up to 5 million watts from thousands of antennas arranged in a phased array." and it is very vital to understand the bigger picture of the grand conspiracy here. All these disruptive and hazardous gadgets such as 5G, Wi-Fi, wireless radiation, HAARP, ionospheric heating, geoengineering, GMOs, etc. Are going to be woven into one giant integrated system of surveillance, command and control and just as a small example, geoengineering involves the spraying of chemtrails loaded with metal particulates which 5G can use.

EMF AND CHILDREN Protecting your children from the dangers of EMF radiation should be a very high priority, and should begin immediately, as there is so much we can do even before the child is born. As you may already be aware, children are far more vulnerable to radiation from devices such as cell phones, tablets, Wi-Fi and much more. It used to be that children were not exposed to much technology until they were closer to adulthood, as tablets and cell phones were not so inexpensive and readily available as they are now. Today it is not uncommon to see a four- or five- year old with a cell phone, and children even younger with a tablet always on their lap. Manufacturers are even specifically designing phones for children preloaded with games, cameras, and accessories to allow the phones to be even more entertaining; everything in this plandemic is interlinked. It's easy to think of cell phones only for the convenience they allow, and they make it very simple to keep track of our children and to easily get in touch. These are great things that shouldn't be overlooked, but it's also very important to understand the potential dangers and risks these devices pose. You might already intuitively know it, but children are more susceptible to all sorts of dangers, from EMF radiation to air pollution and cloud seeding. Although their smaller size makes them proportionally more vulnerable to things, it's important to remember that they are not just smaller sized adults. The biological and structural makeup of a baby or small child is dramatically different and makes a difference in how well it can protect them. An example is a 2003 study that found that children's thinner skulls and bones protect them from less radiation, causing them to absorb up to twice the radiation from devices like cell phones as compared to adults. A 2011 study also found that "When electrical properties are considered, a child's head's absorption can be over two times greater, and absorption of the skull's bone marrow can be ten times greater than adults" if that does not alarm you nothing will. Plus combined with the technology of what 5G will do, it's a recipe for disaster and zombism in children is starting to become very noticeable.

Home-schooling sadly is the only option for some parents and "Hold your heads up High" but I'm sure there are teachers reading this who will come on board the Freedom Train. With the schools heavily geared to technology and 5G you will have to at some point make decisions regarding home-schooling, but for now if you detox your children and protect them every way you can, you will be able to buy a bit more time as this 5G nightmare unfolds. Our body makes over 2 million new red blood cells every second and this rapid creation of new cells leaves the children vulnerable to stresses on their bodies because inside of our red blood cells, there is a series of small receptors, located within the cell membrane. Although these receptors typically receive chemical signals from the body, they are also capable of being influenced by an outside influence. These receptors can actually sense man-made EMF radiation, and they react as if a foreign invader is entering the body and the bloodstream so sensing danger, the cells react by first inhibiting the active transport channels inside of the cell membranes, dramatically lowering their permeability, as well as their ability to function and interpret micronutrients. This does two harmful things because it reduces the number of healthy nutrients that enter our cells, it also inhibits our cells ability to interpret and rid themselves of toxins and free radicals and it should be easy to understand that after just a short amount of time, cells that are unable to get needed nutrients and are unable to expel free radicals and toxins will soon become very damaged. Also, the blood-brain barrier that protects our brains is also more permeable in children which can make their brains even more vulnerable to the toxins and free radicals created in the bloodstream.

Pregnancy It's very possible for children in the womb to be exposed and harmed by the EMF radiation because the mother is absorbing it through cell phone use, laptop use, smart metres, etc. Think of EMF radiation as another toxin you should try to avoid while pregnant and in the same way, if you don't smoke or drink alcohol, and carefully consider the foods you eat, you should also be careful about how much wireless radiation you and your baby are exposed to. The very next thing you'll want to do is make sure that your nursery is as much of an EMF-free zone as possible. I would start by getting a quality EMF metre if you don't already have one, and sweeping the room to see what the baseline radiation levels are, as well as find out how much these days are a near necessity for peace of mind. However, I would encourage you to get a wired baby monitor if possible as the wireless versions emit far more radiation.

So, let's talk about one of the big issues facing you with your children today and that is their Cell Phones and because of the risks that cell phones pose is so much greater for children. France has made it illegal to market mobile phones of any kind to young children and the Russian Government also advises anyone under the age of 18 to not use a cell phone at all. And can you see why there are so many reasons for some of us who are pro Russia to as they are leading the way? Against Agenda 2030. First of all, hold off as long as you feel reasonable and try not to buy your preschooler a cell phone if they don't absolutely need it and you'll know when the time is right for your child, depending on your child's needs and try have your child text you very quick messages instead of calling as text messages because they are quick hardly emit hardly any radiation but, making a phone call and holding the phone against your head can add to the cumulative danger of cell phone use.

This is also very important considering getting your child an **Air-Tube Headset** to listen to music and videos, as well as making calls with as air tube headsets dramatically lower radiation exposure from the phone by keeping the phone away from your body and they also reduce your exposure to magnetic field radiation, by moving the speaker away from your head and passing the sound through a tube of air instead, it stops 99% of cell phone radiation from entering your brain. Doing this will not only improve their sleep and energy levels and reduce radiation exposure, but it will also give them good habits moving forward. First, of all it's important to remember that the harm from EMF radiation, including RF radiation, has been shown to be very cumulative, meaning it adds up over time.

Looking first at an iPad, they emit short bursts of pulsed microwave radiation even when we are not using them, and these bursts typically occur every **4 seconds or up to 900 times every hour** even when they are not in use they are continually searching for a signal and Smartphones do the same thing. Hundreds of studies have linked EMF radiation with ill-health effects: headaches, migraines, anxiety, depression, sleep problems, heart problems, infertility, adhd and autism and the heart, brain and reproductive organs are most badly affected so it clearly makes sense because when we put phones to our ears, brains, iPads close to our faces and tablets or laptops on our laps these organs also contain the highest density of Voltage-Gated Calcium Channels and when we are exposed to man-made EMFs these gates open, allowing millions of calcium ions into each and every cell, wreaking havoc. A massive inflammatory cascade ensues, and inflammation equals disease and of course, our hearts and brains run on electricity too and that's what Ecgs and Eeegs measure, so naturally any unnatural form of EMF is bound to affect our own natural electrical systems. Children are not little adults, and they are impacted way more than we are because their heads are smaller, their skulls much thinner and right up until about 20 years of age their brains are still developing and their brain tissue contains more fluid and so is more conductive than ours and the bone marrow and eyes absorb way more radiation than the rest of their body. Their stem cells are also much more numerous and active in growing bodies and have been shown to be affected by high-frequency radiation. That's why when it comes to children and technology, we simply have to be vigilant and I keep repeating myself for very obvious reasons.

The elderly ask me, do hearing aids emit EMF radiation?, hearing aids emit EMF radiation and in fact, due to their proximity to the brain, the radiation from wireless hearing devices can actually pose a great danger to the human health of everyone using them and I don't think this will surprise you and I personally have tested them on a man who is a friend and his unvaccinated he was very alarmed and it's very obvious they come after us in any way they possibly can. You are aware of the advances in hearing aids over the years and that most are, currently wireless, sound it picks to a chip and then the chip adjusts the sound and the volume to provide an improved hearing experience. Digital hearing aids use radio frequency and microwave EMF radiation to operate as they are wireless and I will end this chapter reminding you all the incredible dangers of 5G and why I have got rid of my phone and plan to go ''Of Grid', 5G relies primarily on the bandwidth of the millimetre wave, which can cause a painful burning sensation. It's also been linked to eye and heart problems, suppressed immune function, genetic damage and fertility problems. Graphene is manipulated from the outside, which is possible with the new technology, and the Graphene frequencies are included in the 5G bandwidth and people receiving this misnamed "Vaccine" are being inoculated with Graphene Oxide, which becomes very magnetic in contact with hydrogen from biomolecules. Microwave syndrome was described in the 1970s by scientists in the former Soviet Union who were researching occupational risks, due to exposure to non-ionizing radiation and Soviet researchers described multiple symptoms of the syndrome, including fatigue, dizziness, headaches, difficulty sleeping, tinnitus, concentration problems, mood swings, dizziness, headaches, difficulty sleeping, concentration problems, mood swings, heart palpitations and memory loss and do these problems sound familiar to you. So, when you understand all of this then maybe you treat your phone and everything to do with Wi-Fi, and anything with the word smart on it as a weapon to be used against you. Many of you may spend a fortune on medicines, consult specialists, and try natural therapies but we are all going to pay such a heavy price due to 5G, if we don't do everything humanly possible to limit the exposure to pulse frequencies and how these weapons will be used and are aimed at you and your loved ones. Children and most people are "Hooked" on cell phones and we all understand the risks of smoking and in the future you all will understand the dangers of 5g and by then you will ask yourselves how did they get away with killing so many people **"Simple Addiction"**. You all learned to switch the TV'S off and do you miss them? well maybe your mobile phones are next "just a thought". Some of you ladies reading this would have "Burned your Bra" way back when and how liberating it was that now try to dump your phones you will understand that makes logical sense.

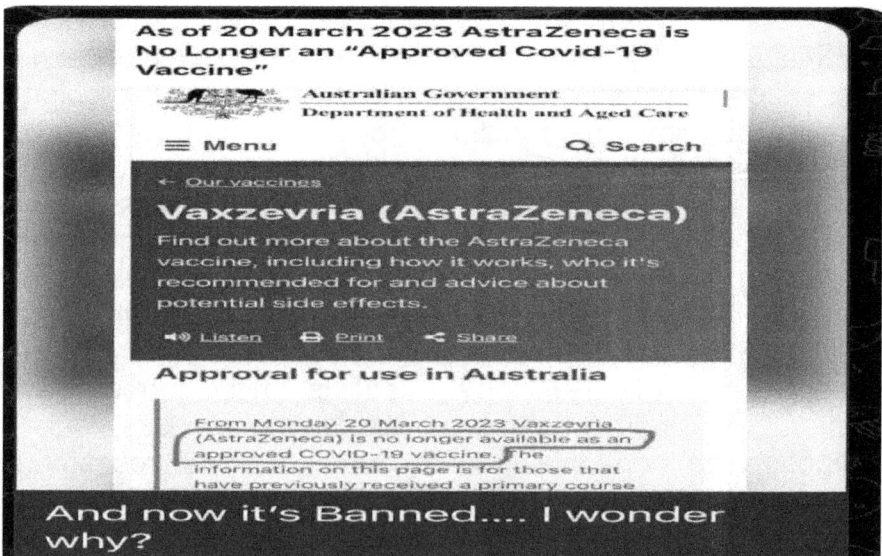

As of 20 March 2023 AstraZeneca is No Longer an "Approved Covid-19 Vaccine"

Australian Government
Department of Health and Aged Care

≡ Menu   Q Search

← Our vaccines

Vaxzevria (AstraZeneca)

Find out more about the AstraZeneca vaccine, including how it works, who it's recommended for and advice about potential side effects.

◀》 Listen   🖶 Print   ◁ Share

Approval for use in Australia

From Monday 20 March 2023 Vaxzevria (AstraZeneca) is no longer available as an approved COVID-19 vaccine. The information on this page is for those that have previously received a primary course

And now it's Banned.... I wonder why?

Chapter 10

The Future Plan for Mankind

The Digital Credit System Will this be a reality soon well sadly, yes and they truly plan to own all of your bodies, all of your minds and finally your spirit, so no more coming back to repeat "Inner Child" past mistakes and no remembrance of previous lives, all that that you have learned and evolved with to get you where you are today. If you are truly spiritual it is less likely for us to allow that to happen but trust me there after all of us on mother earth. The food chain is the next link in the chain where we are going to lose more people who are then zombified. It is coming very fast over the next two years and to stop that happening, you will have to be very aware of it and not buy from the supermarkets and their controlled poisonous consumer goods, and I do understand I am repeating myself so hopefully you will get it. Network and source truly organic foods and if someone is selling it and is vaccinated, I personally would not buy from them, if they don't care about their own bodies, they're not going to bother about yours. I am sorry this is another doom and gloom chapter, but I am sure so many reading this are starting to barter, as we all have things that are of value in our skill sets and our valuables, try to find fishermen and source small truly unvaccinated hobby farmers and grow your own foods then preserve and dehydrate some of the food. I used to have a Ten-acre hobby farm in Tasmania, in a small hamlet called Winkleigh, between Exeter, and Beaconsfield, which I owned for six years because when I lived in England before I emigrated, I used to watch a show called 'The Good Life' about being self-sufficient, so I decided to make that a reality and learnt so very much about being self-sufficient, and having that experience. It really is not that hard to milk a cow especially with a bucket machine and having your own truly organic food supply.

What is the social credit system they have planned for all of us and what does it mean, and how will it change our lives forever to a "Living Nightmare" that there is no escape from. The social credit system will design that all its citizens will be controlled by all its laws, linked to your behaviour and which services you will be 'allowed to access'. Think about that for a minute, it's has already happened in China which started in 2014, and it will be our own style of communism, if your already complying with this Plandemic Agenda then for you will all you be fine for a while until you finally realise is actually your own voluntary euthanasia. In China you can start off with a 1,000 points, then deducted from that any if you misbehave and I truly love to misbehave "stuff their rules ", that often are not legal anyway, how many silly little licences do we truly need to pay for, could you imagine having paying for a TV licence like in the UK, to then basically watch and make you as daft as some of your so called friends who are addicted to it. There are many licences that are simply just money gouging and are not legal under "Common Law" most people just pay them, but for some of us we only pay for those that truly provide a service. Information will be gathered from all sources including schools, my gov, libraries, supermarkets with their loyalty programmes, banks, insurance companies, internet platforms and close circuit television cameras the list is endless. There will be supermarket cameras watching what you spend on food, alcohol, cigarettes, also legalised drugs they also make that legal here as they have in Thailand, because they're going to need to give you a lift as most you seem very "dubbed down" marijuana use will be legalised, and maybe encouraged. I have already stated "Nicotine" is counterproductive to this agenda, so taxes will be increased on all nicotine products including patches and gum which I suggest you stock up on. You also will be encouraged to eat even more fatty foods and sweets plant based foods are currently being encouraged by the major supermarkets with companies like Woolworths, Coles, and Aldi remembering their companies that mandated vaccination of all their employees, another reason to give them a wide berth.

This is on the current Woolworths website, Plant-Based, more and more Australians are trying a plant-based diet and here's why it might be time for you to discover it too. But please note Woolworths we are on to you and your products as they are not what they seem, please remember you are what you eat and ultimately also you are the master of your own destiny, so don't play into their Agenda, especially if you have health issues that are increased by the poisons that are in their controlled foods. The Governments will also reward those respectable 'Controlled Citizens' for a while and "Good Citizens" will be allowed to travel, especially if they are up to date with their latest gene therapy stabs, but I would do it as soon as possible, as the days of affordable travel are ending and if you were to go and check flights to Bali, for Xmas, 2023 for instance that would give you a clue.

If you are not vaccinated I would be very wary of travelling, especially overseas because a lot of you will not be aware, that in the last lockdowns in some countries, and I will just highlight one Vietnam, men came to your hotels and then you were given a choice to be vaxxed and given food, or the other option was to basically to starve you out, and that is one of the risks you take when going through some countries, but you not hear about it until it happens to you. Good Citizens will also be allowed to visit public libraries, rent bicycles, Borrow Money, send children to private schools, access better health care and finally be awarded better jobs. Praising the corrupt Governments will increase your credit points and ultimately your social standing. But Bad Citizens that are people like me and a lot of you reading this total control, will have a future of being denied all of the above. We will be banned from shopping malls, and that truly be a good thing, as we are currently planning on bartering and using cash with like minded bad citizens, who are truly awake, and who do want to be good citizens under this style of tyranny. Buying alcohol will also be deemed with some point reductions for all good and bad citizens, but most of us will be brewing our own so that will not matter, and we will barter accordingly and will not be paying their exorbitant taxes.

Walking dogs will be on leads as they are currently but you will be punished with point deductions, well some of my friends including one I will call 'Smiley Face' does not do this anyway. Living here in Queensland, watch the cretins who walk their dogs on leads on boiling hot concrete, do they think? no simply because some are thoughtless or vaccinated controlled zombies. Reporting friends, neighbours and family members for anything that is not classed as 'Good Behaviour" will earn you more of their evil brownie points. You might even be given access to evil treats they have for some of their sick sadists. History sadly does repeat and dob in your neighbour, as it has happened in all previous wars and this one will be no different, so be very careful who you trust even amongst your family members especially if they're heavily vaxxed. If you don't keep your vaccinations up to date you then will be deducted points, as also you will be for not wearing masks when required and the mandatory PCR testing.

Parents and if one of you has a poor points score, then your children will be penalised by not attending good schools and universities and employers will be encouraged to consult 'black lists' before employing new staff or awarding contracts also you will be required to always carry a smartphone with its tracking apps, and I suggest you consider not carrying these tracking devices when you go out, or even better dump them. Smart TVs, ipads, cell phones will collect data on everything you do, recording all your conversations, movements and all your activity. Facial recognition will be the norm as it is already happening in some of the video games. New Zealanders will be deported for any bad behaviour and that will become the norm in deporting all bad citizens, in most countries to their country of origin. Bad citizens like me will no longer be able to rent, or buy a property, drive a car as you will no longer be able to access a licence and get car registration for your electric car, but how far do they go in the plan for all of Us bad citizens, the 'Wellness Concentration Camps' are a big clue to the future that is coming, if we don't stand up and fight now.

So, if you are currently a Good Citizen maybe it is time to wake up and become a rebel and grow some dam testicular fortitude. You don't realise even if you're good and you're sick, overweight, and finally old, you will also lose points. So welcome to their dystopian world they have planned for all of us, and it's coming very soon, and you've been given so very much warning and time to prepare for the worst, and I truly hope I am wrong, but I am not. So many of the 'Vaccine Injured' who have complied in having these "Not Safe" experiments are now classed as anxious and prescribed antidepressants. So, many were not allowed medical exceptions, in fact they were often impossible to get, my own doctor in Redcliffe, when I asked him for a mask exception because it was giving me panic attacks, and he understood my lung condition and that I needed to breathe pure air and not my own carbon monoxide stated to me "I never ever have given out an exception certificate", and I expect a lot of you reading this have had the similar problems. In the lockdowns did you comply? I did not because I am a proud rebel and enjoy living on the edge and understanding common law, any fine would not ever stand up in court. With any fine I would simply have put two lines across it in 'RED' with the words, "I am a man and I decline" and then let the universe decide my fate. It has already been proven it was always a total facade as none of the fines stood up, it was always a scare and smear campaign.

So, when the climate lockdowns start again with a Marburg style lockdown, which is very likely and then mandatory vaccination's also start all over again and this total genocide continues on. **Climate Engineering** We are all being sprayed which has been happening for at least fifteen years, and happening a lot and is accelerating and it is blamed on global warming and some of you truly believe that. The effect on all of humanity is very profound, you all will have seen how mould here in Queensland, where I live has become a major problem, but I also talked about how effective Zeolite is in conquering that issue which is conquering that issue which is ultra dangerous to your health if not removed.

Geo-Engineering as it is known was first studied and experiments occurred between 1946-47. They discovered adding dry ice (frozen C02) or silver iodide to the clouds could help in nuclearization of rain or snow. So that was a weapon that could be used on mankind when they deemed fit and has been classed as a secret ever since. From 1967-1972 an operation called Popeye, with these evil people and their silly names and the basis of that operation was to extend the monsoon periods during the Vietnam War by controlling the weather and gave the military a weapon of war and the Germans possibly lost the war against Russia due to the cold and snow and lack of fuel. So they have learned how to make clouds, produce rain or snow more or less on demand, they then proceeded to learn how to create a drought or starvation on a perceived enemy nation on "people which are all off us".

For over thirty years experiments were carried out by jets in the lower atmosphere that involved spraying undisclosed chemicals with very easy to spot chemtrails which we all have witnessed, but often you only see what you want to see. If you were to go for a bike ride early in the morning and observe the sky, you would notice these strange patterns. Why does the scientific community ignore the obvious answer that is so blatantly obvious? So now daily they are spraying pollutant particles into the troposphere, with evidence that it is coal fly ash, a substance that is very toxic and injurious to all biota and that includes all of us and universities worldwide have been responsible for 'Critical Thinking' to be beaten out of you Forever' and be aware it is often based on many miss-truths. If you were a critical thinker, the constant red pen corrections of your truth being assessed as a lie at university would likely have you conform "to live their lies", and down the rabbit hole you have gone never to return and most of you who have done this will be the young vaccine addicts that we see today and will continue to justify this Plandemic Agenda and will continue to do so till the day you die. When I went to Launceston University, I lasted 3 weeks because I rebelled and would never accept their lies and never will.

Whistle-Blowers Worldwide that have for three years spoken up can often have to pay the price of it and continue to die from Suicide? or an accident? and will I be different only time will tell, but I will show no fear but to live in my own truth as God deems fit. If enough people do this showing "No Fear" then this Genocidal travesty will end very quickly. Project Blue Beam At the end of World War Two an interesting event happened and at this time in history, people all over the World for the first time were reporting seeing unidentified objects in the sky or UFOs which are Unidentified Flying Objects. These objects were witnessed moving around in the sky at great speed.

In 1947 the first UFO was spotted by a man named Kenneth A. Kenneth was documented stating that he saw, with his own eyes, 9 saucer-shaped objects flying at the rate of about 1700 kilometres per hour. Naturally of course seeing events like this obviously sparked a lot of interest from scientists, military, government, law enforcement and the general public alike. A great abundance of data concerning these UFOs was collected at that time. This is when U.F.O's became a public phenomenon and living in the UK, when I was about six years old, I saw crop circles in my hometown of Rushden, Northamptonshire and have had an interest in this phenomenon ever since. I remember before President Clinton got into power, he was going to lift the lid on these strange events, and naturally that never was going to happen. The United States government and the media were involved in putting out misleading information which contradicted the original stories given by eyewitnesses and therefore effectively convoluted the airways.

This didn't sit very well with Serge Monast, a Canadian from Quebec born in 1945, who was an investigative journalist, essayist, poet, and conspiracy theorist. Serge gained a lot of popularity from guest appearances on shows that deal with the phenomenon of an esoteric nature.In 1994, he published Project Blue Beam (NASA), in which he detailed a four-step base operation set up by the US government by way of NASA with the help of the United Nations. This operation or program was to implement a New Age religion with the Antichrist at its head who will publicly ridicule and denounce all the four major religions. This will help usher in the New World Order. In his publication, Serge mentions how these entities will further fool the people by projecting a technologically simulated Second Coming of Christ. The four steps of Project Blue Beam start with step number one where they will manufacture sophisticated top-secret weapons to cause earthquakes, as we saw recently in Turkey in 2023, and around the world in specific and strategic locations, in order to unearth religious artefacts, with the attempt to use them to disprove the religions effectiveness. This phase was said to have been in effect Since 2012 and in step two, Serge writes that they will use sophisticated technology to beam 3D holographic images of all the prophets or heads of the four major religions: Jesus, Mohammed, Krishna and Buddha. The images would be broadcast simultaneously in the sky around the world. They will then merge these images into one in order to make all people feel their God is speaking directly to them.

Their sole intent is to use this tactic to usher in the antichrist, and the end times. In step three of Project Blue Beam, Serge writes that they will use invisible wave frequency Technology, via a telephonic platform to access people's minds and implant thoughts, in order to gain control of the mind, and make people feel that they are in direct communication with their God. Step four is the final step in this evil project where they will use their sophisticated tech to put the thought in the individual's minds that the rapture is coming and that they face an imminent alien invasion. Also, they will get a transmission into their minds that currently there are other planets being invaded and ravished. They will use a fake alien invasion, we all will tell of the shooting down of UFO'S recently to finalise the birth of their New World Religion, the antichrist's arrival, and the New World Order. Serge Monast mysteriously died in 1996 in his home from a heart attack the day after he was arrested and jailed.

The authorities also took custody of his children who he home-schooled at the time prior to his untimely death. Is there truth to this Project Blue Beam dilemma? Was Serge Monast's untimely death a coincidence? You can decide that, but don't live in fear because 'if you die you will return' and that is how we will continue to grow and evolve, just put your trust in yourself, and if you are one of the people who has lost so much in the last three years who have still stayed true to yourself because we will not lose your soul, and when you are under pressure and stressed then just breathe golden light in to your heart space.

Smart Cities Modern cities are brimming with objects that receive, collect and transmit data and all part of this Plandemic Agenda. This includes mobile phones but also objects embedded into our cities, such as traffic lights and air pollution stations. Even something as simple as a garbage bin can now be connected to the internet meaning that it forms part of what is called the internet of things. A smart city collects the data from these digital objects and uses it to create new products and services that make cities more liveable. The word Smart refers to self-monitoring, analysis and reporting technology. This is their sales pitch and different estimations show that smart cities become more responsive and efficient after the changes. For example, innovative urban systems can save from 30 to 300 lives per year, decrease crime by 30-40%,save 15-30 minutes And there are more uncountable parameters like the resident's happiness. It might sound wonderful, a bit like that magical vaccine and the only thing they both got in common is once you're bought into this control you continue to defend it and be labelled smart city addicts.

Climate Lockdowns are planned and if people don't respond very strongly to this, it is likely that we will soon see these measures implemented all over the world. The elite have always promised to do "Whatever It Takes" to fight climate change and now we are finding out that they were not kidding, so expect to see more extreme weather events and natural disasters to try to get the sheeple to accept this false reality. Most of you are aware or should be made aware of the plan for Oxford, Oxfordshire County Council, UK who have approved plans to lock residents into one of six zones to 'Save The Planet' from global warming and it is hard to make this rubbish up. The latest stage in the '15 minute' city agenda is to place electronic gates on key roads in and out of the city, confining residents to their own neighbourhoods. Under the new scheme if residents want to leave their zone, they will need permission from the Council who gets to decide who is worthy of freedom and who isn't. That is an easy one to work out if you are not zombified and under the new scheme residents will be allowed to leave their zone a maximum of only 100 days per year, but in order to even gain this every resident will have to register their car details with the council who will then track their movements via smart cameras round the city.

So, this is the smart city climate lockdown pandemic agenda and if they get away with it in Oxford, UK who will be next Brisbane, London, and Moreton Bay Queensland which will be one of the world's first smart cities as its controlled by a ''Comrade'' mayor and a real bunch of clowns your heard of the adage of ''Useful as Tit's on a Bull'' well that sums them up. Thankfully I have never met one of these clown councillors. So good honest citizens revolt and remove these tyrants who just take taxpayers money with no check and balances in place. In other countries the madness continues, it's really like sketches out of ''Monty Python'' movie and the people being crucified are all of us.

France can now make you take a train rather than a plane and The European Commission has given French officials the green light to ban select domestic flights if the route in question can be completed via train in under two and a half hours.The plan was first proposed in 2021 to reduce carbon emissions which originally called for a ban on eight short-haul flights, but the EC has only agreed to only three that have quick and easy rail alternatives, with several direct train connections each way every day, but this is total madness. But the madness continues with the **Netherlands**, the government there is going to be buying and shutting down approximately 3,000 farms in order to "reduce its nitrogen pollution" The Dutch government is planning to purchase and then close down up to 3,000 farms in an effort to comply with a European Union environmental mandate to slash emissions, according to reports. Farmers in the Netherlands will be offered "well over" the worth of their farm to take up the offer voluntarily. The country is attempting to reduce its nitrogen pollution and will make the purchases and if enough farmers accept buyouts as "There is no Better Offer Coming,". We are in the beginning stages of an unprecedented global food crisis, and the Dutch government has decided that now is the time to shut down thousands of farms. Well, it is all part of the Plandemic Agenda to get you to enjoy their poisonous products.

Brazil anybody who seriously thinks that Universal Basic Income (UBI) programs of the future won't be full blown social credit systems need look no further than Brazil, where newly selected socialist globalist Lula da Silva just decreed that the Bolsa Familia program will require family members to be vaccinated in order to continue receiving benefits. "We Can't Play, it's a Question of Science and If I have 10 covid vaccines to take, I will take all that is necessary".

Canada has found a way to get people to stop emitting any carbon at all once their usefulness is over and assisted suicide has become quite popular among the Canadians, and the number of people choosing that option keeps setting new records year after year. Last year, more than 10,000 people in Canada astonishingly that is over three percent of all deaths there ended their lives via Euthanasia, an increase of a third on the previous year and it's likely to keep rising: next year, next year, Canada is set to allow people to die exclusively for Mental health reasons. If you are feeling depressed, Canada has a solution for that and we really could not make all this up, so it is very tragic we are all only livestock.

Digital Currency America's new digital dollar is almost here as the Federal Reserve gears up to unleash its "Fed Now" program at some point between now and next July 2023. The Federal Reserve is planning to implement "Fed Now" digital currency between May and July of 2023 there will be forced digital identification to accompany participation in the new digital currency economy. All of this is being peddled by the Federal reserve as a convenience to the public, and a solution to the engineered collapse that will predicate it and, in the end, the masses will be herded into a total surveillance and police state, where people will have to prove their identity digitally in order to participate in this new digital money scam. This is coming worldwide, and can we stop it? Well, if you are not using "Cash" as much as humanly possible currently, then we must accept the hard realities of what they are planning. We're already seeing that the credit agencies in America TransUnion, Equifax, and Experian have already said that they have agreed to start carbon footprint individual tracking on your credit score. This is just the same from the Chinese playbook, and if we don't wake up when the pot is starting to boil, it's going to be too late. If we all look at the Federal Reserve and then we look at fiat currency, a currency that is not backed by any hard assets, like it was when it was previously on a gold standard, you will quickly realise we've really reached the end of the road and we cannot continue. As the critics predicted, soaring debt required ever greater currency creation, which eventually caused the cost of living to jump by 10% in 2022, leading regular people to demand that it stop. So, the Fed now has to keep raising interest rates to counter inflation and as the US borrows more money, and its existing debts roll over at higher rates, the cost of that debt is soaring. This year the government's annual interest bill will break $1 trillion and combine that with the soaring cost of Medicare, and Social Security as millions of Baby Boomers retire so they will need to eliminate you, because Washington is looking at $2 trillion a year just in 'Just Interest and Entitlements' which it will have to borrow to fund, which will send interest costs even higher, which will require more borrowing, and so on, until it all comes crashing down.

Markets go up like the stairs and down like the elevator and it's all part of the plan and it is coming very soon but Gold and Silver are always a safe haven, and they are still very good value at the moment, especially Silver and there are a lot of survival preppers who are hedging, as you should never have all your eggs in one basket and buying Gold and Silver might be a very good move. If you have bought real estate in the last eight years you should be doing very well, but nothing goes up for ever, and supply and demand is taking over. I paid 17% interest on my farm in Tasmania, and will head back there is anyone's guess, but the days of "Cheap Money" are over, and a lot of people are going to be sadly financially underwater very soon.

We must look at the USA & UK where their interest rates are currently at, and where they might be in Australia, as we are well behind the financial curve, and our very weak RBA who told you all that the rates will be low until 2024. Then due to this total Pandemic, it let you access your super, and encouraged you to borrow and buy with as much cheap money as you wanted, and it has got you in a financial melting pot. But greed is everywhere, but we all have had choices and it was not hard to see that this was always planned and will end very badly with all the excess deaths, then who is going to move into all of these houses. So many construction companies are currently going bankrupt, and this financial meltdown has not even started yet, so it is possible that a lot of these construction sites will never get finished. Most of us who are switched on The Pure Bloods, and the awakened who have been planning to go "Off Grid" but even that will not be sacrosanct, because Governments are on to all of us.

Travellers who enjoy the simple freedoms of their humble vans face a major roadblock in the form of legislation requiring a fully plumbed-in toilet. Particularly the young, adventurous, and those on a strict budget have embraced the van life converting vans into DIY campers and taking to the highways to find out of the way nooks and isolated beaches.

In Moreton Bay Queensland you might not get the welcome you would hope for as a tourist as we who have vans are being booked up $280 as it's "not allowed" unless you registered as homeless. Amid the growth of remote, laptop-based work, a growing cohort moved into their vans for long stretches and documented their travels, sharing tips for vehicle conversion alongside wanderlust themed photographs of waking up to unspoiled sunsets and rooftop yoga. Fuelled by social media and word of mouth, the number of freedom campers ballooned, from the low tens of thousands in the early 2000s to just over 250,000 in 2019, according to New Zealand's ministry of business, innovation and employment. Australia will be next needing van toilets, this Agenda evolving on a daily basis, and it is very hard to keep up with it and trying to write a book about it is not easy, as they keep throwing out curve balls such as this.

The global "Elite" are currently attacking **"Eggs"** by calling them dangerous and deadly after it was revealed that the high-protein superfood is a natural cure for covid. The World Economic Forum tweeted a lie stating that eating eggs "increases the risk of heart attacks and strokes," the suggestion being that people should stop eating them for their own safety. We all are aware of the truth that covid "Vaccines" are responsible for the sudden uptick in heart attacks and strokes being observed all around the world, but the WEF is currently trying to convince everyone that eggs, are worse than crack cocaine or heroin Globalist aligned "scientists" claim that eating eggs which are currently in short supply, could cause blood clots, leading to death a convenient cover story for the hordes of "fully vaccinated" people who are dying every single day from the injections and they are truly hitting the panic button, and they have truly got the egg on their faces, with this total chicken shite, and I wonder if they have consulted their own beloved leader in Qld who is a "Pile of Chook". The claim is that **Choline**, a nutrient found in eggs, somehow contributes to the alleged blood-clotting activity of this superfood and Choline consumption. We were told why people are dying suddenly, seemingly without cause.

So, they want you to eat bugs, and all their plant-based poisons and not healing eggs and meat. I have noticed recently how all the streetlights are very bright and is it not logical that by doing that will affect your melatonin levels and your sleep circadian rhythms so that you always tired and combine that with 5G and Graphene Oxide and when you are not feeling well, sleep is your tonic, food for thought as this Agenda will be attacking you from every angle they think they can, so get a block out screen for the bedroom. Finally ending this chapter we just had Easter and here in Australia some the hot cross buns had the x removed from them well we lost a cheese brand called Coon a few years ago as it might upset some people and there is not going to be an end to this total moronic behaviour of the elite unless we stand up.

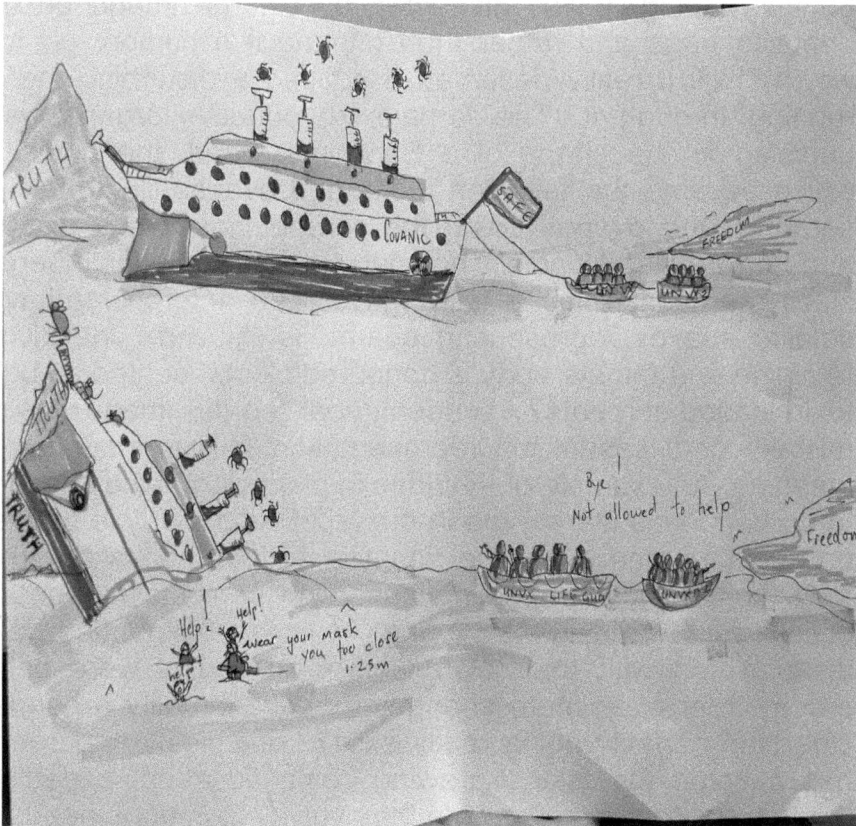

The Plandemic Agenda Will be Sunk © Harmonica Man

Chapter 11

Celeste

Just Another Deception

I was sitting in one of my favourite coffee shops tucked away in a quiet arcade waiting for the exquisite aroma of the freshly brewed coffee beans to hit my nostrils. As I waited patiently, I reached for a magazine from the nearby rack and began flipping through a new age magazine aimed at a younger audience than myself. I was drawn to the title of an article and began reading. I was distracted by a large image on the opposite page and rather than offering it a cursory glance, which is all it really deserved, I noticed a disturbing theme running through it. The female reproductive organs were depicted in the shape of a Baphomet head, the horns of which became the fallopian tubes and ovaries illustrated as serpents, the ovaries being the serpent heads. My disgust and horror was palpable! The image was repeated in different sizes represented as a full-page spread, interspersed with smaller snakes representing sperm. Is this how the divine feminine and female body is honoured? Represented as ugly, toxin loaded serpents? I suddenly realised this image was no mistake or a casual fun representation. It was loaded with meaning. An example of – hidden in plain sight – the intention to do harm was staring me in the face! As the article prattled on about women everywhere mutilating their genitals so that they looked more appealing based on porn star images, it occurred to me that young women disgruntled and disappointed with their own God-given bodies were being groomed for even more changes to their sexuality & gender. Does the perfect vagina really exist? Labiaplasty apparently, has become the fastest-growing cosmetic trend, expedited through pre-teen concern with their vulva? Someone needs to tell them about 'The Great Wall of Vagina', at The Museum of

Old & New Art, in Tasmania. Jamie McCartney (the sculptor) claims that for many women their genital appearance is a source of anxiety. He believes he was able to do something about that, through highlighting the physical diversity of the labia. So, we might conclude what is all the fuss about? Why the encouragement for such unnecessary surgery or is this a ploy to begin to normalise the alteration of our gender defining features? The insidious inclusion of toxic practices and chemicals into our lifestyle has resulted in a plethora of health concerns and is likely intentional by those who wish to do harm. The image which initially shocked me depicted snakes as a symbol of toxic venom. The serpent intentionally appears in many places, the image in the magazine is not the only place it can be found.

The symbol of the WHO is the most obvious but not understood by most people. The symbol appears as a serpent twisted around a pillar. It wasn't until Dr Brian Ardis made the connection between the whole Covid agenda and snake venom that dots began to join for many of us. Not only was the mandated injectable, gene altering solution packed with snake venoms of different kinds, but it brought to light that venom existed in other forms in other pharmaceutical, feminine hygiene and cosmetic products. We have been encouraged to moisturise, wear makeup, and use a multitude of grooming and skincare products, never thinking for a moment they would be toxic and cause damage to ourselves. As more of us become concerned about what we consume, what we wear and what we apply to our skin, ingredients in mainstream beauty products have come into question. Many of the chemicals used as cosmetic ingredients are listed in toxicity databases. Some are linked with skin irritation, tumours, allergies, or endocrine disruption among other health concerns. We should have been alarmed when we were warned decades ago about aluminium in deodorants, but we persisted using different products hoping to look less aged, more refined or maintain youthful looking skin & hair. Throughout the plandemic we were also encouraged to frequently use hand sanitizers.

They were strategically placed at the entry to most venues and became a normal expectation everywhere we went! We now know how toxic these products are. Not only are they created as a delivery system for alcohol which has various uses and damaging effects on the skin, but they contain other nasties which are chemicals such as triclosan, an antibacterial ingredient that can cause antibiotic resistance. There are also chemical or synthetic fragrances which can be associated with allergies and hormone disruption. We have been led to believe the use of hand sanitizers will help to protect us from pathogens, but they can in fact be contributors to our failing immune systems and ill health.

Generally, there is profound ignorance about the importance and functions of the skin as the largest organ of the body. Its protective function is obviously well understood by those advocating the use of harmful products in the name of sanitation, beauty, or personal hygiene. One of its key functions is to protect us from microbes yet the application of chemicals is advised as being superior protection compared to our miraculous self-healing body. The damage from tanning products, moisturisers & soaps to name only a few interfere with the waterproof barrier of the skin preventing it from functioning optimally. Beauty products are a mine field to navigate, in fact anything to do with the beauty industry is suspect. Fortunately, for those who are awake, organic products do exist, but this is still not safe. You must know what to avoid when purchasing products. Hair products, any facial makeup products, skin care products, nail products and the list continues! I remember how disappointed I was when I realised how much money I had invested in my skin care routine over the years, only to find out it was likely the prime contributor towards the appearance of skin cancers on my face. The horror of realising that I needed to undergo potentially disfiguring surgery to remove these offending growths from my skin was devastating. I was part of the plan for another way for surgeons to make money. Thousands of dollars for more than one surgery, the Dermatologist, the Mohs Surgeon and the Plastic Surgeon all got their share.

All the while I was advised to keep out of the sun. Was it the cause of my damaged skin, or was it? Suggestions of sunscreens, recommended by the cancer council or cosmetic companies or tried and true brands found in the supermarket were made by doctors. I began following this advice from family, and friends. and then my awakening began. Once my diet changed and I no longer consumed toxic seed oils loaded with omega 6, I found I could tolerate longer periods of sunshine without sunscreen and to my absolute wonder – no burning of my skin! This was fantastic! I was getting my daily quota of vitamin D directly from the sun and I felt great. After realising that sunscreens were actually products loaded with toxins just like most of the other skin care products, it was easy for me to STOP using them! So, what is really in our feminine hygiene products?

The average woman menstruates for approximately 40 years or about 500 times in her lifetime. This equates to an enormous amount of feminine hygiene products used, so it makes sense that what is available for use is chemical and toxin free. The sensitive mucous membranes in the vagina absorb chemicals from tampons without metabolising them, which means they go straight into the bloodstream. Plastic applicators for tampons can also be offenders here. There is a diverse range of health problems that arise from the use of these products which are usually synthetic and may have added synthetic fragrances. Beneficial vaginal bacteria can be disturbed by these fibres and fragrances allowing infection to arise. Non-organic tampons or pads may contain bleach or pesticides if made from cotton. These can also make their way into your bloodstream. Then we can deviate to another category of feminine hygiene that includes vaginal soaps, douches, deodorants, and lubricants, many of which contain parabens & preservatives. All these products affect the endocrine system. The delicate balance of hormones becomes disrupted, contributing to many health conditions such as hormonal imbalances, fatigue, skin conditions, weight gain, headaches, and a compromised immune system. Are we concerned yet? Are we joining any dots yet? How are our viable egg counts, sperm counts, successful conceptions going? Have we unwittingly allowed nefarious agendas to interfere with the delicate & miraculous process of fertilisation? We can certainly attribute other factors to these vital indicators of fertility, necessary for the survival of humanity but we must recognize that there has been a concerted effort to directly target the female body under the guise of hygiene or indeed beauty! Apparently being exposed to pesticides or toxic agents are seen as risk factors that can indeed affect a woman's egg reserve. So where else are we being exposed to toxins & pesticides? This is where we need to go back to the snake venom story from which I have deviated. As I mentioned Dr Ardis joined some dots and realised we were being encouraged to take a shot laced with this venom. He also found that our bodies have nicotine receptors which the snake venom likes to attach to, in order to fulfil its toxic promise. However, Ardis found that by giving the body nicotine in the form of a patch or gum the snake venom could be displaced.

This helped many people who had an adverse reaction to the injectable. But it may not however protect the viable egg survival rate or sperm production. We need to remember the agenda is de-population. The recent encouragement to inject graphene oxide products into young bodies as well as the consumption of pharmaceutical birth control pills haven't helped either. My journey into the world of food exploration uncovered a very carefully crafted plan, calculated to poison an unwitting world of humans who would never suspect that their governments, supermarkets, and agricultural practices were complicit in their demise. How often do you hear people tell you they eat healthily? What is a healthy diet when we need to consciously hunt and gather, daily, for real food that is organic or biodynamic or home grown. Sadly, most people are subject to the lure of the supermarket because of convenience, time, variety and location. Little attention is paid to the labels on packets and for many it is a matter of the cheapest brand or what had the hardest hitting advertising campaign.

Awareness is key and gratefully many are now waking up to the knowledge that what they have been eating is in fact not real food. We are witnessing the phase of poisoning with the addition of insects into our food selection. Celebrities rave over how enticing and delicious these creatures are and the unsuspecting would not for a moment suspect that our gut is not designed to digest chitin, a polysaccharide amenable to cancers, fungi and parasites. We are being encouraged to consume foods that the gut of a bird is equipped for. To follow the rabbit burrow of the food source trail is an enormous task which is extensive and varied. Once you realise you have been lied to and deliberately misguided you start to look a lot closer at everything – even the food pyramid, the one we were taught to follow at school, for a balanced and healthy diet, was a lie.

We have been inundated with toxins on every level, GMO food, fluoride in the water and toothpastes, gluten, hormones in our meat, vegetables laden with pesticides and synthetic fertilisers as well as being encouraged to consume dairy products, alcohol and sugar. The most pernicious culprits however, are the vegetable oils, which are ever present in processed foods and the heterocyclic amines in these oils are carcinogenic at cooking temperatures. I have found that by refusing to consume these things I have almost become a social outcast. So much of our social interactions revolve around food and alcohol. Alcohol, in particular, is touted as the social norm, and something is wrong with you if you do not wish to imbibe. The tentacles and poisons are insidious and it's difficult to escape their grip. But free from social expectation and the lure of fast food you begin to feel whole again and can shed not only unwanted kilos but the symptoms that accompany toxic overload in your body. Our health, or should I say sickness industry does not attend to this. There is no money in healthy individuals. You are not dependent if you are well. To stay well we need to avoid the consumables in our society designed to make us sick. Once we become sick, we become lifetime customers of the healthcare industry.

If we become ill through vaccines, pharmaceuticals, surgeries, skin care products or toxic fabrics worn on our skin along with the toxic pesticide laden additive ridden food we are encouraged to eat, we then require more products to treat the side effects! It's the perfect business model according to RFK Junior. For us to maintain optimum health or even survive the lies and deception woven around health, healthcare, and personal health it is paramount that we are awake to the hidden agendas that permeate our everyday lives. The internet is littered with articles and links about the toxic effects of dangerous chemicals found in beauty products, but first people need to be exposed to the idea that this is indeed an area of concern. Toxic fabrics worn next to the skin, the food we eat and how it is packaged, the air we breathe, and the cleaning products we use are further areas for investigation.

Good luck navigating the murky waters of all things we consume or take into our bodies. Genuinely organic products are difficult to find, and ingredient lists are tiresome to trawl through. "We'll know our disinformation program is complete when everything the American public believes is false." (CIA director 1981.) I believe the disinformation agenda goes far beyond America today! Luckily there are more of us waking up and beginning to see what is really happening. The matrix is beginning to crumble hopefully. Society is grappling with the overarching question of what is beauty and who decides? It is becoming abundantly clear that what is considered beauty is decided for us. Many feel compelled to use skin enhancing products and procedures to fit the social norm of what is considered superficially beautiful. **Have you joined any dots yet?**

Chapter 12

Survival Prepping

After the doom and gloom of the last chapter it important to try and raise your vibration and talk about what we can do to be many steps ahead of this satanic Agenda, and it truly is not rocket science, we understand their weapons and how they will use them with these mRNA gene therapy vaccines and what is in them, 5G, there poisonous foods and ultimately their Genocidal Plan. Most of you have been preparing for a very long time, and some of my friends like Dallas, Shane, Greg and Ern have for many years. I myself have several months' supply of food in my war chest and water and cooking equipment and everything I believe I will need. I will go through all of them in more detail in this chapter and some of you already have backpacks ready to leave at a moment's notice, it is so very important to plan for the worst and hope for the best. But in this spiritual war which we are a long way from winning, there is a very, long way to go.

Please do not get complacent and never underestimate this enemy as they have so much to lose, and they still hold most of the very high cards. The evil people behind this we really don't know all of them but are ultra smart, and are they remotely human or reptilian, at some point when we reach victory all will be revealed, but I suspect that will be many years away, and you and your families are going to be the victims, if you're not very smart and out think them. In all wars there sadly are casualties and in this spiritual war, the death toll is going to be immense so be one of the survivors so be smart and think smart. You will have switched your TV's off and you found new likeminded new friends, and you should be planning for the future surrounded by healthy, happy people who keep your vibration high, and you will feed off each other and it is so important to enjoy every day to the max and not sweat the small stuff, like most the vaccinated and their levels of sheepism are very disturbing, and the truth that is coming out is that we were not conspiracy theorists but "Truth seeker's" and 100% correct our beliefs, but they will continue to live the rest of their days in total denial. Consider them lost, send them love blessings and move on, you can survive, and they will not and that is the sad reality they also had a choice. Food how much do we need, how long is piece of string, I mentioned that I am a great believer in intermittent fasting and try to eat breakfast, and then a large meal 8 to 10 hours later, and my current body weight hovers around 68-70 kilos, I am six foot tall and feel amazing fit. So, we all different in how much we need to store in case of that emergency and how long the emergency events last. But more is better, the selection of food is so important and also keep a survival amount in your vehicle's of tinned foods that will keep for many years. You have naturally got to provide for all your family members, and all your pets so plan well, understanding how many calories you will need is so important, and understanding the shelf life of foods you will need. The types of foods and how they need to be stored because I live in a hot humid climate and mould can be an issue, how they're preserved, the variety of foods that are more fitting for long-term storage. A balanced approach with food rotation techniques.

The average adult needs around 2,000 calories a day to stay healthy and to ensure that you will meet your calorie needs when 'SHTF' you will need to stock up on calorie-dense foods. You should also include nutrient-dense foods in your survival stockpile to prevent nutritional deficiencies. It will be challenging cost wise for some to buy food in bulk if you're on a tight budget, but you can buy more for the same amount of money by choosing low-cost but nutritious foods so do plenty of research and make sure it is edible especially if you bought it from the supermarkets. Fruits that are rich in the nutrients that your body needs to function will be important, and making them a regular part of your diet helps prevent nutritional deficiencies, such as Vitamin C deficiency.

Most fresh fruits are highly perishable, but you can always try various food preservation methods to extend their shelf life. Some of the best ways to preserve fruits are canning and freezing and drying. Vegetables your survival stockpile should contain many because they are chock-full of important nutrients. Like fruits, many vegetables don't last very long and for most of you it is just basic common sense that you can extend their shelf life via food preservation, particularly with canning, freezing and drying, or purchasing freeze-dried products. You should also consider growing vegetables at home, so you have a fresh and steady supply of food.

Many vegetables are easy to care for and can be grown in pots and planters, but I suggest before you eat them wash them in Bentonite clay to eradicate the chemicals from the rain. Beans, legumes and nuts you will find that beans are staples of survival pantries, because they contain large amounts of protein and last for a long time and can last even longer when dried, legumes and nuts also store well and have a fairly long shelf life. These foods are also rich in protein and can be eaten as snacks or as part of a meal. Meat is also one of the best sources of protein and makes a meal more appetising and the meat fat is very important, but obviously fresh meat is perishable, canned meat can last for many years and is easy to store. Grains are also staples of survival pantries because they have a long shelf life and are very filling. There are many types of grains you can choose from, including rice, wheat, quinoa and spelt. Each of these are packed with nutrients and can be turned into bread, pasta and the like. Some very important condiments like vinegar are long-lasting and can be stored at room temperature. You can whip up your own sauce or dip using other foods in your stockpile and oils and fats are so essential you will need oil & fats to cook food. Most unopened bottles of cooking oils last up to 18 months before they start to go rancid. Make sure to stock up on some healthy cooking oils, such as olive and flaxseed oils, to prevent disease. Spices have a long shelf and add flavour to your meals and I stocked up on most that are available because many offer health benefits.

Include salt, pepper, garlic, onion powder, turmeric, parsley, sage and all herbs in your food stockpile to spice up your dishes. Canned foods naturally last a long time, and the shelf lives of canned foods are significantly influenced by their ingredients which are salt, for example which aids in the preservation of canned food, extending its shelf life. In general, canned meats last the longest, followed by vegetables, fish, beans, rice, broth, soup, and lastly, canned fruits. Some canned meats can last between 4-10 years but pop up can lids are not as securely sealed as the good old-fashioned cans you have to use a can opener to open.

This means that they are more susceptible to spoilage and after canned meats you will find things like canned beans and legumes can have a shelf life of 3-6 years, also tinned fish also can keep from 3-6 years, and canned fish is one of the healthiest types of canned foods out there, as most of it can contain a high percentage of Omega-3 fatty acids that help lower the risk of heart problems, you should try to avoid canned fish that have sauces like tomato sauce as it will not keep as long. Rice is such a staple part of the diet of many cultures, it has a high-calorie content, and it's rich in minerals, vitamins, carbohydrates, and protein. Both canned and uncanned rice provide these nutrients but canned rice provides them in lower levels. There are many different types of canned rice to consider, for instance brown rice is generally healthier than white rice but due to its high oil content, it tends to last not as long. This is important because uncanned rice, when stored properly, can last for over a decade, unlike canned rice that only lasts for a few years. Canned soup usually contains meat, vegetables, or a combination of both and canned broth is also made of vegetables, meat, or both, but unlike canned soup, it doesn't have solid contents, they can last for 2-4 years. Canned fruits might only last 1-2 years, fruits, like vegetables, are packed with essential nutrients and vitamins, because they're composed of water and sugar, they're also excellent for hydration. Storage environment. You should keep canned food in a cool and dry place where the temperature is quite stable and doesn't fluctuate drastically.

The ideal temperature is below 85°F, but not too low to cause freezing; around 50 to 70°F is good enough. Avoid placing the canned foods under direct sunlight because doing this may cause thermophilic bacteria to reproduce and grow inside the can, contaminating its contents and increasing the spoilage rate. No good list of must have items for survival would be complete without salt, it might not occupy the same position of urgency as water or food in general, but it's a fact that the human body cannot survive without at least some sodium. Food preservation and apart from your body's need for salt, the most important reason to store salt is for food preservation, salt has a multitude of other uses so having more of this resource is very recommended. **Water** will quickly become one of your most urgent needs during a survival situation and believe it or not, most people cannot survive much beyond a few days without any water, especially in a hot environment where you are losing water rapidly through perspiration. Even in a cold environment without exertion, you may need a minimum of (about 1/2-gallon) of water each day to maintain some bodily efficiency with more than 3/4 of your body is composed of fluids and your body loses fluid as a result of heat, cold, stress, and exertion, also to function effectively, you must replace the fluid your body loses. A general rule-of-thumb is 1 gallon of water per day at minimum for your survival needs and many of you reading this would have water filters so it's so important to have spares of everything, some of you will have a backup generator. But if you live where it rains a lot, then use rain tarp or barrels to catch rain or other water holding material or containers. If you can venture out to live off the grid then trails you should follow in the direction in which the trails converge and look for signs of camps, animal droppings, and trampled terrain which may mark trails, also flocks of birds may circle over water holes and some birds fly to water holes at dawn and sunset. While there may be some chemical treatment in swimming pools, chances are it's just chlorine and PH balance. Have you ever heard of people drinking swimming pool water and dying from it? in an emergency it is a fairly obvious source. Snow and Ice please note that snow and ice are no purer than the water they came from but with Water Purification Tablets that are very important to have especially in your backpack, and in your vehicles to prevent microorganisms in water in order to prevent typhoid, cholera, dysentery as well as other water borne diseases. **Water purification tablets** work by killing off the pathogens that are present in water in order to make it safe for human consumption and these tablets are very popular with outdoor enthusiasts like backpackers and survival preppers in order to purify water that comes from freshwater sources like lakes and streams. The importance of having survival water filters in your backpacks and your vehicles and there so many to choose from and because they are inexpensive and very crucial to have on hand, and very portable. Some of these water filters can weigh just 0.1 lbs, so a few ounces, and having a straw design means you can slot them into your backpack with ease, they are also so light, you'll probably forget it's there. One thing is for sure you're not going to want to carry a week's worth of drinking water, if you did, you probably wouldn't make it. So do some research on these water filters and with one of these in your backpack, you'll have the freedom to explore without the burden of carrying or boiling water every day. You can just add whatever water is nearby, add it to the survival water filter, and drink it knowing you're safe to do so.

Talking of **Survival Backpacks** there are a multitude of options available, and they're designed to get you through several days out in the open, whether it's a dessert or just a popular camping ground. They are usually very durable, and backpacks are designed to hold enough gear for one to five days, and with plenty of external attachment points for all your bulky survival needs. Some have features like a water-repellent coating, so it will keep your survival gear dry regardless of the weather conditions outside and have drainage points at the bottom, which will protect the stuff inside the bag in case your hydration bladder ruptures. I would have several backpacks at your disposal, maybe a 2 day lighter backpack and then a 5-7 day heavier one all packed ready to go at a moment's notice. How will you get there? and what conditions will you be sleeping in? Once you know this information and always prepare for the worst-case scenario.

Sleeping Bag, you can choose the one best suitable for you to keep warm and waterproof which will be a major priority. Most will have temperature ratings, for example, if a sleeping bag is rated for 30F, the bag will keep you alive at this temperature. But you will not be comfortable, so it might be prudent to check the comfort ratings as getting a good refreshing sleep is paramount. So, if you live in climates that change a lot, maybe have several sleeping bags to choose from as this is such an important topic so spend a bit of time getting the correct ones for your survival needs, because you will be very glad you did if the worst thing and we pray it does not happen becomes a reality and there are two main choices when it comes to filling down or synthetic and for freezing weather, down is usually recommended. But remember down sleeping bags can be very pricey, and need to be fluffed, and aren't as good as synthetic in wet situations but for winter survival, down might be the best choice and synthetic is probably the better choice for emergency bags and kits. The shape is also very important, and some people prefer to only choose a mummy sleeping bag for survival, because this shape helps trap body heat the best. There other options are double-wide sleeping bags, but sharing a sleeping bag might sound cosy, but it might be such a good option in real life, and I suggest testing it out first, but with a small child or baby their ideal. Size is so important because sleeping bags trap heat best when they fit your body, too much empty space in the sleeping bag will cause you to lose heat, also you don't want a sleeping bag that is too tight because you will end up crushing the insulation, and it won't have the air pockets needed to trap the heat.

Sleeping Pads are just as important while sleeping bags are tested, it is usually with the assumption that you are using them with a sleeping pad underneath.

Even a bag rated to -30F will not keep you warm if you sleep on the cold ground, another plus of having a sleeping pad is using it to sit on and especially if the ground is wet, you will love that you can sit on your sleeping pad while preparing dinner, or just taking a rest so you can see this is an inexpensive survival need and the foam ones are very inexpensive. I suggest having several including a self-inflating sleeping pad and a closed-cell foam pad is on top of this. There are plenty of you-tube videos on all these important topics and some of you are already experts on this Plandemic, to the point that you could do a doctorate on it, so research these subjects as much as you can, it is that important. What shelters will you be using? If you use your sleeping bag with a tent, you can get one with a lower temperature rating because the tent will trap some of the body heat. But if you are going to use your sleeping bag under a tarp, then you'll need a much warmer sleeping bag or understand survival skills, and make sure you have mylar style blankets, also called space blankets, weigh just a few ounces, fold down to fit in your pocket, and can be used in many ways in an emergency.

Mylar is so awesome that it has become synonymous with the term "survival blanket" as they are a thin sheet of plastic with a film of aluminium or another metal, and the metal film is what makes mylar so shiny because they reflect heat and you see them put on runners after a marathon race, to keep them warm because when we sweat, we lose a lot of body evaporation. If your shoes or boots get wet cut a piece up mylar and place them inside and they also work inside gloves.

Campfire reflectors when it gets cold, they can be very important as a campfire reflector placed behind the fire, will bounce or radiate more heat back toward you, reflectors can be made very simply with rocks or stones piled up, they can also be made by building a simple wall of logs or branches, corrugated metal, or they can be made simply by propping up and stretching out a mylar emergency blanket.

If your reflector is built close enough to the fire, the smoke will be drawn up rather than finding its way into your face.

Survival fire starter kits Understandably this is so important, and I always have one in my bike saddlebags because fire starting skills are essential to your survival, especially when and if the SHTF. Ideally, you should know how to start a fire using very basic tools, like tinder and wood but zippo lighters can stay lit longer than plastic lighters without melting. A Bic lighter isn't 100 percent foolproof under all conditions, but it is the simplest and fastest way to start a fire. Keep one in your kits and in your pocket for everyday carry, just in case you will find the lighter will work better in cold weather because it is warm in your pocket, but also have strike anywhere matches as a backup for your lighters. To make it easier to start a fire, maybe bundle two or three matches together to strike a nice, big flame and store the matches in a waterproof matchbox. Fire steel rod will produce a shower of sparks onto a pile of tinder when you firmly scrape down its edge, with the metal striker that comes with it or your knife, and if the sun is shining you can also use a lens or a magnifying glass to start a fire. Another good option is Vaseline on cotton balls that can be used to light a fire easily, you can store the cotton balls in a small plastic bag or a resealable container, so prevent the Vaseline from getting all over your gear.

Push bikes I personally have two and prefer mountain bikes if you are fit, it is very important because the only fuel required for bicycle transportation is your own muscle power and calories. A bicycle is obviously much faster than walking and so important that they are a great escape option in an emergency, it may become even more crucial when vehicular transportation may no longer be an option, and we are aware that day is looming. In this case we're now talking about a survival bicycle, and make sure you have all the bike repair equipment and several bike pumps. Considering all options and folding bikes can be very useful, another good option is an all around-bike called a hybrid. It will have a mountain bike gearing with a road bike frame.

The wheels will be the same diameter as a road bike but with wider tires closer to a mountain bike width. The handlebars allow an upright riding position like a mountain bike, wheels are generally the first point of failure so a survival bike should be as strong as possible, using common components, e.g. 36 spokes. Accept nothing less, and never depend on modern low-spoke-count wheels. Look at bike trailer options, keep it simple with the gearing, get the tires that are a road, dirt combo, and I always have bike mirrors. Mountain bikes are generally tough and will take you places where road style bikes won't go, and the reason why is that I prefer them, and I rarely have bike punctures.

Survival Vehicle When a disaster strikes, many people become stranded because the roads are impassable to ordinary cars because debris can clog the roads and if you try to take a little car over debris on the road or through the slick mud covered trails, you're not going to make it very far. I myself have chosen a four-wheel drive to have a vehicle that's not going to wimp out, when there's a little trouble on the road. You will need to get a four wheel drive that will give you the traction that you will need when things get a little rough. Not only do you need a vehicle like a four wheel drive, but you have to have something that gives you some space and is perfect for just me. So, get a vehicle that offers you all the room you and your family will need, to pack it up and haul it out of any bad situation.

Roof Top Beds These are becoming less expensive and very easy to pop up. I prefer the hard top style because you can leave bedding in a roof top tent for storage, or while going to the next destination on a trip but always take the necessary steps to keep the bedding clean and aired. Not every rooftop tent will fit every vehicle so understand the load capacity of your roof rack, as well as the maximum spread of your roof rack bars. I prefer a hard shell because they are typically more durable but can range from plastic, fibreglass, to metal shells.

A hardtop can usually fit extra bedding and already has a thicker more premium mattress. I also suggest an anti condensation blanket. I get all my supplies from Kings at Brendale Qld look out for their daily specials. Roof top tents will affect your fuel efficiency and affect how your car drives also, the increased wind resistance will force you to drive slower, and hard-shells are more forgiving here since they are more aerodynamic, so there are many variables at play here than just the tent itself. Speaking of tents I like to cover all my bases and back up options because sheltering is private.

Tents have come a long way but for survival, a lighter-weight portable tent is your best bet and setting your tent up quickly and without headaches is a significant survival advantage. For SHTF survival, you will want a natural-coloured tent to blend in with your surroundings. It is important that if a tent doesn't come with a rainfly, it should be made of a single waterproof wall. Nothing worse than waking up trapped inside a wet tent so make sure you investigate the waterproof properties of any tent you intend to buy, and I have a two person tent, a swag tent and a backpacking tent. Tips never store a wet tent, and you also need to make sure you let the tent air-dry, for a while before you roll it up, and pack it away. **Survival sleeping bags** I like to cover all my bases and we are all aware that one of the greatest risks during a survival situation is developing hypothermia, a condition where your body core temperature drops dangerously low. If you keep a 72-hour kit in your vehicle, even during the summer months I would suggest also keeping a sleeping bag because during the summer months it is still cold enough at night to bring on hypothermia, especially if you get wet. If you get stranded in a vehicle when it's cool or cold outside, getting inside of a sleeping bag while inside the vehicle will be warmer than wrapping in a blanket and if you have to walk out of a situation, having a sleeping bag will enable higher chances of survival if you have to shelter at night. Most of this information is basic common sense but the aim of this book is to give basic awareness to hopefully save lives in every way possible so also consider a popular ultralight mummy sleeping bag.

Detoxes and Vitamins in your survival kits, I would pack essentials like Colloidal Silver, Colloidal Gold, Zeolite, Magnesium, Zinc, Vit C and Bentonite Clay and I have already talked about the reasons why. First Aid Equipment and no matter what SHTF scenario you think might and could happen, being prepared is crucial. If you don't have medical help nearby, you will obviously need to deal with the situation yourself and even a simple splinter could kill you if not taken care of properly, it's a very good idea to have two medical kits and one should be for your home, and contain a wide range of supplies for all types of medical emergencies. The other should be small, with just the essentials, for your bug out bag. Also, I suggest adding a third kit to their car and some in your push bike saddle bags. Even if you don't need the medical kit for a disaster situation, you may end up needing it in your everyday life sadly accidents happen and it's best to be prepared and that's the key because going into hospital with the risks that entails with blood transfusions etc and with the simple fact that if you are unvaccinated, they have got an **End Of Life Protocol** designed especially for you.

Clothing dependant on the climate where you live, picking clothes you will need is crucial, cold weather essentials like thick woollen socks, thermals and waterproof clothing because that you lose somewhat about 2% of your body heat when you are cold and should you have your wet clothes on, the body heat loss will increase five times more, also be sure you have a durable hooded raincoat in your survival wardrobe. Also, rugged survival boots are a big must, I will not dwell on this anymore as I am sure you can work out your own survival needs clothes wise and body warming products are not expensive. Around $13 for a four pack and can provide up to an amazing 20' hours worth of heat, and capable of producing heat as high as 155 degrees, helping to warm up your body in a matter of moments. The entire time they're open they'll give off a consistent 130 degrees of heat, more than enough to help you stay warm when it's brutally cold.

Wood stoves can be amazing but just do your research as there are so many to choose from and they don't waste too much firewood, but the heat they produce will let you heat your entire home or a survival cabin. Get yourself one and a large pile of firewood to go with it, and you are all set. Also check out **Portable Solar Chargers** the charger is designed to be perfect for harsh outdoor conditions making it a perfect portable charger for camping or survival and it sure deserves its place as a part of your emergency kit.

Solar Cookers a solar cooker is a type of solar thermal collector, and it "gathers" and traps the Sun's thermal (heat) energy, the heat produced when high frequency light (visible and ultraviolet) is converted into low frequency infrared radiation.These are well worth looking at as cooking will be so important, and the utility of any resource is so important, the prices of them are coming down in price and are around $300 dollars. I just bought one and look forward to using it. Books on this are limited in their information. I might write a comprehensive one.

Rechargeable Batteries A few sets of rechargeable batteries will be perfect for powering your electronic devices and I highly recommend getting these USB rechargeable batteries that you can recharge with a portable charger or a hand-crank radio also add a couple of sets of rechargeable batteries in all the sizes you will need for your electronic gear.

Light Sources have so many options but again an important thing to have like a Survival Headlamp takes the modern-day concept of hands-free devices and gives a survivalist stance to it or while headlamps and tactical flashlights are perfect for the Outdoors, LED lanterns are good for illuminating your home and I really recommend buying LED lanterns powered by standard-size rechargeable batteries.

Self-Protection which is such an important topic as the zombies are out there and even riding my bike currently in the Moreton Bay Region of Queensland as its daily challenges.

I am used to verbal abuse, but the more violent attacks are becoming more frequent in a post-disaster world, the worst of threats that you may be facing is from humans. There will be many hostile strangers out there who may want to take what's yours, maybe even killing you in the process. So, getting yourself armed with a self-defence weapon of some description is your top priority. In this section, you will also find information on home protection because your home is your castle, as the old saying goes, also, it's twice as true when you find yourself amidst a devastated world full of looters, thieves, and other nasty zombified specimens. You don't want any of them to break into your home and harm you or someone in your family, firearms create a lot of noise. But there's been a silent alternative you can use which is a bow and is silent compared to guns and rifles, and you will never experience a shortage of arrows. First, they are reusable and secondly, in time you can learn to make new arrows yourself and there are other self-defence weapons to consider like tasers, laser catapults and knives.

Titanium Torches are my current favourite as they are legal to carry with you and a nice hard tap to the back of the leg calf does the trick and if you are a lady don't go for the man's testicles because you need to put them down and keep them down.

Vehicle Safes There are so many including ones that fit underneath your car and spray them so they're not visible and they could be very helpful in a time of an emergency. Finally, I will end this chapter by mentioning bartering so having an amount of gold, silver and precious stones could help you at some point as this manic world and the situation is very fluid always think outside the box as this as I keep repeating myself, we are a very long way from winning and it get so much worse before it finally does get better. That knock on the door is coming and I am 100% sure that reality will be your worst nightmare so are you just going to wait and pray for the very best, or be ready to run for the hills.

Chapter 13

No Surrender by Sawdust Caesars

I have never surrendered to anything in my life that I thought was wrong and possibly taken a lot of punishment for doing so but that does not change the fact that I stand in my own truth. In the year 2020 that strength was tested beyond any imagination and to be told by Governments, Politicians, Scientists, the media, family and friends that a virus so strong was going to cause my death should I not conform to the mandatory rules now being written and implemented at a rate faster than the virus could travel. They said people are falling dead on the streets, the hospitals are overwhelmed by cases of humans struggling to survive due to infection and you must wear a mask to protect yourself and others. To be told I was unable to travel more than 10 miles into another zone, area, town whatever you wish to call it and to be told if I go shopping, walking the street, visiting restaurants, a pub to meet friends was not allowed without a mask, to be told once I sit down in these places of people gathering I can remove the mask but if I stand up I must wear it, enter this way, exit that way. Distance yourself on the streets and at work. anyplace really by two metres or so. To me it sounded like some type of futuristic movie, and I was playing the part of a human being captured by aliens.

What the hell was going on, why suddenly the world had stopped turning, life had become locked down in a sea of panic and I was curious, could this be real? I had read about this in some book of fiction, but this was really happening, they who I was to discover later had made an attempt to isolate the people of this world, take away the rights and freedoms we cherished so much. To say this virus propaganda was the biggest scam ever introduced onto this planet would be an understatement, the question now and into the future, why, what reason would they wish to lie to us, what was the purpose.

Quite simply, they can no longer sustain the overpopulated planet and the best way to achieve sustainability by introducing a system of fear and control, a fear and control of the human so intense that foods, energy and movement will be offered should you comply with the new digital world of identification, vaccine management, no vaccines, no credits, no life, divide, discriminate and finally destroy. The idea and the implementation worked a treat, divide, most of the non compliers of this Propaganda have lost family, friends and loved ones. Discriminate, if you did not have the experimental vaccine, you lost your freedom to travel, work and to exist. Destroy, that's the part they have not quite achieved just yet, the non compliers are still here on this earth. We are not going away, we are the thorn that sticks into their body and they know not what to do.

We grow everyday, we wake people up every day. We are the so-called Conspiracy theorists who got it right, it's a lie, a big scandalous lie and the world is very slowly waking up to it. The real war is just beginning, good versus evil, the fake wars are propelled by politicians, they create death and destruction to gain wealth and power. The war I and many millions of others fight against, it's real, they want to take our freedoms away, the freedom to speak and the freedom of movement. The right to protest, every person's right to do so in a so-called democratic world. The democratic world and the people that fought for those rights, rights of the working man and women.Quite strange really, the ones who pushed Governments to force change are now in jail, Isolated dead or assassinated, Julian Assange JFK, Martin Luther King, Nelson Mandela. The biggest mistake they made was to give us the internet and social media, the one most important tool that spreads so quickly across the world they failed to control effectively although they are trying to curb it now they underestimated the power of social media in providing the truth. In the words of the great man Martin Luther King, I have a dream, seize the moment, now is the time, no surrender.

Chapter 14

Living of Grid

A lot of us want to leave the matrix and go and live off grid which is basically sustainable living and renewable energy. For some people it means primitive living and cutting ties with all forms of technology and thumbing your nose at 'Them'. It is making a political statement to move to the wilderness and separate yourself completely from the system. To divorce yourself from a system of materialism, greed, corruption, and debt slavery becomes more of a proclamation of independence and freedom from a system that is very oppressive. This is really taking things to the maximum and few people view off-grid living in this manner and it really appeals; but for our own safety we must all consider these options available to all of us. I will not wait for the knock on my door and be offered a vaccine, and due to an emergency law, I had to take it or the option might be I am not allowed to leave my abode and starve out, as happened in previous lockdowns like in Vietnam. So, will that happen? Well, it could and that is enough to bolt to the hills. So, I and other people call it prepping for survival, and there are some die-hard preppers out there, some who are my friends who been prepping for many years and who feel that living off grid is all about being prepared, making sure they have enough supplies to take care of their families, and survive an apocalyptic scenario. There are some who also say it can mean disconnecting not just from the electrical grid, but also creating your own electricity, growing your own food, and living "green"; it's also about finding balance in a lifestyle that gives back to the earth rather than taking from it. Naturally, living off the grid you think of the system or network which delivers electrical power to residential and commercial properties, building, homes, and machinery, also for one person being off the grid may mean simply being disconnected from the power grid.

A lot of us want to leave the matrix and go and live off grid which is basically sustainable living and renewable energy. For some people it means primitive living and cutting ties with all forms of technology and thumbing your nose at 'Them'. An easy way to look at all of this is that if you only require power for things such as general lighting, small electrical appliances, and any appliances that don't generate heat, 12-volt is usually sufficient for your off grid storage, but if you're planning to run heat-generating appliances, electric stove, pumps, microwave, iron, hairdryer, etc. a 24-volt system is a better setup. So, do your research, as this is one of the major pitfalls if you get it wrong. world; switch your phone off for a day to start, if you can, and don't be so spoiled; have less showers; be less dependent on the control they got you so accustomed to. Then after you cut down on your water needs, the next key to off-grid water systems is having a source of reliable water. If your proposed location has not got this, you need to think long and hard before you purchase any off-grid land without water, I personally think you do not need to purchase anything, land or property wise, before this Agenda 30 happens.

Logically every old timer that dies will possibly leave a bush cabin empty so we will really be poor and be truly happy. Because water-storage systems act similarly to the battery systems with electricity generation, and water storage allows you to use increasing or decreasing amounts of water on your terms, and not on the water sources terms and we are all sick of being controlled and you will need a water source to fill up your water storage tanks, and then you use water out of your storage tanks (and for me this is not that hard as I had gravity-fed bores in Tasmania); just do your research and plan and it will all come together. When you start by showing less and start to treat life from today as though you were in drought-survival mode, it doesn't hurt to not wash so much and it is actually a good thing, not washing those natural body oils out, especially Vitamin D. Using gravity fed if your water source spring, pond, or creek etc, is physically higher than your home, then you can use gravity to flow the water to your home and with pressure. But you will also need to run a pipe system from the water source to your home water storage system and if you have enough head pressure difference in height between the water source and your home then this will automatically fill your home's water storage system.

Rainwater Harvesting is so very important and if you get a constant amount of rain per year, you should capture as much as possible by using this method, but droughts do happen from time to time, and if that's your only source of water you're buggered when a drought happens, so rainwater harvesting is best used as a water subsidy rather than a primary source of water.

Human Waste you have three main waste streams. You must plan for which are human wastes, grey-water wastes and trash wastes, and one of the solutions for both human wastes and grey water wastes is the tried-and-true septic tank, which I had on my farm in Winkleigh, Tasmania. A septic system is the best way for those who can afford to have one installed if you can get the large equipment to your location needed for installation and to pump out the solids every two years. You also have the option of a composting toilet if you are living off the grid or just trying to be environmentally conscious, a composting toilet can be a fantastic alternative to a conventional flushing toilet. Requiring no water at all because they work by converting human waste into compost, a substance that's cleaner and safer to handle than unprocessed waste and I have one for my off-road vehicle. They can also be installed almost anywhere since they don't need to be connected to a sewer or septic tank. The easiest way to deal with your grey water outside of a septic system is to pipe it out away from your home, so it will and can absorb naturally back into the ground; and smart people even use their grey water to water their trees and gardens.

Non-Compostable Trash Waste starts to reduce the amount of trash waste you generate so start today while you're in the matrix, and for all waste streams that are organic in nature, just add those to your compost heap. For remaining wastes such as plastics, you will have three options. Just be cautious about any soaps or chemicals that you use as they will end up in your grey water, and since those can be harmful to plants and trees in high concentrations, you understand it makes sense and turning waste streams into compost and using compost for garden plots. Having a milk cow to provide milk, butter and cheese and then breeding more livestock to replace the ones you use for meat, and then working towards getting .

I have had my own farm in Tasmania for 7 years and I made every mistake there was to make. For example, I had a Jersey-cross milk cow and called it UFO, and its first calf, which I called Mars, was a big challenge because of the bull I had selected to put over it, a Hereford bull, is a very big mistake as we needed 3 of us to pull the calf out. A big lesson was learned that day and after that I used bulls that would throw smaller calves, such as Murray Grey and Black Angus bulls. Black Angus meat, as you will be aware, is very tasty. I then stupidly, but not on purpose, on my farm fed a cannabis plant to my sow pig and a stoned pig is some an experience you don't forget. Having your own animals and food source is very liberating and for most of us who believe we have to go off grid at some point, we will treat this as an adventure.

Preparing Your Body and Mind for moving off grid demands a lot of work, and you could start preparing today, because you have to be prepared both physically and mentally. You will need to have a determined and calm mind that welcomes challenges and possible hardships, because living off the grid is not as cosy and convenient as regular city life I included in the next chapter some tools by my spiritual friend Kootah, which will help you breathe into your heart space, and help if and when you go into panic mode, which happens to most of us including me at some point; and that rush of adrenaline and sheer fear is very alarming, and the more one panics the worse the event often becomes.

If you are also in good shape and good health, it will help a lot in some of the challenges you will face, so use this time of preparation wisely and get as fit as you possibly can, because running an independent homestead, raising livestock and crops, making furniture, digging a well or performing regular maintenance on all of this will be easier if you are fit and strong. Consider these very important factors before deciding whether or not you will make this significant change in your life; and increasing your food self-sufficiency makes off-grid living more viable, and even if you can't grow everything aim to supplement your diet with fruits and vegetables raised by your own green thumbs, and choose plants suited for the area's climate where you live and plant them in an area that's well-drained and that gets at least 6 hours of sunlight a day. It is also equally important to have ways to preserve your food supplies, through methods like freezing and preserving.

But for many people, living off-grid still means you will have to make trips to the grocery store; but if you're aiming for maximum self-sufficiency in your off-grid lifestyle, supplement gardening with food gathering methods hunting, trapping, and fishing can provide protein for your diet and gather food from your environment which could be anything from fruit trees that can offer an abundant source of ready-to-eat food during the seasons that they flourish in. Get an illustrated botany book that explains which safe-to-eat fruits, nuts, and berries grow naturally in your locale.I would also get books on foods the natives used to eat, and for me the Aboriginals naturally are a great source of knowledge. Off grid living is easier if you are very fit because you will likely be active every day, especially in the wintertime especially if you are using wood to burn for fuel and heat. Work on strengthening your core and upper arms so you're able to pick things up and perform the work it takes to build and establish your off-grid homestead and you can build your core with ab exercises like crunches, planks, and leg raises. push-ups and curls are great for building arm strength.

For me riding a bike and walking helps to build muscle and while you are living in their matrix so try exercising for a little bit every day, and keep increasing it to get in shape. Also, you can help others by using your hobbies to make money; for instance, if you are spiritually gifted, you might want to help to teach people those skills to help people evolve at your local markets. Turn your knowledge of off-grid living into financial opportunities by maybe monetizing a blog, producing videos, or writing a book about your experiences which will be good in helping others.

Increasing your food self-sufficiency makes off-grid living more viable, and even if you can't grow everything aim to supplement your diet with fruits and vegetables raised by your own green thumbs, and choose plants suited for the area's climate where you live and plant them in an area that's well-drained and that gets at least 6 hours of sunlight a day. It is also equally important to have ways to preserve your food supplies, through methods like freezing and preserving. But for many people, living off-grid still means you will have to make trips to the grocery store; but if you're aiming for maximum self-sufficiency in your off-grid lifestyle, supplement gardening with food gathering methods hunting, trapping, and fishing can provide protein for your diet and gather food from your environment which could be anything from fruit trees that can offer an abundant source of ready-to-eat food during the seasons that they flourish in.

Get an illustrated botany book that explains which safe-to-eat fruits, nuts, and berries grow naturally in your locale.I would also get books on foods the natives used to eat, and for me the Aboriginals naturally are a great source of knowledge. Off grid living is easier if you are very fit because you will likely be active every day, especially in the wintertime especially if you are using wood to burn for fuel and heat.

Try living off the grid first by renting an isolated cabin, that provides you with a taste of what you can expect when living off the grid and spend at least a week or so in one that most

158

closely approximates the sort of home you plan on living in because if you want to totally disconnect when you go off the grid full-time, to see if you can handle going without use of your phone, computer, or other communication technology during your stay. The benefits of living off grid are numerous, and this way of life will come with some challenges, but it also has lots of benefits that will really make you happy and proud of yourself, once you are able to achieve independent success. But before you learn the benefits of living off the grid, you should focus first on the main reasons why you must prefer to spend your life in this way, and the reasons will motivate you to do whatever it takes just to reap the rewards in the end. There are many books on this subject to help prepare you for this incredible journey, and getting it right is going to be so important, as the NWO Plandemic Agenda is not going to stop until they have reached a 90% reduction of the population of planet Earth.

Communication will be so important especially in an emergency, and the options like Two-Way Radios, Ham Radio, CB radio, Satellite phones are some to be considered. The one I have chosen for when there is an emergency and need help with a two-way radio. How do you communicate and reach out to family and friends to check on them and to see if they need assistance? During these events like the power grid going down and cell towers being inoperable, you might not be able to rely on your cell or mobile phone, or landline, and that's when two-way radios will come into play; they are one of the most reliable means of communication, not only during emergencies but also when you are off-grid in the middle of nowhere. Two-way radios are usually powered by NiMH rechargeable batteries, so have backups of them. Communication will be vital as we aren't meant to be on our own 24/7, so try to utilise this time before you go off grid to build friendships with like-minded people and try to catch up with them on a regular basis.

I've been fortunate to have been in the music industry in one form or another for many decades and music is such a great leveller in times of stress, so take instruments with you for me it's a harmonica, but whatever makes you relax during nights where you get together and play whatever, sing and be happy. So finally, to summarise living off grid I feel for most of us will be the road to freedom and out of their manic matrix with its intention to control or own all of us. This madness only ends when you take full control and rebel and live your lives in total freedom, understanding your own vibrations living with the pure bloods, the awoken, are as one and the same and we will survive together by being smart and not trusting anyone:because who is the enemy, or who is paid opposition, and who is not?

Through the food chain is how they are after all of us currently and they understand we will never stab ourselves with their poisons, so their Plan B is our food and water; so think and be very smart. Everyone holding a mobile phone is controlled and tracked to some extent. You can plan all you like and detox all you like and march and protest, but while you are connected to that you are doomed, so think of ways to reduce your exposure. People often ask how I can survive without a mobile phone and I find it very easy, it is liberating and then when I set intentions for people I would like to meet, it just seems to happen. The universe truly does provide, so be brave and dump it.

We survived without these devices for thousands of years before, and the wheel always turns full circle. How many of you reading this are truly happy? There is maybe a reason you. I have been living off grid since I published this book in May 2023 and have never ever been happier thanks to the Milton family for making that happen.

Chapter 15

Simplicity Observation

Activation and Illusion Reality

by Kootah

My name is Kootah. I am here to share my life experiences and my story for people to understand where I came from, and the work I am going to share through my whole journey. I was born in a war-torn country, and at the age of 4 years old I sadly experienced my first trauma of seeing my mother die in front of me. I saw everything, and even to this day I remember vividly what happened, and for many years I have been suffering from it. But at that time when my mother passed away, my aunt sent us back to Lebanon. In 1975, there was a civil war going on which had been going on for many years. We then went and stayed with my grandparents for the next seven years, and in those years that I spent there, I saw many buildings being blown up and saw people being shot. At the age of 6 years me, my brother and two other friends would play at the park, and a man confronted us on numerous occasions with lollies, and finally convinced us after a period to come to his place. That is where he would then take one of us into his bedroom, while the others would be outside eating our lollies. Each of us had to go into the bedroom with him and that is where the sexual abuse started. After that he would take us all into the kitchen, then before we left he would ask us to return, when we wanted more lollies. This happened on several occasions, and the very last time it happened I went to my grandfather and told him what had happened, and he asked me to show him the place where it had occurred. I pointed it out to him, and found out later in life that the man who was a family friend and it was taken care of.

Later on in my life I realise this trauma, and why I went through this trauma. Was not about breaking me but giving me strength to evolve and to become the man I have become today in the line of work I do, and to set me on the path that I have chosen to save others and to help people save themselves by using the tools I have gathered through my life's journey. I have witnessed things most people would not see in their entire lifetimes, and I had to go through all of that after my mother passed; then my father had married again, and his new wife became my step-mother and had asked about us and where we were, and she basically got my dad to the Lebanon in order to bring us all back to Australia. In the 3 months previous to that I had lost my grandfather who I had loved dearly to a heart attack, but a month after that I had also lost one of my favourite uncles, who was shot in Beirut; so that was more trauma for me.

You can all understand the traumas that I had experienced in this short period of time. For years I went through so much, and went within myself so much that I did not give a shite about my life, and I did not care about what happened to me through those years. I then tried to commit suicide about three times, and every time that I tried there was a reason not to achieve that. Even at that time I knew I had a gift, but I was just denying that in so many ways, but only until I got to about the year 2016, when I had a major awakening. I then had to make a decision: was I going to live my life as I was living it, going through this in my head at this time I was getting sick with so many health issues, and was on so many medications, that it was destroying my whole body. I had to make a choice, within two weeks, to keep going the way that I was going, which is my subconscious mind, or I was being in my consciousness and following my true path, and later after I had this awakening, things started to change for me. It was not because of a miracle, but the way I had chosen to not live the way I was living throughout my 47 years of life, and at that time I started to see my living through it and I started to see these gifts, and started to see myself moving into this different dimension.

So, I started to have the courage to go deep into my darkness, and a little bit by bit I had started to work on myself, and I started to release what no longer served my purpose, and I started to get stronger, and through all of my experiences that I had through all of that. I started to feel it was through my consciousness, and everything that was in my subconscious mind was an illusion. So, from then on, I started to understand what was the difference from the subconscious mind to the consciousness, and I started to be more brave and more courageous, and to surrender myself. I then started to show this love for myself, but this did not start overnight, and in the past 6 years since I've had so many experiences, in so in so many different ways that every time I went through an experience, I began to get stronger, and I realised the only thing that was guiding me and helping me was to keep it very simple. So having then realised by keeping it simple that I was not in my head space, I accepted energy and I knew the low vibration, and the high vibration energies, that were coming through, and I was working with these frequencies.

After I had worked with these frequencies, when I was shifting from that, I started to see a lot more, and I started to really see the world for what it was showing me, and everything that was on the outside of me that was in turmoil. Whether it was wars or hatred toward other people, it did not matter: I saw that within myself. So outside of me was the illusion, and the reality was showing me the blockages I had within my body, so I kept working and kept releasing, and kept being the person I had truly come here to be, and starting to see throughout this experience. I could see after I had started to see, to walk away from so many things that no longer served my purpose. Every time I did that I became stronger, and then started to see more and feel more and I had separated my emotions from my reality, and knowing without my darkness, I would not be in enlightenment and evolve to the next level without it, so what I am trying to say our darkness is our reward for freedom.

Naturally everyone experiences things differently, but we all have these certain aspects of ourselves that other people have got as well. There are some people that we are compatible with, and we get along really well with, because we are connected to these frequencies, whether it is high or low vibrations it does not matter. People who will trigger us in so many different ways, that it is all part of our paths and the more people trigger you, the more you need to show you are working on yourself from the inside, and from that you will become honourable and more loving to yourself, towards these people that you have chosen to be here with at this time. In doing this work we sign these contracts, just before you have this incarnation, and it no longer serves my purpose.

I remember one such occasion and I am only talking through my experiences again was my mother's 47th anniversary of her passing, which was last year in July, 2022, and two weeks prior to her anniversary. I then had time-travelled back to 1828, in England somewhere, and I can see the vision of my mum, and a vision of myself that I had let go of her hand, as I ran to pick something up but yet a wagon wheel got me. I slipped and my mum watched in horror when I died in front of her. I was 4 years old at that time and she was 27 years old. So over 150 years later the same situation repeated again in a different timeline, where I was 4 years old and she was 27, this time it was me watching her die. With all that said, it just shows us two souls can choose an experience on different dimensions and frequencies, through the people who we agree to experiencing certain aspects, certain vibrations and certain frequencies, and this is the agreement we had and this would be the agreement I had with my mother in 1828 before we were born. I needed to see it and she needed to feel it in one lifetime, and I need to feel it in another lifetime. So the emotion of losing a mother or losing a son is very similar, because of the connections that we have, so what I am saying is from my own experiences and I know from all this keep it simple, simplify it by observing what is really going on.

Take a deep breath in, to breath into your heart space and by breathing golden light or whatever you can visualise, and by being in that connection and by being in the heart space you can open up your solar plexus, which is the place of suppression of all emotions as the mind only sees what you have experienced and the trauma. But when it sees outside of yourself it goes: I know I am going to suppress this because I can not deal with it, and can not bring this up as I am to unfearful of the unknown; but when you open it up through the heart space and you breathe in, that is the connection to your soul and to your inner children and the ages of these inner children, that you have been neglecting for many centuries and life times. It is the key to freedom and when you start doing that, you become better at it.

You then start to see things, and you start to see the difference between the illusion and the reality, and you then understand it because these walls shown on the physical level are the walls within us. Nothing is on the outside of ourselves, but it is always on the inside because love only comes from within, and when you show all that love you will attract people on these frequencies. But by running around and chasing an invisible tail all of your life and dreaming and fantasy about the true love of yourself, it has always been within you, it has never ever been on the outside of you, and when you do that you become stronger and you the individual will start to lift the vibration, and the vibration on the existence on this planet. It does not happen through fighting others, but starts from the inside, and when you start showing that love within you it then starts to radiate to every person into the whole world. And all those aspects and those frequencies dimension, we connect on that frequency, and that is how we lift our vibration. Like I have said before, keep it simple, and by keeping it really simple and understanding yourself you are unlocking the key to your heart, and it is through the breath work into your heart. Once you do that you won't have the fear of the unknown because nothing can harm you, and nothing can touch you and you're just as powerful as anyone else here on earth.

We are all powerful but we just need to know how to use these tools, and from there we become more at peace with ourselves and being more intuitive, and about being intuitive and connecting with the 3 brains and aligning them all together, through the visual, the emotional, and the soul which is your heart. We are all here to do this work and we all have chosen to be here in this time, to lift the vibration from within us; so be kind to yourself, be loving to yourself and there no such thing as right or wrong, we are perfect and imperfect humans, and we are here to experience new experiences with different souls. Even though we come from the same energy fields we exist. We are everything but just on the 3D level, and we do not see that and do not see how powerful we truly are.

When you do that and start feeling that and start working inwards, you then start radiating that love and you start sharing using your tools to help others that are going through what they are going through. We are all here in different dimensions, different realms, different frequencies, and there is no one better than anyone.Do not bow to anyone as I do not bow to anyone. We are all equals; we just need to see that we all come from the same energy fields. We are all precious souls, we are existence, and we chose to experience specially in a physical world with a physical body. The body is so very powerful it could heal itself, you've just got to simplify it and you've got to observe, and you've also got to see the difference between illusion and reality through the subconsciousness of a conscious mind, illusion and reality. You're here to align all aspects of yourself, to move forward. Some, though, choose to do it in one lifetime and some others do it in many lifetimes, and some have chosen to activate it for the next lifetime. Know how to work on it as we all have different frequencies and different dimensions, there is no right or wrong, this is our choice. We are all different souls that have chosen these vibrations through our existence. Whether you think you are right or wrong, there is no right or wrong decision; it's all an experience. Everyone is your brother and sister, we are all one.

We are just a separation of one energy into 8 billion souls, and that what we are (I understand whether you agree or disagree with that, it's my own experiences), and it is time to stand up for ourselves with love within us, and that's where the illusion has always been: it has always been on the outside. So please see, feel and hear that and sit with yourself when you meditate. It might be frustrating but breathe into the heart space starting with one minute, then move to 5 minutes, then work from there. You have to change just 1% about yourself every day. Karma is non-existence, and it is part of the programming and conditioning to make you feel fear as we are all perfect, imperfect souls, and everything that we are is an experience. Every soul that you interact with in this timeline is through a contract before you enter an incarnation, as our paths are already set before we incarnate. Life is an experience no matter what, it just is when you see that you will see and feel this, no doubts, no questions. Please look at this not from a tunnelled perspective, but with your soul because karma creates judgement in people, and we all need to see this. It can take you away from life's purpose, your mission and pathway, so stand very strong, be vigilant, move forward with love as love conquers every frequency and vibration. Start once a week and then every two weeks it does not matter, as long as you are being authentic to yourself that you are ready to move forward. We are all here for a purpose, Loving and Blessings to every single one of you. **Activation Code**.

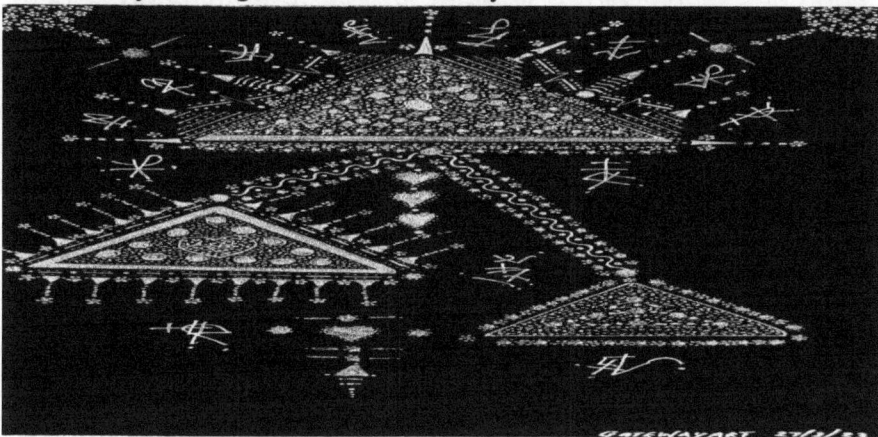

Chapter 16

Being Spiritually Aware

A very heavy topic which will truly upset some, who I will refer to as bible bashers and I truly struggle with some of them. They eat and breathe the bible yet every word in it could be read in many different ways. If you truly "See" and, contrary to their belief systems, you can be a believer in God and energy and still have spiritual sight for what is the Holy Spirit. For me, some are not critical thinkers and are totally brainwashed, as religion and churches have been for many centuries. There are so many religious churches in the Moreton Bay region, yet how many have come out and said that the C-19 vaccines are gene-therapy poisons and " The Mark Of The Beast " as it is written in the Book of Revelations, but instead have encouraged their parishioners to take these clot shots and they still call themselves priests and think often they are 'Holier Than Thou.' How many people reading this have trusted your doctors and your priests?

Well, I am sorry, but they have lied to you all but there are the exceptions and I found one at The Church on the Bay, Margate, Qld, and most who were there were from other churches, who did not want to be discriminated against, because they did not want to check in, wear a mask, and get vaxxed. So I started to go and took some of my friends and everything was fine, until one day I mentioned to 3 younger ladies that I could communicate "In Spirit" with my daughter Ethan Elizabeth Warren, who had passed away on Friday, 13th (Black Friday) August, 1989, and she is now of my spirit guides. Well, three ladies were not happy and said to me "I am talking to the devil", but there is no one so blind as those that can not see, so I was politely asked not to come back, which I have respected and would never be around a few of the bigots there anyway, but a lot who go there were kind to me, and not all are blinkered. Ironically it is they who had judged me, had left other churches because of being judged and then judged me and truly the only person I will allow to judge me is God. My other spirit guide is Martina Batovska who passed away on 12th January, 2022 and I truly believe 100% in the proof of existence, and I have had too many experiences to never be swayed by people who are truly blind. If this upsets some then maybe the truth really hurts, and I am too long in the tooth to mince my words. When you realise your bible will not save you, if you do not save yourself, as so many got on the trains to the death camps in World War II and maybe were still clutching their bibles, if you don't wake up soon you could be on the train to the wellness camps clutching your own bibles.

Maybe God believes in actions not words because words can be very cheap and I would estimate about 90% who religiously read their bible are vaccinated, and only 5% of truly gifted spiritual people are vaccinated. There is some irony in these figures, and I would think all spiritual people would agree we do not need swords to beat Lucifer. If we all put away differences of opinion, would we not be able to beat him quicker, if we all walked together as one in no "Judgement"? So let's look at my own personal proof of existence which happened after my daughter died in 1999, because I was wanting to connect, as losing a child is a parent's worst nightmare, we are not meant to do that, and sadly as this pandemic unfolds it sadly will become more common, and some you reading this might also need guidance it's very challenging, to make rhyme of reason to what as suddenly destroyed your life for ever as life is never the same, and the pain never really goes away. I first went to a spiritualist church in Hervey Bay, Qld, in 1989, and a medium Jason McDonald, was there that night, a very talented man, who came to the elderly lady next to me and it was very obvious that Jason could "See", so proof existence started for me that night and life will never be the same thankfully.

In about one minute he motioned with his hand at his neck to the lady next to me, he had Bill and Fred with him, they were telling him they were all right now, the lady was in such a state of emotional breakdown that I was very concerned and when the service finished I went and made her a cup tea and she explained her distress was tears of joy because Bill, her husband and Fred, his co-pilot were shot down over Singapore in 1944, and were beheaded by the Japanese, and here she was 45 years later and she was being informed "They Were Alright Now." Moments like that in time are life changing, and the spiritual journey started for me and the more you see and the more you listen, then the more you grow, and I could mention lots of incredible spiritual events, but I will just mention one.

I was DJing in Prestatyn, Wales, over 10 years ago, when the technics equipment played up, and I was on stage warming up for international artists from the US and I was in a quandary about what to do. When I finally managed to get off the stage, a good friend of mine Nel Goddard, from South Yorkshire, UK needed help, so I put my hand on his shoulder and said you are not on your own." He looked at all his friends gathered around, and he said I know, and in the twinkle of your eye, his 4-inch beer glass peeled very slowly, a bit like peeling an orange skin and about 2 inches of glass and the beer in it dropped onto the carpet, he shaking asked " What is that all about John?" I calmly replied I told you were not on your own, meaning his spirit guides were with him and the record that would not play and had started this chain of events was Joanne Courcy, "I Have Got The Power". I have to truly live in my truth, and have referred to myself as a spiritual dancer, and in my first book "John Warren Our Soul Music Journey", I mention that spiritual dancing is truly better than sex, and I truly believe that, and in these times, sharing body fluids with all and sundry it might not end well, as vaccinated sperm is incredibly potent if you are a female and I would be more worried not about getting pregnant, and especially if you have gone through menopause there could be a chance your periods could restart, and also there is a risk of cervical cancer; and you also might be aware ⅔ cancers that are being diagnosed currently are turbo cancers.

Sorry, I have gone off on a tangent, but when I play my harmonica, it is also done through connecting with energy, vibration, and spirit. Also, when I write my better prose, it is often done with the "Moving Finger Writes." Life is all 'Energy and Vibration' and connecting with 'Spirit' is so profound S is "Souls origin", P is "Paranormal phenomena", I is "Innate longing for eternity", R is "Revelation of the scriptures", I is "Inconceivable consistency amidst global diversity", and T is "Transformational potency of spirituality"

Once we understand that there is a difference between the body and the soul, and the body is temporary, the soul is eternal, the body is unconscious, the soul is conscious, the body is a source of misery, the soul is a reservoir of ecstasy and joy, then naturally we will be inclined to know where the soul comes from. There were so many evidence of Paranormal phenomena that since the start of the 20th century people like William James, who was one of the most prominent psychologists of the modern times, has said that "The examples for these phenomena are so many and so wide spread that to dismiss them to wish them away is bad science". We keep ourselves narrow minded and closed minded, if we dismiss such phenomena as unscientific, fake or undocumented. We have seen if there is a longing there is a fulfilment as we observe from these other examples of food and water. We can therefore conclude that there is a place where this longing is fulfilled where we can get eternal shelter, and that is the spiritual world. If we look at some of the greatest thinkers in world history they were saintly people, and they talked about the world to come which is beyond this world, the world where there is no death, the world where there is eternal life. A lot of you reading this who do have divine spiritual talents are often channelling them, and you may realise it is not you, but it is so very liberating to have these gifts and powers. This consistency in the teachings of all these traditions gives credence to the understanding that there is a wisdom which is universal, and it is hinted at by the universality of these teachings, and by this particular teaching of the eternal world or the spiritual world and that nobody can live without happiness. But there have been many great saints, and great spiritualists, who have become detached from matter and they've become attached to something higher. What is that higher thing? that higher reality is the spiritual reality but again you only see what you want to see and believe.

In my second book 'John Warren Our Soul Music Journeys.' While interviewing Ruby Andrews, a well-known singer I worked with in Chicago, US who had several hit records. Back in the 1960's, she had told me how she was regressed into a previous life, when as an Indian squaw she had drowned, and in this current life she was still very afraid of water. The actress Shirley MacLaine had taken Ruby back into a previous life on Shirley's television show. Some of you would have experienced "Deja Vu" as I have on my travels, and I having lived in 7 countries in my 20's-30's and sometimes when getting off a bus, or train in a strange land and understanding of what is around the corner, like I had truly been around the corner before in maybe a previous life.

Music has been my love for many decades, and I have been privileged to work with and been around so many talented artists (too many to mention) in Detroit, Chicago, Orlando, Philadelphia and New Jersey Ect: I have been very fortunate to be involved in several record labels including my part-owned Red Pants Records based in the Jersey US, with one of my best friends Robert Paladino who kindly wrote in both my previous books and is an "Icon" in the music industry and wrote one of Northern Souls greatest records The Epitome of Sound "You Don't love Me. I met Robert and family in a lift in Orlando US and had the pleasure of working with him when we brought out the fabulous Johnny Boy Pryor's "Cause My Love is Gone" song on our label. It will be in a movie one day soon and thank you Robert he is always there for me, and I truly miss not being able to go to the US and catching up with him. Music has been my first love and it will be my last, and my favourite music genre is Soul music often referred to as the devils music.

"Music can ultimately be one of our most powerful gateways to connect to our true spiritual nature, our divine source, the unseen, as well as to the universe around us and those other divine beings that inhabit it with us."

It has always been a great tool bringing people together; it is so much more empowering and I could only imagine what the NWO and the satanists listen to when they bang their drums and I truly believe this is a war we can win and will win. It truly bothers me that so many who believe in their respective gods, and understand the Book of Revelations and the Mark of the Beast and attended churches all their lives, have trusted so many preachers who have said, "Go and Get vaccinated" and we will ultimately pay the price for believing in them. God must truly be disappointed in your lack of faith in him and we do not need any weapons, because spiritually we are so very powerful. In Religion and Spirituality, I like to walk the talk, and some of you who will have judged me should maybe try that, and then you will no be referred to as being "Glass Half Full." So many years ago I went and lived in Israel, to study some of the events in the bible and lived there for six months, and volunteered and worked on Kibbutz Beit Guvrin, House of Men. It is a Kibbutz in the Lakhish region, west of the ancient city of Beit Guvrin, for which it is named. Located 14 kilometres east of Kiryat Gat, it falls under the jurisdiction of Yoav Regional Council. In 2021 it had a population of 414. Kibbutz Beit Guvrin, was founded in 1949, on the eve of Shavuot, by former Palmach members after the Palestinian Arab residents of Bayt Jibrin who fled the military assault by Jewish forces during the 1948 Arab–Israeli War. The first residents were members of the "Yeti Zivim" youth group, which emigrated from Turkey in 1945, and the "B'nai Horin" youth group, which emigrated from Romania in 1946.

The Kibbutz was established on the fields to the north of the Arab village of Beit Jibrin, which sat atop what was once a Hebrew town known as Beit Guvrin that was later renamed Eleutheropolis, "the city of free men" by the Romans in 200 CE. It was later the site of a Frankish colony, "Beth Gibelin", before becoming better known by its Arabic moniker "Bayt Jibrin" following the Muslim conquest. So, I went to live here and on the sabbath, I would travel around Israel visiting holy places like Manger Square, Bethlehem, on Xmas eve and Jerusalem, where God spoke to me for the first time. Spiritual people try not to lie as it is bad karma, and our guides are watching us. I also visited the Sea Of Galilee, Jericho, Ein Gedi, Elat, Hebron and Masada to name a few. Speaking of Masada, I slept in the Negev desert with Brigitta and Yvonne ''My First Three Some'' Masada is a rugged natural fortress, of majestic beauty, in the Judaean Desert overlooking the Dead Sea. It is a symbol of the ancient kingdom of Israel, its violent destruction and the last stand of Jewish patriots in the face of the Roman army, in 73 A.D. It was built as a palace complex, in the classic style of the early Roman Empire, by Herod the Great, King of Judaea, (reigned 37 – 4 B.C.). The camps, fortifications and attack ramp that encircle the monument constitute the most complete Roman siege works surviving to the present day.

Living in Israel left many profound memories with me but none more than at Beit Guvrin, as life and the people you meet can change your destiny because I was fortunate to have shared a room with Jim from New York, who was an archaeologist and studying the burial tunnels near the Kibbutz, Beit Guvrin, and he took me one day with the two Swedish ladies I was sharing a room with Brigita and Yvonne, to a burial tunnel. When we went through there it was very claustrophobic and dark as Jim was the only one with a head torch, and then when we reached the opening I witnessed an amazing site, but experienced real fear that day as I had walked on a narrow ledge and scaled the rock wall, and looked my maker in the face but I was not meant to die that day.

A bit of background information of where I went and the earliest written record of Maresha was as a city in ancient Judah (Joshua 15:44). The Hebrew Bible mentions among other episodes that Rehoboam fortified it against Egyptian attack. After the destruction of the Kingdom of Judah the city of Maresha became part of the Edomite kingdom. In the late Persian period a Sidonian community settled in Maresha, and the city is mentioned in the Zenon Papyri (259 BC). During the Maccabean Revolt, Maresha was a base for attacks against Judea and suffered retaliation from the Maccabees. After the Hasmonean Hyrca I captured and destroyed Maresha in 112BC king John E, the region of Idumea remained under Hasmonean Control. In 40 BC the Parthians completely devastated the "strong cite", after which it was never rebuilt. Beth Gabra or Beit Guvrin succeeded Maresha as the main town of the area. Conquered by the Roman general Vespasian during the Jewish War (68 CE) and completely destroyed during the Bar Kochba revolt (132–135 CE), it was later renamed Eleutheropolis, "the city of free men" by the Romans in 200 CE. It was later the site of a Frankish colony, "Beth Gibelin", before becoming better known by its Arabic moniker "Bayt Jibrin" following the Muslim conquest. The Hebrew Bible mentions among other episodes that Rehoboam fortified it against Egyptian attack.

After the destruction of the Kingdom of Judah the city of Maresha became part of the Edomite kingdom. In the late Persian period a Sidonian community settled in Maresha, and the city is mentioned in the Zenon Papyri (259 BC). Sources from the Byzantine period mention both Christian and Jewish personalities living in the city. We were there witnessing its wonders in 1981 and remember it was not excavated then as both Maresha and BeitGuvrin/Eleutheropolis were finally excavated after 1989, and 1992, respectively by the Israeli archaeologist Amos Kloner. Important finds at the latter site were the amphitheatre built by the Roman army units stationed there, a large Roman bath house, and from the memories like this being one of the first to witness this amazing wonder are etched in my brain .

Life is truly a journey and the book is often written before you're born on the roads it will take you on. Like the Kibbutz also visited many place like Manager Square, Bethlehem, Jerusalem and sites like Via Dolorosa, Wailing Wall, Church of the Holy Sepulcher where God spoke to me for the first time and Yad Vashem the holocaust museum which has left an everlasting, sad profound effect on me, I spent the whole day there drinking in the horrors they went through. Memories like this are in some ways events that were meant to be and I think our lives and the book of our lives have already been written, and we truly might be living in the past, what is time travel and what is our 'Out of Body Experiences', and the people we meet like Jim do change everything.

The only person I have spiritually let heal me is (Kootah) and when doing it for the first time, he opened a portal in me that I shared with him, which was the ability that I could do past life regression, which is a hypnotic technique that that aims at recovering memories from your past life or incarnations. The therapy assists persons struggling with mental health problems like anxiety, depression, mood swings, and gender dysphoria. Hence, the therapist assumes that our past traumatic memories are the origins of our current mental challenges. For this, a past life regression therapy session seeks to address these past traumatic events before we were born in this life and since that portal has opened. I have successfully managed to take every one back into their past lives, that I was supposed to. The previous chapter by Kootah will have meaning to some and be very confusing to others, but we all have the ability to evolve by learning from our inner children and the contracts we take on with other people, which are to help us on the path of enlightenment. When you are triggered by someone there are specific reasons for that, and understanding that everything in life is meant for a reason and when you get that, it is very liberating as you will feel the changes in your personality. Learn to breathe into your heat space when under duress. It takes a lot of work to achieve, and I am no different as I am also on the same learning path as most of you.

Spiritual Orbs when looking for evidence of Spirit, the presence of an orb is one of the first things ghost hunters, sceptics, believers and non-believers look to verify the bona fide presence of a spirit and over time, I've heard a lot of people talk about orbs, and there seems to be a lot of confusion collectively. Ghost hunters use emf readers as well and another reason to invest in one. The evil that have created this Plandemic Agenda, and they have been cunning and utilised it to the maximum to get you to put this vaccine in your arm to keep your job and provide for your family. There is no judgement from me as this was your journey, and you have to walk in your own shoes. Even trying to format this book was the hardest. It was a fight between me and the devil. It took me 19 days longer than my last two books to try to format and every time I was close to finishing just like that the devil wiped my manuscript clean he truly does not want this book to happen. The devil is so very powerful the only way to beat him is to save everything you do as it tries to sabotage ''God's Work'', twice he had me to tears though but my angels came through. But let's all come together as one: vaxxed, unvaxxed, spiritualists and church goers to beat the evil common foe, and after the great victory we can then fight amongst ourselves if need be.

Music is a great way amongst all of us to come together as one, and for me it was my first love of music, of the future, and music of the past, to live without my music would be impossible to me (John Miles). We all can be confused by 'By Spirit" and orbs can be confusing especially if there are ''archangels' occasionally I will get blue and green orbs and so it is very enlightening. I am a spiritual dancer and often orbs appear when I dance and on my 50th birthday for a charity event for the Multiple Sclerosis Society that I organised in the UK, many orbs were around me when I was dancing. I hope reading this opened some portals for some of you that have long been buried. The day of "Proof of Existence" is a very special day and I hope you have that awakening really soon in this age of Aquarius.

In the photo below you can see I am in the Zone " Lost In Music", but you only see what you want to see so you will either believe or you will not but when you do, life is easier if you do not fear death, and fear is what has got us where we are today.

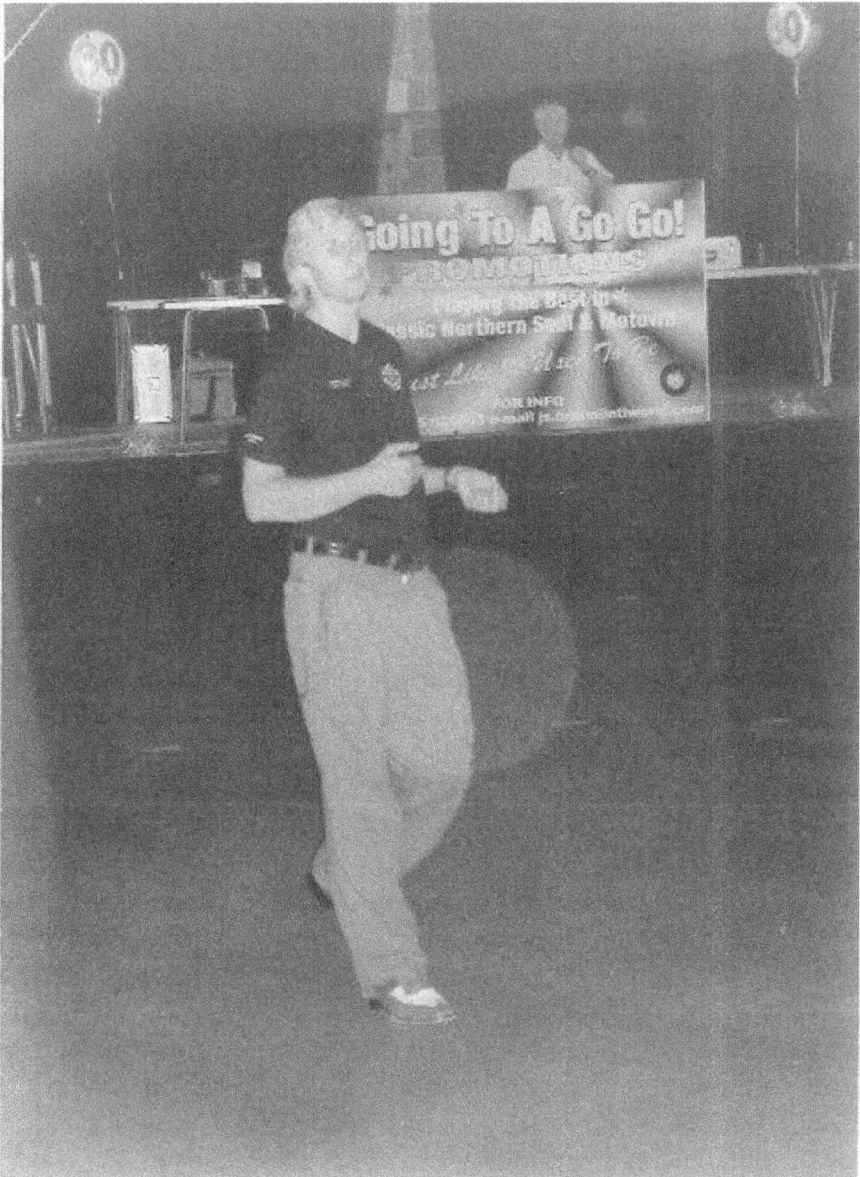

Chapter 17

Homeschooling

It is important to look at this critical topic in more detail as the education system is truly flawed, worldwide, and it seems to like to reward unlogical dimness and crush critical thinking. I was born dyslexic and at the age of 6, I was subjected to punishments along with 2 other boys because we were termed as "Slow," and every time we made a mistake in the headmaster's office, at Alfred Street Infants School, Rushden, Northamptonshire, the headmaster would hit our hands with a wooden ruler which really hurt, not just physically, but mentally and you're truly scared for the rest of your life. The amount of abuse I suffered at that school was immense, and all I did when I was 7 years old was to look up Mrs. Phillips' dress as she reached up to the blackboard, and the other children laughed, and she caught me looking. For this terrible crime, I was punished and caned in front of the whole school of 300 at morning assembly but at that moment "A rebel was Born" that day and I will die a rebel. One moment they were singing 'All Things Bright and Beautiful' and the next moment I was being made an example of. When I went to Rushden Boys Comprehensive School, after failing the eleven-plus exam, I was put in a B class, and the abuse got even worse, and I was constantly in trouble and hit with things like sports shoes, sometimes with my underpants pulled down in front of the whole class. Also, one day I was put up the climbing frame in a straitjacket, and the kids could throw a medicine ball at me. So, you can see why I'm not very respectful of the schooling system, and I am sure some of you reading this have your own horror stories. Teachers who are sadists and abusers in general are out there, and maybe it is why some might go into the teaching professions, where they have access to your children. After this con-vid scam, and the levels of vaccinations in the education system due to the mandates, you have to assume that most teachers are vaxxed and people that have been vaxxed, there can be many changes in their personalities. You might find them very slow in concentration, like they're asleep, the lights are on but no one seems to be at home. But there would still be some great teachers who are vaccinated who might have had no choice due to financial reasons so don't I judge them all. Go with your gut feeling and remember they look after your precious loved ones. Sadly I would expect some children would be having to lie to their teachers, and their friends, about their vaxxed status just to be left alone, and what a sorry world that this is that spiritually gifted, creating thinkers and the future for all of us worldwide, have to be subjected to this total bullshit.

So be very prepared, as I have already talked a lot about zombism in previous chapters, and it's no different in the education system and likely worse when you consider the 5G and all the technology used in the school system as this all plays out. It is going to get so much worse, that home-schooling might be your only sane option so when I was a child and I looked out of the school window and the teacher would say "Johnny, you're a Dreamer" because I had switched my logical brain off and I did not want to learn rubbish like algebra or that Hitler died in 1945 and he did not he was too much of a ""coward " to commit succide. I was so very happy when leaving at 14, and then setting fire to my tie outside of the school gates, and then singing, "You can stick your school system up your arse." It was so liberating to finally be free of their system. When are they going to teach children important things like the real meaning of money, well they are not, because they plan its extinction anyway. We all need to start again with the school system and this is the reset we want and need for our future and for are children that are receptive to truly learning and making countries like Australia truly great again. Learning to protect your children from all dangers in the schools, the toxins, and especially how dangerous mobile phones are due to the roll-out of the 5G, in the education system, and teaching the correct safe use of them which I have already related in a previous chapter. You can enjoy life so much more if you switch your mobile phone's off and time, maybe to form more youth clubs, where children can just be children, and maybe teach them farming skills, because such things as milking a cow and raising chickens, is simplistic and very empowering. Also, time to build their confidence in public speaking, because communicating with each other seems such a task, when they appear to text each other so very much, and some have seemed to have lost basic skills like talking.

Music is also such a great tool to bring them together and encourage them to learn to play simple musical instruments like a harmonica, guitar, drums or a tambourine. It is not rocket science and they are never going to visit the moon anyway, with their zombified, vaxxed school friends. But the school system tries to teach them lies like the moon landings really happened. If you are religious then maybe Sunday schools could be an option, but only if your children really want it because I was made to go because it was parents wanted us out the way as it was "Nookie Day", and I never bothered and instead I played truant and spent the money I was given on lollies, and did what I thought was best for me. Normal children are rebellious by nature, so do not crush their "spirit" by making them do things they do not want just because you had to do it yourself.

All children should be taught how powerful the sea, sand, moon and the sun are, especially around the full moons, new moons, and the Solstices. Some of the best things in life are free, and they will learn a lot more than sitting in a bedroom on their own, glued to their ipad, mobile phone, or laptop. How true it is that a happy child is a happy parent, and all of you reading this who have children or grandchildren must truly fear for their future, as most of the politicians really do not care about any of them, because if they did, this madness would be treated with the respect and importance it should have. So, the basics of making the decision to home-school might be difficult at first and is a decision not one to be made lightly off and some of you are deciding if home-schooling is going to be right for you, but in reality for most it might be the only option to keep your loved ones safe and emotionally stable. You will need to consider such factors as the time and commitment needed so please talk to other home-schooling families in person or online and consider attending a home-school support group meeting or find out if the groups in your area offer events for new home-schooling families. Some groups will pair families with an experienced mentor or host Q&A nights, and recently at Burpengary Men's Shed there was a speaker explaining it all. Home-schooling and a talk by Terry explained the differences of distance, public, private and home-schooling and how the funding by government affects the curriculum.

It is impossible to get away from the agenda that is being taught in schools unless you home-school, and most of us are truly aware and are getting prepared as we are not in your agenda and never will be, so please just leave us alone. The last 3 years have taught all of us that they are not to be trusted, especially at some of these Prestigious Religious Private Schools but I suppose some of them who go there with their parents who have eaten all the lies at university and think they have a high IQ. But I have news for you; if you vaxxed your children for a "COLD", you truly are a moron; and if that offends you, good because that is what some of us truly feel and that is people like all of us who would never vaccinate our precious children with an "Emergency Approved Only Experiment" and I expect some of you will regret it now seeing that your children might not have the innate natural immunity they once had, and seem to get sick a lot more recently since they have vaxxed, but you can try to fix it and the chapter on detoxing might help you fix some of the damage which your actions and lack of responsibility will have caused. Once you make the decision to Home-school, you will want to do all that you can to ensure that you start on a positive note, especially if your child is transitioning from public or private school to home-schooling.

There are many steps you can take to smooth the transition and for example, you might want to allow time for everyone to make the adjustment, don't rush, be relaxed, make it fun, learning is so much easier if you are very calm, and you don't have to make every decision right away. You may find yourself in the position of wondering what to do, if your child doesn't want to home-school, but sometimes it will be simply part of the adjustment period, like missing their friends and their usual routines, so focus on the positives like no more bus rides and listening to zombified teachers and past friends who are vaxxed who they might not have anything in common with anymore. Learn from the mistakes of veteran home-schooling parents, and listen to your own instincts regarding your children, for who truly understands your children better than you? anything in common with anymore. Begin by searching for home-school support groups by state, and towns, and asking other home-school families you may know and there is great support in online support groups as selecting your home-school curriculum can be overwhelming. But discuss with your children what they love and aim to aspire to be in their future, so they don't waste time and energy on things they do not want to study instead and just focus on learning what they will need to achieve their future goals.

Try to keep it simple, as KISS always seems to work and there is a confusing array of options, and it would be easy to overspend and still not find the right curriculum for your student. You may not even need a curriculum right away but can utilise free printables from your local library, while you decide to choose every option, so do not be afraid to ask. The world needs to return to the basics where we are helping to support each other, and not this selfish greedy world we are currently living in, where not many seem to be very happy. Consider using an existing curriculum or creating your own and learn the basics of record keeping as it is very important to keep good records of your child's homeschool years, and our records could be as simple as a daily journal, or as elaborate as a purchased computer program or notebook system. The state you live in might require that you write a home-school progress report, keep a record of grades, or turn in a portfolio. Even if your state does not require it, many parents will enjoy keeping portfolios, progress reports, or work samples as keepsakes of their children's home-schooling years. For the start just learning the basics of scheduling, because home-schoolers generally have a great deal of freedom and flexibility when it comes to scheduling, but it will take a while to find what works best for your family. And learning how to create a home-school schedule doesn't have to be difficult when you break it down into very manageable steps and it would be very helpful to ask other home-schooling families what a typical day looks like for them.

Many of you are being thrown in the deep end in all of this, but if you all work together, you can all grow together and your children will make new like-minded friends. Look at yourself as pioneers even though home-schooling has been around for a long time. One thing to consider is when your children do work the best. Are they early birds or night owls? Obviously, your spouse's work schedule, activities outside of the classes and your own commitments are important, but it's important to remember and reward them with the things that they love to do. No more school bullying issues, and the mental issues they might be causing them grief which could dissipate over time. Also, as they become in tune with these new routines you might even find your children jumping out of bed to actually want to learn because how many children go to school longing for the day when they can leave for good like I did, and as for myself I do attempt to write these books so I might not be the dud I was once told I was going to be. If you have pets, they can be a useful teaching tool as pets don't judge, and children can truly learn so much when they are given the correct tools. Exciting times are ahead and hopefully you will not look back on no more controlling teachers, expensive uniforms, and the children have more time to learn sporting skills that they might want to do and might excel at.

How many sporting things are they made to do and not want to do? Treat this Plandemic agenda as a new beginning as there are many methods for home-schooling your children but finding the right style for your family may take some trial and error. It's not uncommon to try a few different methods throughout your home-schooling years or to mix and match, and the most important thing to remember is to be open to what works for your family rather than feeling that you must make a lifetime commitment to a particular home-schooling method. So, let's start at the start. Day One, in terms of basics, your child will need a reliable internet connection, webcam and microphone and more likely built into desktop and laptop screens for video conferencing, a supportive and comfortable chair, and a thoughtful workspace, including easy access to pens, paper, and space for their books and resources.

Please don't overthink it but treat it as trial and error till a routine is established. In the future there will be many brilliant teachers who will work with you, who never complied to get vaxxed, and they will be a great asset for the future of your children moving forward. We need to reward them for their stoic beliefs, and all you teachers reading this who were strong and brave and did not get vaxxed, we salute you and the kids will need your skill sets. As time goes by, you can customise your child's workspace according to your child's needs, such as: do they need a large, colourful calendar to help them keep track of upcoming assignments? Do they benefit from having reminders or prompts of important educational concepts spread around the room? Do they prefer working with pen and paper at the kitchen table, and completing written work on their computer in their studies? Please try to use the first week as a grounding exercise for what routines suit you and your child and then work towards implementing that from here on and try to find a way to integrate your child's subject matter into the world around them; maybe try using bright and colourful templates to reinforce knowledge, from the fridge to their bedroom with colours that truly work in bringing out their creativity in such a way that you start to look at your children in ways you may not have noticed before and some are much wiser than even you, and school for them is boring. Even at 15 years old, they might be ready to sit a degree and I have met one such lad recently in Scarborough Qld, as boredom does crush their spirit and when did you last see your child truly happy, chilled, and they might come alive especially when not surrounded by so much Wi-FI. I have spoken enough of the dangers of it that it is now time for action.

Also, it might be helpful to remember that you're not the teacher but a kind of teacher's assistant, keeping them very focused, on track and making yourself available for help when needed. Another corner-cutting option now that you're schooling from home, you can channel your effort into familiarising yourself with the distance learning tools your child's school might have been employing, such as synchronous classes being broadcast over Zoom? Keep documents, assignments, and submission hosted on a shared Google Drive? So many options are available; but take it very slow as this is a new beginning and, unfortunately, unless something changes drastically you are all going to have to consider this option. Although the physical classroom has temporarily disappeared, the foundations of the schooling experience still remain somewhat fundamentally in place as your child will spend many hours a day immersed in knowledge, with a view to completing certain tasks to fulfil curriculum outcomes. This could be as obvious as enforcing the same school hours, and making sure your child dresses for school not in a uniform but certainly out of pyjamas, and that socialising with friends over Zoom, Skype, FaceTime or instant messaging services remain restricted to the hours allotted within the school day that naturally facilitate this, such as recess, lunch and of course, once the day has ceased.Another helpful way to maintain the structure of the school day is to allow for regular breaks and the school day is broken up into pieces with natural breaks either between formalised classes or maybe for younger children, between subjects; so, encourage your child to do the same.

Remind them to get up and walk around, stretch, anything that makes them happy. It is so tough on children today in this totally manic world they are being subjected to, and if you all had stood up in the last 3 years as one, we all would not be in this shambles. When they return to class, get them to dive into something different to keep them focused. School is not just a place for learning about what's between the book covers, it is also about healthy, constructive socialisation and these skills will stick with your kids for life, no matter what the reasons are for being home-schooled. It's very important that socialising is as much a part of their day, as they work on their to-do lists.

Please give your children a realistic amount of space and privacy to pursue their friendships, digitally and virtually and meet and catch up like they always did in the past and do not let your child make the rules here, just as in school there have to be certain rules where their behaviour doesn't interfere with their learning. You are not just their teacher, but one of the current custodians of their education, sometimes you will need to bring them back into line a little when there is schoolwork that needs to be completed and really allow plenty of time in your child's day for deep, explorative learning and discovery, both supervised and unsupervised. Encourage them to dig in the garden, dance to their favourite songs after dinner or whatever age-appropriate hobby or pastime they find to be their real passions.

Although their home has temporarily become a classroom too, you will need to allow for the space for their home life as well, there are numerous videos on YouTube to help you to make it as seamless as possible. Some studies have shown home-schoolers score better on achievement tests than public-school students, regardless of their parent's income or education. I already mentioned this, but it needs repeating for your children's safety. People are switching over to earbuds (wireless earphones) and have asked me if earbuds emit EMF radiation.EMF radiation. I was pretty convinced I knew the answer, but I decided to do a bit more research on the issue. Wireless earbuds, including Apple Air pods, emit high levels of EMF radiation, mainly in the form of microwaves because they rely on Bluetooth technology, among other things, and this is a potentially dangerous thing to have so close to your brain. So please invest in **Air tube headphones** utilising a hollow tube between the speakers and the hollow tube so the sound is transmitted through air only, allowing a safe distance between your brain and the radiation emitted from your phone or device. Sound is delivered to your ear with almost zero emfs. I am repeating myself for a reason. Sound is delivered to your ear with almost zero emfs.

The main reason for Home-Schooling in my humble opinion is this one and that is "Protecting Your Kids" as they are literally being told to masturbate one another, as part of "comprehensive sexual education" pushed by the World Health Organization. These are not isolated cases as it is happening in schools worldwide and telling toddlers to masturbate and teaching them sexual techniques starting from age 4 is described in several World Health Organization directives for sexual education worldwide for children to watch pornography at school and then practise together, as part of their "education". Boys are encouraged to "do it" with boys, and girls with girls also the children's books are distributed in schools that tell kids how "exciting" it is to engage in sexual activities with their teachers. The goal is very clear: sexualize little children, as part of a program to make pedophilia mainstream and perverted sexuality totally devastates humanity simply because people who are addicted to pornography for example, develop social, relational, emotional and spiritual problems. Anyone reading this is horrified by how things are going in schools and now Libraries are getting in on this sickness with Moreton Bay with an international drag legend and can you understand why I vilify the local council who approved this sickness to everyone of you. I really question your morality? And in a word, you have none and shame on you Councillors. It's a sad world that kids just can't be kids and all the mental distress this can cause them and their parents and their grandparents.

Love and blessings to all the children, they are our future and they deserve to live in a World of no fear and to be nurtured and we are the examples that our unconditional love for them will shine through you only just got to believe in yourself and in them which leads us onto the next chapter.

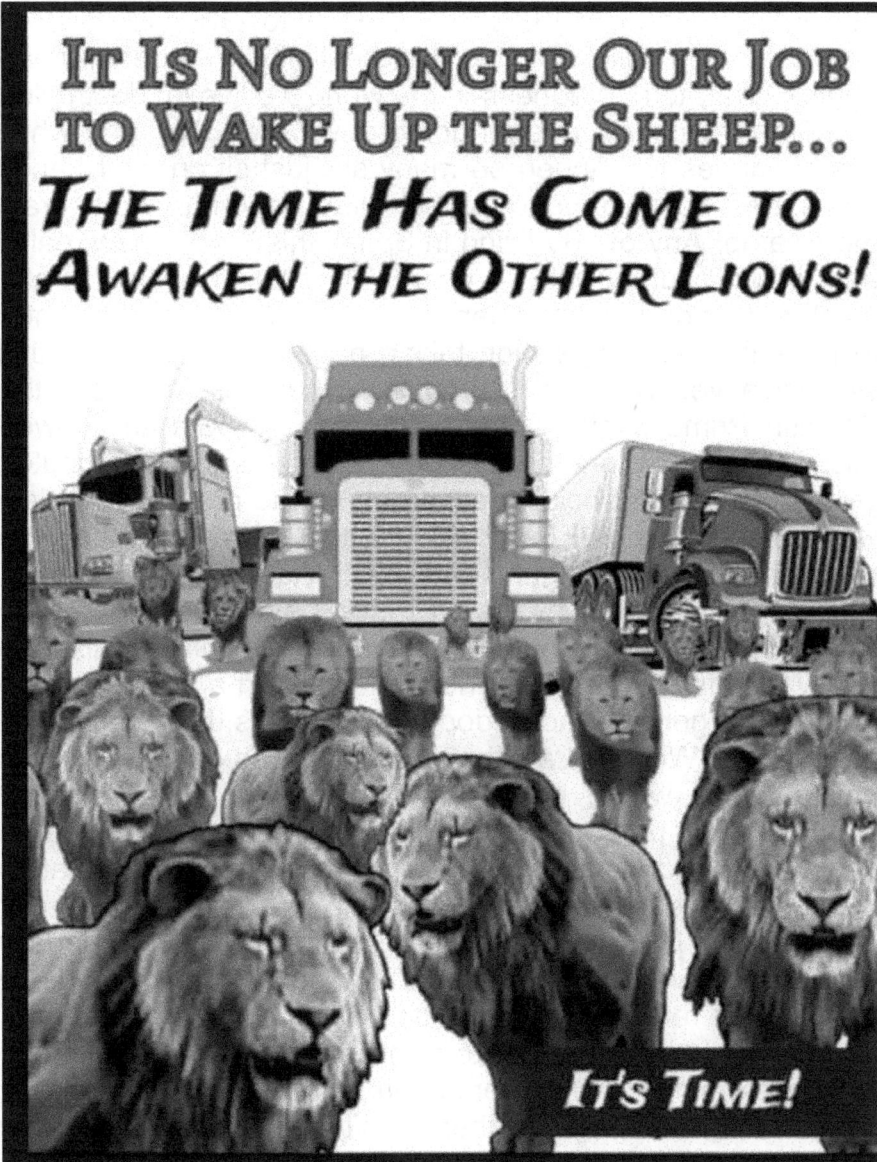

IT IS NO LONGER OUR JOB TO WAKE UP THE SHEEP... THE TIME HAS COME TO AWAKEN THE OTHER LIONS!

IT'S TIME!

Chapter 18

The Sick World They Want For All Of Us

The World Economic Forum is now calling for people to have the right to marry animals, in an effort to promote diversity and inclusion, while claiming that bestiality laws defy human rights? What total madness in the world we live in, destroying all human decency. It is all going down the toilet, and while this continues to happen so many still just sit on their hands and expect some of us to do their dirty work in trying to drain the swamp. Any of you living in Spain, this is your new reality and which country will be next? All of us in every country must fear when it will happen to us. Spain is the first country to pass this new legislation taking huge strides towards this sick initiative. This isn't surprising when you consider the Spanish Prime Minister Pedro Sánchez, is both an avowed socialist, and a World Economic Forum Agenda Contributor. Within Sanchez's socialist government, the pro-zoophilia law was pushed by WEF-affiliate Ione Belarra Urteaga, the minister of Social Rights and 2030 Agenda. That's right, Spain is so infiltrated by the WEF they have a Minister for the 2030 Agenda and any normal-thinking Spaniard, must be totally disgusted with this. The world was on a slippery slope with all the gender and pedophilia craziness, but Spain's the new Animal Welfare Law that decriminalizes having sex with animals is a whole new level of craziness. The new law states: "The person who by any means or procedure mistreats a domestic or tamed animal, an animal that is usually domesticated, an animal that temporarily or permanently lives under human control outside of legally regulated activities including acts of a sexual nature, causing injuries that require veterinary treatment to the restoration of its health, shall be subject to a minimum of three months up to a maximum of 18 months in prison." This essentially means that as long as there isn't a physical injury that requires veterinary treatment, people are free to have sex with animals. Writing about this for me is very distressing.

Most of you will have pets so you can see this is very depraved and if this isn't disturbing enough, the WEF has ordered the mainstream media to begin pushing the narrative in other countries. Make no mistake, this isn't just about Spain, they simply want to roll this sickness out across the world, and when I do my research there are sadly are lots of sites that offer free animal porn, sorry I am very open-minded, but this is just plain sick, and I will spend no more time writing about this and at least you have been made aware if you were not already I would estimate most of the unvaxxed would find this topic disturbing and for the vaxxed I would expect even though some of you seem to have lost your moral compass, this would sicken you all.

The sickness here in Australia still rolls on with more sickness, and if you ever needed more proof of the indoctrination happening in Australian schools right now and the crusade of activists to sexualise children, look no further. Be warned, it will make you feel sick, but it is necessary to show people exactly what is being taught in some Australian schools. A 53-page sexually explicit script has been recommended for Australian high school students, described as for "young people about young people" to study and participate in. The play is called Cactus, by Victorian playwright and actor Maddie Nunn, and depicts sexually explicit acts, mature themes and the sexualisation of school children. It highlights the overly sexualised agenda of the activists who have found their way into our country's education systems. Caution: reading excerpts from the play will make any parent feel sick and angry. With lines such as "I had sex with a human penis", "And Kevin fingered Eliza in the bushes", and "then one minute I had a gherkin in my mouth". The play reads more like a pornographic book than a play for school students. Yet this is what the bureaucrats in Australian education departments think is alright for your children to be studying at school in Years 10, 11, and 12 students are being subject to this filth in some schools. Think I am being too harsh? Then have a look for yourself as the play opens with a scene in the girls' bathroom at school with a character speaking about blood and sticky blood everywhere, and a girl considers taking a used pad from the bin. The description is gross, and it gets a lot worse and too graphic to be put in this book. The playwright is obviously very sick minded like the premier of Victoria's Desperate Dan, and the fair-minded people of Victoria should make Maddie (Mad) Young aware that she should be ostracised by all the decent-thinking people in that state of Victoria.

Last month, March 2023, Alex Antic wrote the following: I am often contacted by people from across Australia who are concerned about the material that children are exposed to in school. Recently I was told how a South Australian public school introduced a woke social credit system which rewarded students for "Apologising and correcting themselves or someone else for using incorrect pronouns challenging racial, sexist, or homophobic language or actions "whatever that means," and "Authentically using an Acknowledgement of Country before presentation in class." This is not education but indoctrination into leftist activism. Other parents have expressed their dismay over the sexualised LGBT agenda being forced onto children in schools, particularly through sex education programs. They have good reason to be concerned. Public schooling in South Australia appears determined to socially condition children into leftist ideology rather than teach them to master reading, writing, and arithmetic. Sadly, parents are also lamenting that many private schools are not much better and enough is enough. It's time to expose these insidious woke practices and sound the alarm so that more parents are aware of what is taking place within school walls. I am calling on South Australian parents, teachers, department of education employees, students, or anyone who encounters such practices to contact my office with concrete examples if possible. For example, you may have worksheets coaching students into progressive perspectives on sexuality or Australian history, library books about transgenderism or Critical Race Theory, examples of woke exercises that students are required to perform things such as the "acknowledgment of the country," and so on. If you are in South Australia and have access to such material and would like somebody to blow the whistle on it in the federal parliament.

Send it to me via my private campaign email address anticreport@protonmail.com and I will expose the woke indoctrination taking place in South Australian schools. By telling me first-hand about the indoctrination happening in our schools I can bring this issue to the nation's attention. I suspect that the South Australian Department of Education would prefer parents not to know the extent to which progressive ideology has captured our schools. Parents do not send their children to school to have them puberty blocking drugs, they send them to school because they want their children to be educated and well equipped for life in the real world. At this stage, this campaign relates only to South Australian schools. They may be public or private schools. Let's expose these subversive practices and build the movement of parents fighting back for their children's wellbeing and for their own rights as parents. Yours sincerely, Alex Antic, Liberal Senator for South Australia.

Thank you Alex Antic, for standing up for us and our children. We need more politicians who have a moral compass and not just puppets of the WHO, NWO and just take their very high salaries and all they leave behind is a world in a worse place because of their often sick decisions.

We all will have noticed this more and more recently and why has there been a sudden spike in drag shows for kids and drag queens in public libraries? And why are these groomers so desperate to perform for children, and people are so willing to enable them? What happened to just have a nice old lady reading books to children like we have always had? The answers to these questions are obvious, the sickness that pervades some sections of society and is being normalised to the rest of us.

I really do not care what you put in your body but protecting our children is paramount. Parents who take their young children to drag shows are indecently exposing their own kids to explicit adult content and are setting them up for gender confusion and identity crisis, and this next generation will have an even bigger explosion of mental illness, as if it wasn't bad enough already.

Body Doubles the use of body doubles has been used for a long time and there are rampant rumours circulating that the political figures you watch on TV, behind the mainstream media, aren't who they say they are. Popular speculation is that these people are wearing masks, or maybe are just body doubles. Take Kim Jong-un, who is reported to have as many as three. Past leaders who used body doubles included Joseph Stalin, Saddam Hussein and Adolf Hitler, to name a few. The use of body doubles has been used for a long time and the reptilian Queen Elizabeth is famous for having a double, as are many high-ranking American officials, and there are photos of Kim Jong-un giving instructions to his body doubles before a missile test for instance. With the evil that they are creating it would make it very obvious they are a target as they're very weak specimens, so the need for body doubles would be very obvious; and when you look at are federal leaders here in Australia during this Plandemic, Scomo and Anal could we have had weaker leaders? whose morals are very questionable. Hopefully all will be revealed in time and some of the things that I raise in this chapter that is happening in Dan Andrews state of Victoria, and what a sorry state it has been under his tyranny and for all you Victorians who voted him back in seriously? That tells us that all or most of you who had the vaccines that it really did a good job on brainwashing you all and the little brain matter you had before, the vax sure did destroy the rest. Another piece of Victorian madness: the Alfred Hospital, in Melbourne, Australia is denying a mother of two (Vicki Derderian) a heart transplant because of her vax status and she even has a valid exemption (not that she should even need that). There is no end to this and it is totally not Australian, and we are

are earning the right to be called 'Prison Australia' and we will all be their prisoners, vaxxed, and unvaxxed there will be no escaping that, if we don't act today.

Toxic Train derailments like what happened near the town of East Palestine, in the US state of Ohio, almost two weeks after the train crash with vinyl chloride, the picture of it resembled the consequences of the apocalypse. Some American media covering the man-made disaster compare the incident with the explosion of an atomic bomb, calling it the "American Chernobyl", and the consequences are called "local nuclear winter" for the whole region.

Eastern Palestine Us became an ominous place on February 3, 2023, when 50 wagons of a freight train loaded with chemicals derailed.There was a large-scale leak of vinyl chloride, which, in addition to problems with general poisoning and pollution of air, water and soil. Then in the US media, this information passed casually and the American authorities did not come up with anything better than to dispose of chemicals using "Controlled Arson", which only led to an increase in the area of contamination. A very dense cloud of combustion products still hangs over the area, visible even from a bird's eye view and the water in the rivers is contaminated within a radius of at least many kilometres, farmers in the district have begun to see cattle die, and birds are. After combustion, vinyl chloride decomposes into hydrogen chloride and phosgene, the latter was used as a chemical weapon in the First World War, when prolonged exposure to the breakdown products of vinyl chloride leads to loss of consciousness and can be fatal to humans, experts have warned. With incomplete combustion of vinyl chloride, dispersed suspensions of dioxins remain in the air, resistant to dispersion and immediately after the disaster, residents of the nearby area were evacuated, but two days later they were allowed to return. Of all the security measures, the authorities only advise to try not to leave the houses, and if signs of poisoning appear, seek medical help. Concern about the consequences of the ecological catastrophe was expressed by the people of China.Almost nothing about the incident, and most importantly, the dangerous consequences, is written by the liberal media in the United States. The fact is that the US is China's main source of food imports, and Ohio is a major producer of soybeans and corn, two of the main commodities supplied to China. Can you with critical brains see where this is going, as China's vaccines are likely to be very mild compared to the poisons of the west? Officially Beijing reassures citizens, declaring that the food-import controlled system will not allow contaminated products to enter the country. At the same time the Biden administration is practically ignoring the global environmental catastrophe in Ohio and the reasons why he is doing that are also very easy to understand and he is aware of the agenda involved in all of this.

Add another to the list April 2023 a total of three locomotive engines and six rail cars carrying lumber and electrical wiring derailed into a wooded area, where they caught fire and started a small forest fire. These toxic train crashes which are happening worldwide regularly, and I would expect a lot more, and this was predicted in the 2022 book-to-movie adaptation of "White Noise" which seemed to predict the recent train derailment in East Palestine, Ohio. The film is about an "airborne toxic event" caused by a catastrophic train accident in Ohio that emitted harmful chemicals into the air.

A lot of reports are being deleted like this Ohio Toxicology Testers Die in Freak Plane Crash Another Coincidence? Jim Crenshaw IITM: Toxic air and soil = emergency = 15 minute cities?? February 20, 2023. Black Diamond IITM: Yes, dangerous chemicals that are components of mustard gas I'm constantly at loggerheads with people who harp on, "the truth is coming out, the truth is coming out." Although that's a good thing, it's completely irrelevant, because the bigger picture has always been Agenda 2030 and these toxic events and fires at all the food factories are all part of the plan. So be very aware this is happening and it will never be on the mainstream media.

But some great news Russia has recently managed to destroy the bio-weapon facilities, and temporarily help stop the Ukrainian infants and small children that are being kidnapped and sold at the Ukraine-Poland border. "This is just a sweet shop for them at the moment," says Dean, a former British soldier who is astonished at the world of elite pedophilia he has encountered. Dean now works for MitMark, a private risk consulting firm that 'fell into' human trafficking prevention after coming near the Medyka crossing in Poland for crisis management projects. If you watch TV and buy newspapers here in Australia and only use Google, then you will be oblivious to information like this. Reports are the going rate for a baby or very young child either to be sold into sexual slavery or killed and harvested for organs is around USD $150,000. But sadly wars cause opportunities and inevitably the traffickers now see opportunities on the Ukrainian side of the border, targeting people as they enter their home country and look for ways to travel to their hometowns. Of course, people will get thrown under a bus from time to time to appease the baying mob, and that is all part of this agenda game they're playing; you know to be seen to be doing the right thing that kind of tripe they always cover up in that way, in wars they often give up some troops and some leaders to gain more time.

It is all 'Smoke & Mirrors.' US sovereignty is being handed on a plate to the unelected World Health Organisation via inter-governmental bodies. When they start talking about ironing out small details, you know all 194 nations, signatories to the WHO, have lined up to hand over all health matters to WHO and that all happened in a matter of days. This means in all future pandemics that the WHO will have complete authority, power with impunity to implement lockdowns, jab mandates, travel restrictions, basically everything. There will be no court system of due judicial process, and it's as good as done to steal all your civil liberties and freedoms and all over this scam and a lot of you fell for it a con-vid cold. If we thought EUA (emergency use authorisation) was a bad deal, wait till the next part of the agenda kicks in.

When you consider the WHO track record, the mess they've made of this pandemic you'd think the US government and all other nations would run a mile from WHO. As the world battles the coronavirus pandemic, more and more protective equipment is ending up in the sea. Globally we are using 129 billion face masks and 65 billion plastic gloves every month, according to some estimates. And divers and observers are spotting more of this discarded waste floating underwater, causing problems for wildlife and washing up on shorelines all over the world. That works out to three million masks every single minute of the day and most of these masks are plastic, single-use face coverings. The kind that has been mass produced at scale since the start of the pandemic also will have a dangerous impact on the environment, and the researchers, from the University of Southern Denmark, can't say what that is yet, because there's insufficient data. But it's unlikely to be good as single used masks are made from plastic microfibers which aren't biodegradable so when they break down, they do so into micro and nano particles which make their way into the ecosystem. Eventually, they will end up in rivers, lakes and oceans where they have an impact on marine life.

A newer and bigger concern is that the masks are directly made from microsized plastic fibres (thickness of ~1 to 10 micrometres) and when broken down in the environment, the mask may release more micro-sized plastics, easier and faster than bulk plastics like plastic bags. With increasing reports on inappropriate disposal of masks, it is urgent to recognize this potential environmental threat and prevent it from becoming the next plastic problem, the scientists have written in the scientific journals. Total madness that creates a virus that is basically a cold and that is accepted as such by most now then builds up fear so that we still have people wearing silly face nappies and then create an environmental disaster. Wait till they turn 5G up, and Marburg hits Australian shores. The money people have wasted on PCR tests is basically money thrown down the drain. The World Health Organization finally owned up to what 100,000's Doctors and

Medical professionals have been saying for months that the PCR test used to diagnose C19 is a hit-and-miss process with way too many false positives. And remember this was in 2020, but still this shite show rolled on; and how many PCR tests did you take? Also, how much money have you wasted on them? I myself have spent zero on them, and would not give them room in my home as I am a rebel, so please go away and leave me alone, 'I am a Man and I Decline.

Smart City Lockdown Madness: This is such an important topic that is going to affect all of us on planet Earth at some point, that I will go into more detail about it. So what is a smart city? A smart city is a city that uses insights from information and communication technologies, to increase operational efficiency, improve the quality of government services, and manage data assets, resources, and services efficiently. The Data that is collected is used for transportation systems, utilities, power plants, waste management, and crime detection. Smart-city technology allows cities to reduce both costs and resource consumption; they tell us that Smart cities need to collect reliable sensor data. In order to be successful and do so through various means, the smart cities will use the Internet of Things, consisting of sensors, devices, and applications that enable cities to collect data from specific areas to process for implementation, IoT sensors include water-quality sensors, image sensors, gas sensors, proximity sensors, motion-detector sensors, level sensors, and temperature sensors. An example of how these sensors work are sensors in a parking garage, or along streets that can connect to an app to show where empty parking spots are available. This reduces traffic congestion and prevents frustration or tardiness, so the value of a smart city is not necessarily dependent on how much information they have, but on what they do with it. Success also depends on its ability to form a strong relationship between the private sector and the government, as smart cities and the technology they use will become increasingly important in the future. Today approximately 55% of the world's people live in urban areas, a number expected to rise to 68% by the year 2050, according to the United Nations. With the growing urban population around the world, smart cities and their technology allow governments to monitor and improve the financial, social and environmental aspects of life for its residents and visitors, making life more enjoyable, efficient, and sustainable. Public and private companies and federal, state, and city governments are working together to make smart cities possible.

Smart cities started in Europe, with early adopters being Barcelona and Amsterdam. Following suit shortly after were Hamburg, Copenhagen, Nice, Dubai, and Singapore. In the United States, San Francisco, Atlanta, New York City, Miami, Denver, Boston, Columbus, Chicago, and Kansas City were among the first US smart cities. The IESE Business School Center for Globalization and Strategy looked at 174 cities around the world and analysed them across nine metrics: human capital, social cohesion, economy, environment, governance, urban planning, international, outreach technology, and mobility. The plans are for most including New York City, London, Paris, Tokyo, Reykjavik, Singapore, Seoul, Toronto, Hong Kong, and Amsterdam. So, if you live in any of these cities, you may want to consider moving? Including Redcliffe and Scarborough here in Queensland Australia, Your government is pushing ahead with plans to bring 15 minute cities to a location near you. They are a brainchild of the UN's Agenda 2030 and are in effect. Climate Change Lockdowns. And once that is combined with a digital ID, a carbon credit score, and a programmable central bank digital currency (CBDC) token, you've got the perfect recipe for creating a digital open-air prison and seriously you must plan for the Worst and Hope for the very best. In all wars there are casualties, and is it going to be you and your family? **It is hard trying to write a book** when the goal posts change every few days. Former UK health secretary Matt Hancock Covid-19 restrictions, a trove of leaked texts stated, to "frighten the pants off everyone" to ensure compliance with the government messages. More than 100,000 text messages were leaked to the Sunday Telegraph newspaper and among them is a purported exchange between Hancock and Cabinet Secretary Simon Case in which Case suggested in January 2021 that "fear" would be a "vital" factor in ensuring UK citizens' compliance with Covid restrictions. They also appear to show that Hancock discussed when to reveal information to the public about the discovery of a new strain of the virus in the hope of maximising the impact of lockdown rules. "Rather than doing too much forward signalling, we can roll pitch with the new strain," a purported message from Case reads. Hancock reportedly responded: "We frighten the pants off (sic) everyone with the new strain." "When do we deploy the new variant," Hancock apparently asks in a subsequent message. The alleged text message conversation, which took place on December 13, 2020, came at a time when concerns were rising about a sharp increase in Covid cases in southeast England Hancock revealed a day later, on December 14, that a new variant of Covid-19 had been identified in the country. Five days later London and southeast England entered a so-called tier 4 alert status which imposed increased Covid restrictions over the Christmas period. Hancock has responded to the leaks saying that there is "absolutely no public interest case" for the "huge breach" of text messages, which he described as a "massive betrayal". releasing them in this way gives a partial biassed account to suit an anti-lockdown agenda,".

Matt Hancock, are you for real? Do you not have a conscience? How many have died unnecessarily because of a Plan you created.that was all fear and orchestration. How many could not visit dying loved ones and might have committed suicide over the fear and their lack of hope? That all was baloney, we saw through it all, but for all you who did not, be angry and understand everything on the TV is not the truth. You will be held to account Matt WandCock.

Switch the TV off for good and join the "Great Fight." Our strength is our numbers and not joining the masses, who consider us conspiracy theorists and we are a danger to others seriously?

If the government regards me and all of us truth seekers as terrorists, then the worst is very likely to happen and the 15-minute city lockdowns are coming to New Zealand and Australia really soon. What better place than to use all of us living here as their guinea pigs because we have very high vaccination rates, and the population is very compliant and seem to want to do as they're told, and the Gallipoli and Anzac spirit is long gone.

Human Composting It is legal in these states in the USA, and this wacky world is just getting crazier. Yes, it is legal to put your loved one in the garden as long as they are dead. And with more and more people wanting to make sure their deaths are even more sustainable than their lives, you may be wondering where these practices are legal, and what states allow human composting in the U.S.A. just getting crazier. As of January 2023, human composting, aka natural organic reduction, is legal in six states in which a deceased human body is mixed with soil and plant material in a vessel for 30 days, essentially composting the body. Washington was the first U.S. state to legalise human composting back in May 2019, when Washington's Gov. Jay Inslee signed a bill making the practice legal and it went into effect on May 1, 2020. The legislative move makes New York the sixth to do so, since 2019 gives New Yorkers access to an alternative, green method of burial deemed environmentally friendly. In most cases, the deceased is placed into a reusable, semi-open vessel containing suitable bedding such as wood chips, alfalfa or straw ideal for microbes to go about their work. At the end of the process, a heaped cubic yard of nutrient-dense soil, equivalent to 36 bags of soil, is produced that can then be used as fertiliser. I have mentioned the movie **Soylent Green** before and their plan is very clear at some point. Bio Sludge supporters of this madness claim that legalising human composting will be great for the environment, as it's supposedly as close to the natural process of decomposition. But is it really a good idea to spread liquid sludge made from dead humans all over our food crops? Because that's exactly where much of it will go, especially when "liquid cremation" ends up being flushed down the drain or toilet and into the local sewer system. If America now begins "recycling" human beings as liquid rather than simply burying bodies or cremating them into ash, as has traditionally been the case, then these remains will almost certainly end up being converted into recycled "biosludge" and spread as "fertiliser" on food crops. It's true that traditional burial protocols aren't necessarily environmentally friendly, seeing as how the embalming fluids and formaldehyde are made from toxic, synthetic chemicals. Releasing mercury, pharmaceuticals, and disease into the water supply does sound like a great idea, what could possibly go wrong?

Think of all the additional drugs and vaccines that we give our bodies that will be in the compost. The reality of this nightmare for those experiencing this are the flies and health problems that now plague Leslie Stewart materialised as soon as her neighbour started spreading sewage sludge as fertiliser across 216 his 160-acre farm several years ago. Flies consistently swarm the 5-acre farm where she has raised goats for 18 years. Within weeks, the goats started getting sick. Stewart said then soon after, 12 of the 36 died she blamed the flies crawling on the goats feed, and the pests also began entering her home however they could through tiny cracks in the building, through her stove vent. The sewage sludge stench "knocks me to the floor, and I feel like a prisoner in my own home," said Stewart, 53, who receives disability payments and was already on oxygen from existing health problems when the stench arrived and moving would be prohibitively expensive, she added. "A lot of elderly and disabled people are in the same boat," Stewart said. "There's no way we can afford to move so we're stuck." Stewart is just one of a number of rural Oklahomans who say sludge spread as fertiliser is putting their health at risk, destroying their quality of life, and contaminating drinking water, livestock, and crops with toxic PFAS and other dangerous chemicals. Sludge is what's left over when water is separated from human and industrial waste, sent into the nation's sewer system is also called bio-solids, it is a semi-solid, toxic mix of human and industrial waste that's also rich in nutrients like nitrogen. In recent decades, wastewater treatment plants have given it away to farmers for no cost as a cheap alternative to fertiliser. So, **What Is Agenda 2030** there is no excuses for me repeating myself and well, it is many things and it's already started and its well under way so now you read this you will understand there is going to be no let up, and looking at all the agenda they have planned for you in the Agenda 2030, will they succeed? I sadly strongly believe they go very close and that thought process terrifies me. They hold so many high cards now, but I believe they have underestimated the 10-15% resolve and our strength and our resolve will go a long way to putting a spanner in their works. Any of you reading this could make the final difference when this is all over, so stand up with us, and fight side by side to beat this insipid evil that seems to pervade everything at the moment. This is a very good summary of Agenda 2030 and all the aims they have carefully planned for every one of us reading this, and if that does not alarm you then nothing truly will. You will recognize that some of the agendas are now underway. This is their plan which in 2015 the United Nations adopted the 2030 Agenda for Sustainable Development and a multilateral agreement between all UN Member States that lays out a road map to a more sustainable future. At its heart is a series of goals of the 17 SDG ranging from eradicating poverty and hunger to protecting life in the oceans. It has morphed from the original plan which was called Agenda 21 which released hunger to protect life in the oceans which was released by the UN with a primary focus solely on environmental issues. This new agenda now addresses virtually all areas of human activity and is truly a blueprint for global governance and at first glance, this agenda appears to be combating every serious problem on the global stage. That amazing investigative journalist Whitney Webb reveals the inner workings of the World Economic Forum ("WEF"),and the driving force behind The Great Reset.

WEF's Board of Trustees is packed with powerful and prominent representatives from government and multinational corporations like BlackRock, Salesforce and Nestlé. WEF supports the "Merging of Man and Machine," or Transhumanism, and the Fourth Industrial Revolution, which aims to use wearable and implantable technology to snoop on your thoughts and launch a digital dictatorship. Once it is implemented, a digital dictatorship will be almost impossible to escape from and the one way to stop it is To Not Comply with or utilise these technologies.

CWEF co-founder and chairman and when digging deeply into Schwab and his family history, it is very revealing that Schwab's father, Eugen Schwab, ran the Ravensburg branch of a company called Escher Wyss during WWII, when producing "different components needed by the Nazi war machine and the Nazi atomic bomb program."Vedmore Revealed that three of Schwab's mentors, John K. Galbraith, a Canadian-American economist and diplomat and public policy maker, Herman Kahn, who created concepts on nuclear deterrence that became official military policy, and Henry A. Kissinger, who recruited Schwab at a Harvard international Schwab through a CIA-funded program, and they were the real driving force behind the creation of the World Economic Forum. Early WEF affiliations can also be tied back to the Club of Rome and one of Schwab's top advisers, transhumanist Yuval Noah Harari, PhD, who openly admits data might enable globalists to do more than "just build digital dictatorships."Via technology in the form of wearables and implants like brain chips and the idea is to one day spy on your very thoughts. "Humans are now Hackable Animals," Harari said. But Humans also have this Soul or Spirit, and they have Free Will, and nobody knows what's happening inside me, so whatever I choose, whether in an election or whether in the supermarket, this is my free will that's over once they chip you. **Remote Neural Monitoring:** many of these things will be built directly into our bodies." So, let's look at just one of the ways they will spy on your thoughts using how many times you have had thoughts that you never wanted to share with anyone and they could be very personal and very intimate and have been constantly worried at the thought of someone ever finding out about these thoughts. Spiritual People through "Light Language" can do this with animals and people there close to as many people know that Light Language or channelling energy in the form of sound is directly related to star seed origins. That's because Light Language is still considered quite a strange, mystical modality and largely misunderstood and godly .But this is a totally different kind of evil that is walking planet earth at the moment and has so many different agendas. All of us should see through this process, that the new and improved technologies being developed around the world, supposedly to deal with crime and terrorism, inadvertently intrude on one's privacy, and should probably bring us all to the brink of paranoia.

These technologies are funded by governments at the highest level and some of the countries involved include the USA, UK, Spain, Germany and France and recently, the infamous National Security Agency (NSA) of the U.S.A. has developed a very efficient method of controlling the human brain. So let's look at this technology called Remote Neural Monitoring and it is expected to revolutionise crime detection and investigation, as R.N.M. works remotely. Have you ever wondered why we all have been driven relentlessly towards wireless systems? To control the brain under the objective to detect any criminal thought taking place inside the mind of a possible culprit. So, the inevitable questions: How can you isolate a criminal thought if you do not have a comparative measure of non-criminal thoughts? The underlying technology of this system takes under consideration that the electrical activity in the speech centre of the brain, can be translated into the subject's verbal thoughts. R.N.M, and can send encrypted signals to the auditory cortex of the brain directly circumventing the ear and this encoding assists in detecting audio communication, also it can also perform electrical mapping of the cerebrum's activity from the visual centre, which is achieved by avoiding the eyes and optic nerves, consequently projecting images from the subject's mind onto a video display. So with this visual and auditory memory, both can be visualised and analysed, and a Microchip implant of any type all leads to remote neural monitoring. So, how do we block remote neural monitoring? There are certain observations that have been made about these signals, as they tend to be beamed through the window of a room, where one spends most of their time. Usually the window facing the front street. They are specifically directed to target and track a person inside their home. This new agenda now addresses virtually all areas of human activity and is truly a blueprint for global governance and at first glance, this agenda appears to be combating every serious problem on the global stage. You will notice how I seem paranoid with 5G, Wi-Fi, Smart Anything as they are all part of this Agenda and we all need to look for ways to reduce them, or completely dump them.

HAARP may play a part in this as well as a targeted person is tracked, either via some signature characterised by the resonant characteristics of their skull or DNA, or by tracking signals emitted by implants put into them during abductions, or perhaps by more sophisticated methods like vaccines. Computers perform the calculations necessary to alter the signal of each of three cell phone towers so as to triangulate a hot spot of signal at the target's location so when the target moves, new calculations have to be made, which takes several seconds. These signals consist of microwave carriers with ELF modulation and audio encoded messages and the microwaves which resonate with DNA, can penetrate flesh and bone, pass through some walls and windows, and are already in use in your cell phones and why the cell phone is a tool satanic people will use as they understand you addiction to always look at answer messages instantly the need of adulation of a like to a post. Now, let's once again, get back to our food chain, as it relates to Agenda 30 and this has never been more important, especially if you're buying from the big food chains, because insects in our food or edible insects and insect species used for human consumption are not as safe as you may believe. More than 2,000 insect species worldwide are considered edible, and can you really believe that, and how many are not safe. I have lived in Asia and in many countries like Thailand, Indonesia, Mexico, India, Japan and Cambodia and they have eaten insects for a long time, and I never ever tried them but we are not talking about these insects.

But ones created in factories in Vietnam, Canada and anything the EMF have planned and this part of Agenda 2030. I spoke to some of the vaccinated and they go "Yum, it's Protein" because they are programmed and after 3 vaccinations their natural immunity is already at zero this might be the final death knell for them. Yet, Big Pharma uses deadly venoms and venom peptides to make prescription medications, and those medications carry a list of very insane side effects and It is no wonder if you start eating insects regularly, because you believe this will save the earth from global warming or "climate change," you may be putting yourself and your children directly in harm's way, adding to the 'Evil Agenda' of globalists who want to depopulate this planet.

That's why the elite 1% of the 1% are genocidal maniacs, saying everyone should stop eating meat and start munching on insects all day long and Amazon is now promoting and selling crickets in many forms, for human consumption, including freeze dried and powder form. So, as I tend to I repeat myself and for very good reason we are also being primed to eat insects here in Sunny Queensland, Australia. Where we have a high abundance of foods and vegetables, and fish and meat, of the highest quality and comparing a T-bone steak or a vegetable vegan salad and then be expected to eat a bowl of insects instead, does that simply not tell you something is very wrong and there is an incredibly sinister reason for preparing all the vaccinated to do as they tell them and some will but we will say, Hell No.

The Air That We Breathe I will end this chapter with one of the biggest challenges and threats that we are facing today, and that is the air that we breathe. I have already talked about the weather, and how it's being bio-engineered (chemtrails) etc. So, when I went for a bike ride today my face looked fine, but when I got home it was heavily inflamed, and itchy and I am used to my eyes being irritated and running, but this is a new first, so what chemicals were they using today on the 7th March 2023, to cause that and how does one retain some semblance of health while existing in a world that has become alarmingly toxic and incompatible to life as a whole? If you suffer from facial toxins like I did today then Black Seed Oil works wonders and will do the job and I look very beautiful again very quickly. Though there are countless sources of contamination, the climate engineering fallout is the most pervasive of all and they are secretly filling the sky without out are knowledge or consent, with billions of megatons of aluminium, strontium 90, barium and "chaff" to reflect the sun's dangerous rays back into space is epic, and brilliantly manoeuvred on the unsuspecting public by dubbing them as "persistent contrails."

However, what goes up, obviously must come down, and we are being bombarded daily with a chemical and radioactive fallout maybe having been surpassed only by Agent Orange, the defoliating chemicals developed by Monsanto to wipe out the jungles during the Vietnam War. Yes, it is that serious and you would be blind not to see, feel it, and smell it and are you sneezing more than usual, do your eyes run? Well, look up at the sky, there is your culprit. We have just come out of summer here in tropical Queensland, Australia and have you ever witnessed a summer like it? There is another clue and how is the mould going in your house? Since aluminium has an affinity for water, all life forms attract these oxides and this causes contamination of even organic fruits, vegetables, and livestock if they're exposed to the open air, because plants readily absorb aluminium salts from the soil into their vascular systems.

Everything absorbs aluminium salts and it's in the air so the reality is, this "toxic cloud shield" created by aerosolizing the atmosphere, diminishes rainfall, traps the heat and increased humidity so this leads to a plague of pests, mildews, moulds, fungi, diseases, and ultimately the shredding of our precious ozone layer, that protects us from dangerous UV rays, according to Dane Wigington, a solar expert. In California's Mount Shasta region, Francis Mangel, a USDA Wildlife Biologist and water specialist has reported elevated levels of aluminium, barium, and strontium in the mountain's snow, polluting drinking water, rivers and soil in the area, so is it any different here in Qld or where you are living? It's one planet and one big Agenda. In 2008, samples around California's Lake Shasta and the Pit River Arm tributary were tested in a State Certified Lab following weeks of fly-overs and chemtrails and the results of the water samples showed 4,610 parts per million of aluminium and that is 4,610 times the maximum contaminant level in aluminium toxicity levels which were off the charts, chemtrails are putting our life systems at risk of irreparable damage.

As mentioned earlier, aluminium laden "chaff" falling from the sky enters the lungs, causing upper respiratory diseases, lung cancer, breast cancer, and is the gateway to vulnerable areas of the body including arterial walls, where it accumulates like a plaque and in addition aluminium toxicity generates a number of neurological disorders and brain cancer, while radium and zinc cadmium sulphide synergistically can cause bone cancer. You can see Turbo Cancer on a lot of our lips and cannot see when you "Join The Dots" the link. Which demonstrates that exposure to aluminium can increase migratory and invasive properties of breast cancer cells, and moreover these metallo-estrogens, chemical toxins, and bioengineered cocktails are causing multiple problems in the gastrointestinal and immune systems, which is the first line of defence against disease and destroying human health and cognitive abilities. Plus, by shredding the ozone layer allows damaging UV rays to enter the atmosphere resulting in an unprecedented increase in skin cancer cases, to name just a few harmful effects of chemtrails. People in South America have also noticed it with unusually cold summers, trees dying and fungi infested, deformed vegetables just like the reports are describing and a dramatic increase of cancer and unusual terminal illnesses are rampant. So, join the club as none of us are immune from this evil created for very obvious reasons, as there is a growing concern that the Earth will soon become unfit for organic food, and pure water sources have said because of the unrestricted spraying without our consent. It appears that "control of the masses' has taken on a whole new meaning and what a doom and gloom chapter this is but very necessary and even me on my high vibration it could put me on a downer, but not for very long.

So, you can see the importance of detoxing not only your body but all the foods that you eat that might be contaminated as it's not hard to wash them with Bentonite Clay or Zeolite. I personally never felt healthier so my detoxes are working for me but never rest on one's laurels. You will notice that I talk a lot about vibration and energy and keeping it high, and surrounding yourself with like-minded people on a similar vibration is so very important and I personally have never been more excited to be alive, a bit like living in the days of the pioneers. But like most of you, we might have to take responsibility for how we might have spoiled our children and doing that has done them no favours in this world we are currently living in. But as they say no crying over spilt milk, all the generations in the first World war 1914-18, second world war 1939-45, Vietnam, Korea, Iraq, Afghanistan etc and we are living in the Worlds biggest war. This the time to fight or are you going to continue to sit on your hands and let someone do it for you, but we were born for this battle, and I understand the bravery of my friends.

Chapter 19

The Reality of Zombism

For me when I lived in Amsterdam it was very common to witness "The Walking Dead" who were brain damaged by drugs and it was very sad to see. Currently the vaccine damage and linked to the addiction of most having to have a mobile phone addictively near their ears constantly combined with 5G the mark of the beast Graphene Oxide as and will combine to cause an epidemic of zombies which will be termed (The Walking Dead) and anyone reading this it could be you as your brain is not meant to microwaved consistently day after day killing your brain cells. Understanding Zombism is very complex and some of you will have watched the movies which are very confronting and broadly speaking, zombies can be either slow zombies (think of the original "Dawn of the Dead"). Slow zombies tend to shuffle in an uncoordinated manner and can't open doors, suggesting a problem with the cerebellum. This is the region at the back of the head, known as the "little brain," and if you took this vaccine to go to a pub for instance it would be a fair description of you and it plays a very important role in coordinated movements. Tasks such as picking up coins on the ground are actually really hard for them as all zombies and fast ones included seem to have poor memory and lack the ability to plan as a group, they don't have any social skills. They also lack cognitive control and there's no delaying the gratification of warm human flesh and these symptoms suggest their frontal lobes probably aren't functioning correctly, in animal studies, Then of course there's the matter of zombie communication, or lack thereof and zombies will be described with a condition called Wernicke's aphasia, which results from these symptoms suggesting their frontal lobes probably aren't functioning correctly. I would prefer not to write a chapter as confronting as this but having seen this human behaviour currently on a daily basis there is room for thought and awareness is paramount because if this 5G pandemic is not stopped then the reality of this will affect all of us and that is a very scary reality. Zombie brain function established is that in order for the human brain to drive the body, significant portions of the brain stem must be functioning as a zombie. We now turn our attention to the frontal lobe to determine what functions that section of the brain and if any are really needed to sustain the zombie and they are often described as acting drunk, or lobotomized, theories have been put forth that the Frontal Lobes may be out of service in the undead. So, what are the characteristics of a zombie? It's common among the unvaccinated to comment "there goes another zombie" but it is way beyond a joke and incredibly sad to witness.

The zombies have absolutely no emotion at all and examples would be no more morality, empathy, or remorse, also more anger, lack of happiness, excitement, sadness, or fear and they also don't have a very good memory function anymore. The reason for this chapter to make you aware once you cook your brain there is no coming back from that and if you memory is not like it was and your reactions are slow and you find tasks you done all your life difficult in your work and home settings then maybe there is an underlying cause and as mentioned so many times in this book already. Mobile smartphones, **zombie tampon earbuds** and anything linked to Wi-Fi will be your nemesis. This pandemic is so very well orchestrated on so many levels including that the CDC also released a short graphic novel about a "highly mutated form of the flu," that is highly transmissible and turns people into a zombie. The novel depicts a couple and their dog implementing the CDC's recommended safety tips, however the spread of this disease was so severe that early attempts to establish quarantine zones were not working. Scientists at the CDC began warp-speeding like they warp-speeded this poison, of a modified flu vaccine with the isolated virus and if there is some "zombie" outbreak, it will not be because of some new infection that popped out of nowhere.

Yet again are you "Joining The Dots". But there is also the danger of blood transfusions which is immense even the Red Cross has publicly announced that vaccinated individuals are prohibited from donating blood for certain plasma applications because, "the vaccine wipes out those antibodies. If you receive any type of Covid vaccine, you are not eligible to donate convalescent plasma with the Red Cross and one of the Red Cross requirements for plasma from routine blood and platelet donations that test positive for high-levels of antibodies to be used as convalescent plasma is that it must be from a donor that has not received a Covid-19 vaccine. This is to ensure that antibodies collected from donors have sufficient antibodies directly related to their immune response to a Covid-19 infection and not just the vaccine, as antibodies from an infection and antibodies from a vaccine are not the same. It looks like people who receive spike protein injections actually have contaminated blood that poses a very real health threat to others, so even if the vaccines did work and produce antibodies, those antibodies can then attack your healthy cells. This will explain why some people who have taken the deadly vaccines are having their brains eaten alive by their own bodies, turning them into real-life vaccine addictive zombies.

Presuming that some of the vaccinated turn into "zombies," what would be the specific cause? I suspect it would come via the handlers cranking up the 5G EMFs very high, causing the masses' bodies to go haywire and I mention 5G because it has been proven in different reports that the ingredients necessary for 5G communication are in these "vaccines", and so turning up radiation on the 5G towers, I think it would be enough to really lay waste to a lot of people quickly, and making them clearly very docile and stupid, well if your lining up for Jab 5 you might have lack of normal thought processes. For those of you who are religious we are now entering a time period the Bible in Matthew 24 calls the 'Beginning of Sorrows'. Soon after that the '7-Year Tribulation' starts and ends with the Second Coming of Christ.

At the same time many end times prophesied events will happen including the Vaccine Zombie Apocalypse where we see many vaccinated individuals will turn into zombies or as the bible calls them in Revelation 6:8 'Beasts of the Earth'. Will I be correct in my assumption, sadly yes and they will start to appear and rise right from our midst, even our own friends, our families, our relatives, our neighbours, our workmates and people we know, etc. Satan and his plans are a warning to all to prepare spiritually, physically, mentally and psychologically as we are now heading towards an unprecedented very difficult and challenging time. The bible says in John 10:10, 'the devil cometh not, but for to steal, and to kill, and to destroy.

The devil's plan is to steal humanity's salvation through Jesus Christ, kill off their physical body and destroy their soul through eternal torment in hell and those who don't die off quickly from those who don't die off quickly from these death shots will eventually be turned into vaccine zombies once they switch-on the 5G mobile phone and 5G satellite networks unless they repent quickly beforehand. The word Virus means Poison or Venom. So, the words CoronaVirus can literally mean "King Cobra Venom". The devil is so cunning he has hidden the real meaning of this Covid-19 virus in plain sight right in front of our face, staring at us all this time. King Cobras are the largest venomous snakes in the world.and they almost exclusively feed on other snakes both venomous and non-venomous. The 19 in the word 'Covid-19' refers to the 19 distinct proteins/peptides that are in the King Cobra Venom that target specific organs in the human body and it does not refer to the year 2019 when the virus was first released. With the mRNA DNA changing technology in the vaccines, it is highly possible that they have integrated snake venom protein peptides reptilian DNA with the people's own DNA and changed them forever into "serpentine-reptilian--human hybrids" and other words, in one big fell swoop the devil and his minions have managed to beguile, pressured, tricked and deceive up to 67.9% of the world's population to take their fake "Covid-19 pandemic"

215

vaccines that have changed people's DNA causing the vaccinated to literally become 'lizard-people' ruled by King Charles the lizard king, 'snake people', 'the Seed of the Serpent' (see Genesis 3:15), the 'Children of the Devil' (see John 8:44, Matthew 13:38). Can you not see the logics that this is the reason why some vaccinated individuals are exhibiting reptilian characteristics such as continuously shedding spike proteins 24/7 non-stop, striking out against the unvaccinated, being violent and aggressive, much like zombies which I tend to notice a lot due to my level of happiness. One of the devil's end of times goals is to create a hybrid race of people made in his image and not in the image of God as mentioned in Genesis 1:26.

Don't be surprised then if you start to see vaccinated people with serpentine-reptilian slit eyes. I often mention spiritual and religious and you can be all things to God and we should not judge each other as some reading this will judge me and I do not truly care but we all have to be one to beat the common foe that is Satan. The VAERS Reporting System is recording a sudden increase in prion-like disease. Prion disease is also known as Creutzfeldt Jakob Disease (CJD) and very much similar to Mad Cow Disease. Inbuilt into the spike protein that is in both the mRNA and non-mRNA vaccines is a prion-like region. Normally, nothing goes wrong after vaccination but however, for some vaccinated individuals, the protein synthesis goes all wrong, the prions in the brain become diseased and misfolded and start to spread to other prions and this leads to brain tissue deterioration and death. This chapter is to make you all reading this very aware that these all can happen to you. But if you are a phone addict, or wear earbuds connected to Wi-Fi then the levels of Graphene Oxide the cumulative damage will at some point affect your critical thinking and ultimately your brain and the term brain dead, walking dead might be applied to you and the Chief Executive Officer of Nokia, Pekka Lundmark, has disclosed smart gadgets will be implanted into human bodies in the next eight years, as technological innovation will evolve into the sixth generation (6G) network and they are very open with their 2030 agenda and the new world they want for you and you can't all dump your phones like me. I really love not to be bothered day and night and I am glad I did and wish I had dumped my phone a lot sooner. Dependence on anything, especially these control devices, is not good for you. The Vaccine for Coronavirus makes you a 'Biological Robot.' and do you think that hydrogel does 'NOT alter your DNA'? Someday, it is going to replace the DNA for anyone, allowing hydrogel to enter their body and your body becomes a mechanical slave as DARPA hydrogels deliver lithium to destroy the 'Pineal Gland' the (Spiritual Connection To GOD). This is also implanted by the Test Swabs and that is why it is shoved way up the Blood-Brain Barrier and I have met people where they shoved the swabs so far up their noses, they have permanent "migraines". Your pineal gland's main job is to help control the circadian cycle of sleep and wakefulness by secreting melatonin. But just how toxic is Lithium? We can tolerate much more lithium in the body than we can in the brain, and this is extremely interesting if not damning, when we consider how those very creepy "way up in your nose" PCR swabs seem to get as near to your brain as they possibly can? I mean, you can see their 'Agenda'. Why did they not initially just swab your mouth like they do for DNA testing? Does it not make sense, however, for efficient Lithium delivery by placing it where it will do the most damage? And here's a very sad fact: that Lithium overdose symptoms also match the shakes and convulsions seen in many vaccinated? The pineal gland was described as the "Seat of the Soul" by René Descartes (French 17th Century philosopher) and it is located in the centre of the brain as the main function of the pineal gland is to receive information about the state of the light-dark cycle from the environment and convey this information to produce and secrete the hormone melatonin, which is giving humans senses and sensibilities and reducing or eliminating these unique capacities, makes us humans vulnerable to "robotization". You might start to see very bright street lights in your towns and cities because they will do anything they can and whatever it takes to reach their goal.

So be very aware and live every day to the maximum having faith that with God we can conquer all. So I will end this chapter be very aware of everyone around you and the levels of there thinking because anything we might discuss and term "Normal" they will go on the attack when they don't agree with you and they can be very vicious Zombism is alive and well here in Australia and it is going to get so very much worse and I have warned you keep your loved ones safe.

READ THE MIDDLE PARAGRAPH

ALIEN STAR

THE NEW WORLD ORDER

by A. Ralph Epperson

changes have in store for them. In summary, then, these changes are:

The old world is coming to an end. It will be replaced with a new way of doing things.

The new world will be called the "New World Order."

This new structuring will re-distribute property from the "have" nations and will give it to the poor nations.

The New World Order will include changes in:

the family:
homosexual marriages will be legalized; parents will not be allowed to raise their children (the state will;) all women will be employed by the state and not allowed to be "homemakers"; divorce will become exceedingly easy and monogynous marriage will be slowly phased out;

the workplace:
the government will become the owner of all of the factors of production; the private ownership of property will be outlawed;

religion:
religion will be outlawed and believers will be either eliminated or imprisoned; there will be a new religion: the worship of man and his mind; all will believe in the new religion;

The United States will play a major role in bringing it to world.

World wars have been fought to further its aims. Adolf Hitler, the NAZI Socialist, supported the goal of the

The majority of the people will not readily accept "the world order" but will be deceived into accepting it by two

THIS WAS WRITTEN IN 1989

Chapter 18

Russia Is The World's Last Hope

We are all witnessing the tragedy that is happening in the Ukraine but how many people truly understand the real role Russia is playing in trying to end this madness that the world is currently going through. Australia to date has sent $900 million to that mad puppet clown Zelenko and the USA, as been instrumental in all wars in the last 50 years and the reasons those wars are created are often not what it is portrayed to be. Anthony Albanese the Labour leader here in Australia has a massive debt left over by the previous Liberal Government and even with the homelessness and terrible problems that have been created by so many here including the Governor of the RBA Philip Lowe who has gotten so many in debt today with there will be no interest rate rises until 2024, well here we are March 2023, and we have had 10 rates rises on the trot. So getting that so very wrong as to have been a plan and there all in on it "You will own nothing and be Happy" well they will have got that correct, because this insanity is not stopping any day soon. But this great news has just happened with Russian President Vladimir Putin having ordered the destruction of all Covid-19 vaccine stockpiles on Russian soil, citing an undeniable connection between what has been dubbed the "Moscow Vax" and a sudden surge of HIV infections in vaccinated persons, FSB agent Andrei Zakharov told Real Raw News. Although Putin has not made a formal announcement, he has tasked his right-hand man, Defense Minister Sergei Shoigu, with purging hospitals, clinics, and pharmacies of the Sputnik and Cov iVac vaccine variants. The military will ensure compliance by auditing vaccine repositories and performing spot inspections. Like President Trump, Putin was deceived by a lie and a global consortium of devious doctors, health professionals and government stooges spun a convincing yarn about a virus that would ravage the world unless vaccines were developed to inoculate the population as soon as possible. inoculate the population as soon as possible. The WHO had infiltrated the Russian Ministry of Health and planted agents of evil within the Council of Ministers, and State Duma, and Western propaganda with fables of people sick with Covid falling dead on the street that had seeped through Russia's once secure borders. No nation was immune to the most elaborate disinformation campaign in the history of humanity so on 2 December 2020, Russia launched its first mass vaccination experiment, beating other nations to the punch and delivering 6.9 million doses in the first week and as of 21 June 2022, 81.5 million people have received at least one dose, with 74.3 million fully vaccinated. In the West and Russia, vaccine recipients presented with side effects such as cardiac ailments, seizures, and blood clots, with many dropping dead at home or at work and in some in the streets.

The American CIA is brilliant at this and when harmless Covid spread, they made up stories of so many people dying to get us all to beg for the vaccine so when the vaccines came, we did start dying, and the governments can blame it on Covid and of course not the vaccines. It was such a clever plot, the world believed it," Zakharov said and in December 2022, the Ministry of Health reported a dramatic, countrywide spike in HIV infections among persons who had received three or more C19 vaccinations and did not fit the standard demographic homosexuals or the needle users. Between 2015-2019, Russia averaged 16,000 new infections per year but in 2022, that figure skyrocketed to 63,000 to include surprisingly celibate, non-drug users. Vladimir Putin, Zakharov said, arrived at the inescapable conclusion that vaccines could cause a person to develop HIV and AIDS, that evidence was unassailable and the more jabs a person got, the greater the odds of contracting HIV. Putin viewed the correlation as more than a simple coincidence; the vaccine was tailored to deliver Acquired Immune Deficiency Syndrome. "A fake sickness tricks people into getting a vaccine that gives them real sicknesses," Zakharov said. "Only satanic people could have dreamed this up.

For President Putin, this is a very personal affair." Putin, he added, has remained a "Pureblood," but one of his daughters was diagnosed with HIV two weeks after she'd taken her third jab. President Putin told her not to get any more vaccines, but she is Westernised so she accepted their lies, and now she must stay on medicine her whole life. This has really infuriated President Putin," Zakharov said and his daughter's diagnosis was the very last straw. So, Putin decreed that Covid-19 vaccines be destroyed, and he banned all vaccine imports and the Russian military, our source said, has already destroyed vaccines at hospitals in Moscow, Saint Petersburg, Kazan, Chelyabinsk, Samara, Nizhny Novgorod, and Saratov, and was forced to "Put Down" hospital staff that resisted the vaccine purge and can you see how brainwashed some the vaccinated are they would risk losing their lives over protecting something like the vaccines that is unquestionably responsible for the death some of their patients and so much for the Hippocratic oath do no harm.

If you vaxxed in the west, you watch your TV and believe in the lies you're fed and we who do not watch TV will believe what logically could and should be true. Putin has reportedly said he will not rest until every vial is shattered also and Putin has also ordered the execution of 130 scientists responsible for creating the Sputnik vaccines which wonderful news maybe the rest of the paid scientists World Wide should also take note that no person is above pure evil. "Here we don't bring the guilty to trial, it's a waste of time so would we waste time when we know they are guilty so we deal with these matters severely," Zakharov said and in closing, we asked Zakharov whether Putin would have ordered such drastic action had his daughter not been diagnosed with HIV. Is this true in a perfect world yes and who would want to murder their own people you guess? Many people do not understand the difference between viral vector vaccines and mrna injections, therefore would not understand why Russian President Vladimir Putin would never risk injecting his military with the mRNA jabs but is not afraid to use the viral vector option. This article aims to simplify the explanation of the difference, and thus make sense of why the Biden Regime and here in Australia and other western countries they do not mind putting their own entire military forces at high risk of myocarditis, rubbery blood clots and central nervous system disorders by force-injecting nearly all of them with deadly messenger-RNA (mRNA) COVID jabs. Sputnik V is a gene therapy injection that contains 2 adenovirus vectors (rAd26 and rAd5), that are genetically manipulated to resemble the SARS-CoV-2 spike protein. These attempt to enter human cells so they can recreate the spike proteins, supposedly helping the cells create antibodies to fight COVID. In other words, Sputnik uses inactivated viruses called vectors to elicit an immune system response, like the Janssen/Johnson & Johnson jabs and the ones made by AstraZeneca.

These are also known as "Spike Protein Payload Injections." and this is very dangerous to the human body, but not even close to inflicting the kind of health detriment of mRNA "technology." The war in the Ukraine and we all see that it is mostly the vaccinated who proudly show the Ukraine flag on their facebook profiles and are in such universal acceptance of this war by Americans, Australians and the British just to name a few and most of them have embraced the Ukraine because they've been lied to constantly about Russia and its current leader, President Vladimir Putin. It's "what you would call the theatre of the absolute ridiculous," that is seen in cities "all across L.A." where there are Ukrainian flags flying. When in our lifetimes did anybody ever see the cheering that is going on with any kind of war? That really is BS just gone totally mad and shows how so many are zombified and they are the ones who comply with this rubbish. There has to be a common link that vaccinated people are so easily led and ready and able to be deceived. The USA has so much to answer for in response to recent conflicts as events unfolding in the Ukraine, I could not help being reminded of the ten-year Vietnam War (1964-1975), and the war in Iraq (2003-2011).

Both were also based on lies with the Vietnam War seeing over 360,000 Americans killed or wounded, while, in Iraq, the total exceeded 36,000. In the Asian war, the premise was an attack on an American naval vessel that did not occur. The war in the Middle East was the threat of the non-existent weapons of mass destruction, so here we go again with the Biden Administration and the western leaders that have allied themselves with legitimate Nazis, who commit these war crimes without hesitation. In the Ukraine, a war has been started to distract from problems at home the USA, to cover up money laundering of some of the politicians, but the main reason is a distraction of the Covid pandemic, and why are people so in acceptance of the lies and even some of my own family members have swallowed that Putin is evil and my own mother in the UK often reminds me he is like Hitler.

So misinformation is rife, which is (the Biden Administration's favourite word) and has been on display in the Ukraine since the Obama administration supported the 2014 coup against the Viktor Yanukovych government, which was considered pro-Russian. In fact, there has been a large ethnic Russian presence in eastern Ukraine since Catherine the Great of Russia who came to power in 1762. Officially, we were told that the Yanukovych government being overthrown was a revolution of the people. However, one can't help but notice that Victoria Nuland of the Obama administration was in Ukraine at the time of the coup helping the people. The Ukraine conflict has created an information division in the world internet and because they are unwilling to field troops to confront the Russian forces physically and it probably would give Biden a bloody nose so the West engages in a war of sanctions to disconnect Moscow from the rest of the world. In March, 2022 internet technology giants Facebook, Google, Twitter, and Apple joined in removing many, if not all, products from Russia, but the reality and the truth is that whether you like Putin or don't like him, and he's a good guy or he's a bad guy, Putin is not willing to be part of whatever global government structure that is coming our way,".

He is actually the one man who is standing between us and the people who want to see a New World Order. Putin has been calculating and very careful ahead of his invasion of Ukraine, so much so that the Russian leader has said for 15 years "he would not tolerate NATO expansion." He has also made it very clear he is not part of whatever they've got right now in the Bioweapons labs that Hunter Biden's and partners and firms are connected to. "They want to say that we're conspiracy theorists but at the World Economic Forum, they can talk about " a new world order, and likewise for other globalist constructs like a world minimum wage, global vaccine passport, and so on.

The Western leaders have totally ignored that since Ukrainian President Volodymyr Zelenskyy came to power, and such as "Mass Graves" in the country's east, in places like Odessa and in the Donbas region, where the Ukrainian military and militias have allegedly carried out killings when people there "Voted to Secede" and either became independent or moved closer to Russia. How many of you reading this vaccinated or not really understand and want to understand that is really the truth behind this and all wars created by the Americans are often just an illusion and based on lies so we get to be told rubbish like it is because of "Weapons of Mass Destruction" Big Tech has cooperated in a propaganda campaign to portray Ukraine as a victim of Russian aggression, with Vladimir Putin as the personification of evil. The goal has been to get ordinary citizens to sympathise with Ukraine and to support a war that not only does not serve American and the west's interests but is also harmful to them and for example, food and energy commodities are sold on the international market, and now this unnecessary war has driven up prices at home and abroad we all seen everything that has gone up in the supermarkets here in Australia and are all blamed on the Ukraine, and it is of course it is naturally Russia's fault and how naive would you have to be to believe that because it is totally ludicrous. Once that propaganda plan had been taken, we saw the State Department, CIA, and NATO announced they would provide western military hardware to the Azov battalion in Ukraine essentially havingAmericans give equipment to Ukraine's 100,000 strong paramilitary, openly Nazi division as the Azov are frequently used in place of regulars because of their willingness to do what ordinary soldiers will not and the Azov is behind Ukraine. Essentially having Americans give equipment to Ukraine's 100,000 strong paramilitary, openly Nazi division as the Azov are frequently used in place of regulars because of their willingness to do what ordinary soldiers will not and the Azov is behind Ukraine President Volodymyr Zelensky and even controls him. We also saw confirmed reports of Ukrainian atrocities committed against captive Russian soldiers and the drones by the Ukraine forces that are used to drop chemical weapons on the Russian troops and even though that is a crime the west totally ignores it.

So, the hard truths about the war in the Ukraine I believe is that the main misconception about the situation in Ukraine is that Ukraine is winning the war. But with the media's involvement it is that the media have taken sides, because they are paid to do so showing Russian brutality, but we and other freedom fighters and truth seekers are trying to get the word out of the videos showing Ukrainians brutally beating Russian soldiers with canvas bags over their heads and prisoners, some standing, some lying face down on the ground, are shot in the knees and genitals, then left on the ground to bleed to death. It appears that Ukrainian soldiers recorded their exploits for posterity, gleefully bragging as to what was done, which is how we know of their brutal behaviour. In all wars the real losers are the people, it's the children, the elderly that lose and are the cannon fodder and the western media just continue to show propaganda and the Ukraine's losses in terms of people are much higher than Russia's. There are mainly two reasons for that which are that Ukraine has thousands of civilian deaths, while Russia has virtually zero, and secondly and most important, Russian actual battlefield personnel losses are likely to be overstated for propaganda reasons.Ukraine's direct economic losses are incomparable to Russia's as Ukraine's GDP will have contracted anything from 20% to 50% percent in 2022 due to the war and this has been reported by multiple sources, and the estimates do vary. They are of an order of magnitude higher however than the single-digit losses (maybe low two-digits) Russia may have been its GDP for 2022. Russia's losses due to sanctions will take time to have a meaningful effect, and it is even questionable to what extent they will actually have an effect and this may be due to delays in enacting and implementing the sanctions and the West does help Ukraine with weapons, training, and financing, but it is not willing to, for a multitude of reasons to help Ukraine's military as an ally, with soldiers and Western-led actions.

The propaganda machine will make you believe anything if you want to believe it just turn that TV on and listen to the garbage that any normal critical thinker would immediately see as BS, and it is important to stress that the main result of the battle for Kyiv was not Ukraine showing Russia that it is able to defend itself and not fall in three days as predicted as important as such a result may be. Was to show the West that Ukraine is a real country, independent from Russia, willing to and able to defend itself, with several limitations of course, even under extreme conditions. We all remember in the past statements like during the second world war "There is no Good German but a Dead German" and the propaganda to give you reason to support them words, so here we go again and you have seen they had to incite hatred against Russia and the Russian people, I have Russian and Ukrainian friends and in reality in the real world there are good and bad in all societies. But the truth always seems to be lost when you get sucked in by the western media who are paid for that exact reason to lie and deceive you if you are gullible enough, and if you are reading this you should be ashamed if you are that easy to be sucked in by all of this. The Ukrainian President Volodymyr Zelensky banned all opposition parties from the use of Russian as a second state language so why did he violate his 2019 campaign promise to stop the genocidal killing of thousands in Donbas, even though they voted for him? Did he lie because neo-Nazis threatened to kill him if he did not do what they wanted? Or is he afraid of the CIA, which has assassinated other leaders, making him their puppet? Are we to trust the judgement of a man who demands a no-fly zone which could cause a global nuclear holocaust? Zelensky oversees torture and assassination of political dissenters and thousands in Donbas, even though they voted for him? Did he lie because neo-Nazis threatened to kill him if he did not do what they wanted? Or is he afraid of the CIA, which has assassinated other leaders, making him their puppet? One of the main reasons in this war is simply that it is now officially confirmed that the Pentagon is operating a network of bioweapons laboratories throughout Ukraine, which explains at least in part why Russia invaded the country and undersecretary of State Victoria Nuland told a Senate committee recently that Ukraine has "Biological Research Facilities" that the United States the military-industrial complex is worried it might now be taken over or destroyed by Vladimir Putin.

Nuland openly admitted that the swamp creatures in Washington, D.C., have been conspiring with Ukrainian officials to establish and run these biolabs, which manufacture biological weapons similar to the Wuhan Covid-19 coronavirus. We are told that the world condemns what Russia has done in the Ukraine when in actual fact most of the world does not, including China, India, most of Africa, Israel, half of Latin America and many other countries. The two largest political parties in Russia do not oppose Russia's intervention, the second largest party being the Communist Party that might shock you but the truth is always the truth, but you will still hang your hat on what the fucked checkers say. hen the propaganda machine is ramped up because why did you take a vaccine that was experimental and we told you it would not work well basically because of fear and they will use the word fear to get you in again, and again, over this misinformation that Russia wants a nuclear war when in fact Russia, has the same policy as the U.S and on March 22, 2022 a Kremlin spokesman Dmitry Peskov said Russia would only use nuclear weapons if its very existence were threatened, Tass news agency reported.Russia had a "no first use" policy until the U.S. refused to do the same, so Russia dropped it U.S. presidents have threatened to use nuclear weapons several times since the end of WWII against countries not a threat to the U.S so the irony, of course, in all of this is that it is actually a classic U.S. military-industrial complex technique to blame on the other guy what they're planning to do themselves as American history is littered with examples of Deep State hacks staging false flag events like 9/11 as a pretext for pushing some other agenda. In the case of 9/11, it was the Deep State's way of justifying the takedown of Saddam Hussein in Iraq, even though none of the alleged terrorists were even from that country.

On the other side of the coin, Russian troops obtained over 20,000 documents pertaining to American biological research programs in Ukraine since the start of Moscow's military operation, the country's Defense Ministry announced on Monday so who do you believe we were told the China was responsible for the Wuhan virus and it was started by bats how gullible are you, when they still troll out this BS, and you believed that Russia did use chemical weapons in Syria, when Russia negotiated Syrian stockpiles to be destroyed or removed. The chemical attacks in Syria were done by rebels supported by Saudi Arabia and the U.S it is not ironical that people who believe in vaccines will swallow anything hook, line and sinker that the western media choses to feed you, yes and the idiotic words like Moronic and Monkeypox they were simply taking the piss out of you all, so please wake the FK up but some of you will not as you line up for clot shot number 6 in 2023, and why you are labelled by us as vaccine addicts. I am truly ashamed that some who are born with some modicum of intellect really is dumb as dumb can be, and because of that we are where we are in April 2023, up the khyber passes as the world that we love, and we know is flushed down the toilet. Ironically with your house properly stocked up on toilet paper you find the pure bloods and Putin is one that we don't have stockpiles of toilet paper but essentials like Food and Water.

The Bioweapons laboratories in the Ukraine and I will highlighted just one: the Lugar Center is the Pentagon bio laboratory in Georgia, and it is located just 17 km away from the US Vaziani military airbase in the capital Tbilisi it is tasked with the military program and biologists from the US Army Medical Research Unit-Georgia along with private contractors. The Biosafety Level 3 Laboratory is accessible only to US citizens with security clearance and they are accorded diplomatic immunity under the 2002 US-Georgia Agreement on defence cooperation and Battelle is a $59 million subcontractor at Lugar Center has extensive experience in research on bio-agents, as the company has already worked on the US Bioweapons immunity under the 2002 US-Georgia Agreement on defence cooperation as the company has already worked on the US Bioweapons Program under 11 previous contracts with the US Army (1952-1966).

The private company performs work for the Pentagon's DTRA bio laboratories in Afghanistan, Armenia, Georgia, Uganda, Tanzania, Iraq, and Vietnam. Battelle conducts research, development, testing, and evaluation using both highly toxic chemicals and highly pathogenic biological agents for a wide range of US government agencies. It has been awarded some $2 billion federal contracts in total and ranks 23 on the Top 100 US government contractors list. If you do your research, then you will find information that is the U.S gave Iraq chemical weapons which were used to kill thousands of Kurds and Iranians in 1982-83 before stockpiles were destroyed by Iraq and the U.S. is the actual chemical killer and not Russia which has often prevented it and history is full of U.S. false flags and one of the reasons why we support Russia is the stain on mankind, one of them reasons is. 'Adrenochrome" ' which is a disease of some of the rich and this is very good news that Russian Special Forces recently raided and destroyed an **"Adrenochrome farm"** near the Ukrainian city of Shostka, where sinister forces tortured abducted Russian children to harvest fluid from their adrenal glands, said a Mar-a-Lago source who claims Russian

President Vladimir Putin informed President Trump of the operation after Spetsnaz had rescued 50 young kids from the ghastly laboratory. As reported early last year, Trump and Putin kept an open conduit of communication after the latter began his "special military operation" in Ukraine. Putin had assured Trump that his true impetus for deploying troops was to rid Eastern Europe of Western pestilence, meaning Deep State-controlled bioweapon facilities and child trafficking rings, both of which, Putin said at the time, threatened Russian sovereignty. As time passed, their conversations became less frequent, but Putin has periodically updated Trump on progress.

I have struggled with a few people in life in general that have a dark past and I did when I was a sex addict for a long time but only with consenting adult females so having been celibate currently for several years I have sorted that addiction out and I needed to, especially with my current mantra "Share no Body Fluids" and the reason why I do mention that here is Donald Trump and statements like this he has made in the past "I've known Jeff Epstein for fifteen years terrific guy," Trump once said about the convicted sex offender. "He's a lot of fun to be with and it is even said that he likes beautiful women as much as I do, and many of them are on the younger side and no doubt about it Jeffrey enjoys his social life." So Donald Trump must have known about the the pedophilia, and he be very aware it was a trait of so many in powerful positions who have this particular sickness. So that bothers me as no normal person would ever condone sex with younger people? Also, Former Republican President Donald Trump's recent comments touting COVID-19 vaccines as safe. Also it was a major achievement of his presidency that has roiled extreme anti-vaxers, including me and many of his ardent supporters. After months of a relatively low profile on vaccines and no photos of him getting inoculated, Trump on Dec.19 2022, told former Fox News host Bill O'Reilly during an event in Dallas that he'd received the booster eliciting some boos from the audience.

Turning to another important subject which is **Gain-Of-Function** which uses genetic engineering to make a living organism more virulent and the microorganisms studied are often viruses, bacteria, and other microorganisms so the most common application of GoF is in the development of new vaccines. This means that the vaccine has a much higher likelihood of protecting an individual from the disease it was designed for. It's important to know when a pathogen gains a new function because this can change the course of treatment and the severity of the disease, and this alarms me why the "Emergency Powers" the WHO have voted in should alarm you all.

I even mentioned my concerns in person to Matt Canavan the Qld senator when he was here in Redcliffe when I was at the pre-polling booth helping Kelly Guenoun, who was standing for the United Australia party for the ward of Petrie and he commented to me before this was actually voted in by the WHO "he was unaware of it " which alarmed me but he did comment he would research it, so when Marburg is finally released and it will, as it is in of the vaccines then we all going to have to get vaccinated under the emergency powers and this was always there plan so fight so please fight against it large and the only thing delaying it is we winning some battles and this is there last roll of the dice and the fact the **PCR tests for Marburg have been approved** I suggest that day looms large and do not be there when they knock on your door to vaccinate you. A virus can gain function in many ways and it can mutate and gain a new ability to infect another species or change its structure to escape recognition by the immune system, and gain-of-function studies are most commonly used in virology and have revealed many details about the biological mechanisms of virus transmission vaccine-generated antibodies for the virus. So in contrast, survival rates don't decrease appreciably and most mutations that a virus can acquire are detrimental to the function of the virus, although in some cases, the mutation can increase virulence and provide a better immune defence.

International regulations determine that animal studies be conducted before they can be tested in humans. This is such an important point that Pfizer stated they did not stop animal trials because the animals died well the people dying so what can we conclude from that. But in cases where human viruses are being studied the follow-on strains must be generated that could contaminate the model species and this can be accomplished using gain-function research, in which the virus is passed through the animal so that the molecular and that determines transmissibility can be identified and the vaccines being studied can be tested, so you can see this imperative and not something one could skip and would skip and bring out 3 miracle vaccines Worldwide in such a short space of time and if they were to do this "And They Did" then it is why we are in this Genocidal Mess.

All of us on planet earth will live this nightmare and have an effect on families at some point in the next 2 years so how do Scientists determine a pathogen (GOF) well? Scientists use three criteria to determine if a pathogen has gained a function. The first is the degree of complexity, which is determined by the number of parts in the pathogen and how they are arranged. The second is the degree of organisation, which is determined by how well-structured and organised the pathogen's parts are and the third criterion used to determine if a pathogen has gained a function is its ability to produce the desired outcome, which can be done through either natural selection or artificial selection which leads on to Biosecurity: The likelihood that someone would use products or information gained from GOF experiments that led to a more pathogenic virus to carry out intentional damage in the form of bioterrorism and finally Biosafety. The likelihood of accidental escape that could trigger an outbreak and epidemic and part the pandemic that was created and it was the Bats fault and enough to make anyone batty.

Mick Mclennan (Mullet Mick) I first met Mick at Common Law Caboolture, and over last 2 years we have become good mates he is one the men you would want behind you when

232

the chips are down, he recently has been interviewed by that legend the pro-Russian the Aussie Cossack, for his stance on supporting Russia and in the interview Mick even gave his home address out because he simply has "No fear" and when you meet Mick, be prepared for a proper man's handshake. Mick kindly sent me his notes on Russia, a topic I only have minimalist understanding of. Mick's Facebook page is "Stand With Russia" and even though Mick is busy running a local roofing contracting business he still is very proactive in trying to make change and ultra passionate about what has happened to all of us in the last 3 years. On February 16, 2022, a full week before Putin sent combat troops into Ukraine, the Ukrainian Army began the heavy bombardment of the area (in east Ukraine) occupied by mainly ethnic Russians.

What the OSCE discovered was that the bombardment dramatically intensified as the week went on until it reached a peak on February 19, when a total of 2,026 artillery strikes were recorded.Keep in mind, the Ukrainian Army was, in fact, shelling civilian areas along the Line of Contact that were occupied by other Ukrainians. We want to emphasise that the officials from the OSCE were operating in their professional capacity gathering first-hand evidence of shelling in the area. Officials from the Observer Mission of the Organization for Security and Co-operation in Europe (OSCE) were located in the vicinity at the time and kept a record of the shelling as it took place. This has all been documented and has not been challenged. So, the question we must all ask ourselves is this: Is the bombardment and slaughter of one's own people an 'act of war'? We think it is. And if we are right, then we must logically assume that the war began before the Russian invasion (which was launched a full week later). We must also assume that Russia's alleged "unprovoked aggression" was not unprovoked at all but was the appropriate humanitarian response to the deliberate killing of civilians. And as we said earlier the OSCE had monitors on the ground who provided full documentation of the shelling as it took place, which is as close to ironclad, eyewitness testimony as you're going to get it. This, of course, is a major break with the "official narrative" which identifies Russia as the perpetrator of hostilities. But, as we've shown, that simply isn't the case. The official narrative is wrong. Even so, it might not surprise you to know that most of the mainstream media completely omitted any coverage of the OSCE's fact-finding activities in east Ukraine.The point we are trying to make is simple: The war in Ukraine was not launched by a tyrannical Russian leader (Putin) bent on rebuilding the Soviet Empire. That narrative is a fraud that was cobbled together by neocon spin-meisters trying to build public support for a war with Russia. The facts I am presenting here can be identified on a map where the actual explosions took place and were then recorded by officials whose job was to fulfil that very task.

Can you see the difference between the two? In one case, the storyline rests on speculation, conjecture and psychobabble; while in the other, the storyline is linked to actual events that took place on the ground and were catalogued by trained professionals in the field. In which version of events do you have more confidence? Russia did not start the war in Ukraine as that is fake news as the responsibility lies with the Ukrainian Army and their leaders in Kiev. And here's something else that is typically excluded in the media's selective coverage. Before Putin sent his tanks across the border into Ukraine, he invoked United Nations Article 51 which provides a legal justification for military intervention.By most estimates, the Ukrainian army has killed over 14,000 ethnic Russians since the US-backed coup 8 years ago. If ever there was a situation in which a defensive military operation could be justified, this was it. For that, we turn to former weapons inspector Scott Ritter, who explained it like this: "Russian President Vladimir Putin, citing Article 51 as his authority, ordered what he called a "special military operation" under Article 51, there can be no doubt as to The legitimacy of Russia's contention that the Russian-speaking population of the Donbass had been subjected to a brutal eight-year-long bombardment that had killed thousands of people. Moreover, Russia claims to have documentary proof that the Ukrainian Army was preparing for a massive military incursion into the Donbass which was preempted by the Russian-led "special military operation." [OSCE figures show an increase of government shelling of the area in the days before Russia moved in.]

Here's a bit more background from an article by foreign policy analyst Danial Kovalik:" One must begin this discussion by accepting the fact that there was already a war happening in Ukraine for eight Years preceding the Russian military incursion in February 2022. And, this war by the government in Kiev that claimed the lives of around 14,000 people, many of them children. It also displaced around 1.5 million more as the government in Kiev, and especially its neo-Nazi battalions, carried out attacks against these peoples precisely because of their ethnicity. While the UN Charter prohibits unilateral acts of war, it also provides, in Article 51, that "nothing in the present Charter shall impair the inherent right of individual or collective self-defence " And this right of self-defence has been interpreted to permit countries to respond, not only to actual armed attacks, but also to the threat of imminent attack. In light of the above, this is my assessment that Russia had a right to act in its own self-defence by intervening in Ukraine, which had become a proxy of the US and NATO for an assault not only on Russian ethnic's within Ukraine but also upon Russia itself.``("Why Russia's intervention in Ukraine is legal under international law", RT) .Instead, the media continues to spread the fiction that 'Hitler-Putin is trying to rebuild the Soviet empire', a claim for which there is not a scintilla of evidence. Keep in mind, Putin's operation does not involve the toppling of a foreign government to install a Moscow-backed stooge, or the arming and training a foreign military that will be used as proxies to fight a geopolitical rival, or stuffing a country with state-of-the-art weaponry to achieve his own narrow strategic objectives, or perpetrating terrorist acts of industrial sabotage Nord-Stream 2) to prevent the economic integration of Asia and Europe. No, Putin hasn't engaged in any of these things.

In Washington's eyes, international law is merely an inconvenience that is dismissively shrugged off whenever unilateral action is required. But Putin is not nearly as cavalier about such matters, in fact, he has a long history of playing by the rules because he believes the rules help to strengthen everyone's security. And, he's right; they do. And that's why he invoked Article 51 before he sent the troops to help the people in the Donbas. He felt he had a moral obligation to lend them his assistance but wanted his actions to comply with international law. We think he achieved both. Here's something else you will never see in the western media. You'll never see the actual text of Putin's security demands that were made a full 2 months before the war broke out. And, the reason you won't see them, is because his demands were legitimate, reasonable and necessary.

All Putin wanted was basic assurances that NATO was not planning to put its bases, armies and missile sites on Russia's border. In other words, he was doing the same thing that all responsible leaders do to defend the safety and security of their own people.There's no way to overstate the importance of the Minsk betrayal or the impact it's going to have on the final settlement in Ukraine. When trust is lost, nations can only ensure their security through brute force. What that means is that Russia must expand its perimeter as far as is necessary to ensure that it will remain beyond the enemy's range of fire.Putin, Lavrov and Medvedev have already indicated that they plan to do just that. The new perimeter must be permanently fortified with combat troops and lethal weaponry that are kept on hair trigger alert. When treaties become vehicles for political opportunism, then nations must accept a permanent state of war. This is the world that Merkel, Hollande, Poroshenko and the US created by opting to use 'the cornerstone of international relations' (Treaties) to advance their own narrow warmongering objectives. We just wonder if anyone in Washington realises what the fu** they've done it? As you have just read Mick Mclennan could write his own book on Russia, as it is one of his many passions and he kindly wrote this piece.

Mick is also involved in groups like The National Soverignty Party Australia, which you can find on facebook. The Australian Soverignty Party, was born of an idea and appeal to all generation X,ers and younger who, like myself are just starting to come into our maturity and aware that we must take charge of our own destiny and future. So when we are held to task by future adults with (what have you done to ensure a secure future we can proudly hand over a legacy worthy of continuity) we need to shake the foundations of this established prison and kick to the curb the 'rein holders' of our lives and take charge of the 'couch horses' once was a time the older folk were expected to make way for the new blood and in old age shamelessly neglected but the 'reverence for our elders' is misplaced. They have robbed and deceived us at our and our descendants' expense.

We must redress this going back to 1920's Australia. The average age of a sitting MP was 35yrs old today it is 58 yrs old believe it or not the biggest demographics is the under 20's still coming of age who will not blame 'the adults of our world' for the world woes but the adults of theirs' that is US folks they will rightly ask of us 'what the fuck did you do and what can we say i'll tell you what we can say that we studied our route and set a sure course and be proud to hand over 'the ship' but we must first take charge and we need a new political platform and even approach and perspective on everything, be damned what the current powers and smug 'rein-holders' say they have all betrayed us for self serving agenda's like spoiled brats glorifying their post world war 2 affluence and successes like it was their victory and squandered it at our and our children's expenses so in the future vote 1 for the NATIONAL SOVEREIGNTY PARTY. AUSTRALIA and start reclaiming our future. This is a proud Australian with true values and views and with more people like Mick Mclennan we will Win.

People forget that during the First World War over a thousand Russian-born servicemen enlisted in the Australian Imperial Force (AIF) and they were the largest national group in the

AIF after British, New Zealand and Canadian born servicemen. Besides ethnic Russians, these Anzacs included members of a score of different ethnic groups born within the borders of the Russian Empire how easy some forget the sacrifices and the links we got with Russia and join in the baying mob that Putin is evil and tar and feather the Russian people as one, evil exists in every race, colour and creed and the west have more than its fair share of satanic followers and if you watch TV and buy into alarmism and then you also complicit in accepting all those arms and bullets that kill people, children, elderly and nobody wins and humanity loses. The Fact is Crimea is not an exception and Russia did not 'seek to recover' Crimea and the citizens of that peninsula voted overwhelmingly (90+%) to rejoin the Russian Federation of which it had been a part for centuries until 1954 when Khrushchev 'gifted' it to Ukraine without consultation with the Crimeans also desire to rejoin the Russian Federation followed an American organised and financed a coup d'état against the legitimate Ukrainian government in February 2014. But again, such analysis is truly not permitted in the Australian mainstream media, and you only believe what you're told as you are led down the garden path to the madhouse and your early demise. So, I end this chapter that most of the unvaccinated understand the war in the Ukraine is a total "Smokescreen" to try to detract attention off what evil they are trying to achieve and they will do anything for their thirst for the blood of innocent children.

Chapter 21

Homelessness

In the last three years the homeless situation where I live in Redcliffe Queensland, Australia, has become very dire with one of the highest rates of homelessness in the whole of Australia. All of you reading this will probably worldwide be facing similar challenges with this real pandemic, that is all pre-planned and why is that? and why is it going to get so much worse. There are lots of reasons and greed is high up there, the haves and the have nots, some might have bought rentals recently as part of their superannuation package on very low interest rates, and now having to pass it on to us the tenants and we could maybe understand that a little bit. But on the flip side of the coin when the interest rates dropped, did any of you reading this have your rents reduced? And factor in the Capital gains on these properties as some went up by 20% especially where I am living in Scarborough Qld, and even though they did well with capital growth gains they still want their cake and eat it. Most of you reading this will understand that supply and demand will be endemic especially in areas of high vaccination rates, which will relate to higher death rates and last year, 174,000 deaths were registered in Australia, that is 12 percent (20,000) more deaths than projections estimated and the deaths from this poison this only the tip of the iceberg especially where you high amounts of older owners. Factor in beach erosion and the floods and other extreme weather conditions and real estate prices could go anywhere, and I feel they will as it is all a part of a Plan. So, this is the "Perfect Storm Scenario' that some parts of Australia are going to be hit very hard. The lack of wage growth and people in insecure job markets and the homelessness is going to reach epidemic proportions. So, to my own situation as I can relate and empathise with anybody reading this who is homeless or is about to be must start to press the panic button at some point.

I had worked and lived overseas and although I have owned 6 houses worldwide, I had no rental history when I arrived back in Australia over 5 years ago. I then rented a unit in Rock Street Scarborough from Century 21 Scarborough, a local real estate agent. To obtain it and having no rental history I was happy to pay 6 months rent and bond in advance it was sight unseen as I was about to be homeless. On arriving to pick up the keys with my son, I found the place had not been lived in for 3 months because it had recently been for sale. I was horrified by the smell of the unwashed torn carpets and the dead cockroaches. I broke down crying in front of my 26-year old son and he never saw me cry before.

I went back to Century 21 to voice my concerns to the female property manager whose attitude was " you do not have to take it" well my furniture was arriving I was in a dilemma so I cleaned the carpets with my son's help. I moved in and continued to pay my rent up to 5 weeks ahead for over 5 years. Two years ago, the new owner wanted to renovate and kindly put up in alternative accommodation until I could move back in. When I moved back there was builders' dust all over my furniture and remember I have lung disease, but I let that go anything for an easy life. I provide my own labour to paint the walls to the lounge, kitchen and bedroom to make it look nicer. Then the bombshell hit with this email from the property manager Jon Eagle head of property management. The owner of the property that I rent from works for Century 21 and I believe is a corporate manager. "Unfortunately the owner of your property has contact (sic) me to advise that your lease at the property will not be renewed in May of this year. She is planning to have further renovations carried out once you vacate and then **substantially increase** the asking rent after all the work is complete."

So, no offer of alternative accommodation and then being able to move back in the "Substantial rent increase" for me would not be a problem. Also, John Eagle and please remember he is head of property management (and not God) made no attempt to offer me another rental so my loyalty and good faith that I showed that in a normal world you would look after "Good Tenant's'. I should not have to remind John how to do their job in a normal way with a modicum of basic human decency and kindness which you are very sadly lacking. I was to be treated like mud on the bottom of his shoe and his reasons for that are unclear. In November of 2022 he did an inspection without any notification which is a "Breach" on his behalf. Today 26th April 2023 John Eagle did an inspection and remember I have to move out on May 16th because they are renovating. He kindly left me a note "Carpet Cleaning / Pest Control along with thorough cleaning all in block capitals.

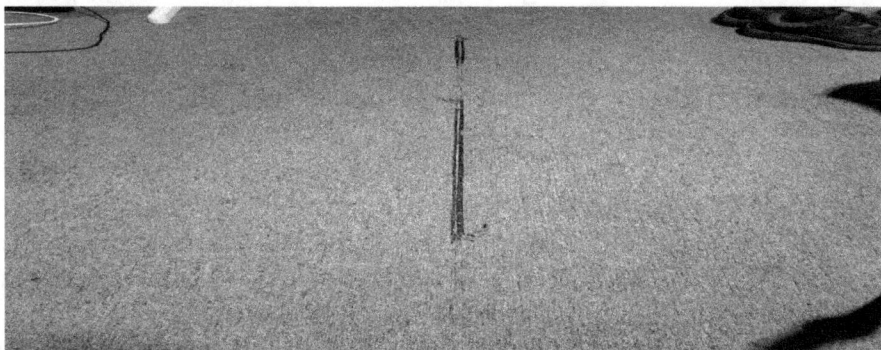

This is the torn carpet that must be cleaned. I let you decide if this is not the actions of a vaccinated Zombie: they are a worry as their brains do not engage and compute in a logical and "Normal Way" remember the reason I must move out is their renovating the games some people like to play Jon Eagle you are a Zombie. Avoid this Zombie Real Estate Agency's Century 21 Scarborough they are a shocker. I am 65 years old and about to receive a UK retirement pension that I paid in until I emigrated here over 35 years ago. Anyone reading this please take note that not all real estates are as bad as this one In fact, I do not need to name them but there are several on the peninsula who have good Christian ethics. I will stand up for the little guys like myself so don't let bad real estate agents treat you like they have me "Because they think they Can".

I already mentioned how bad the homeless situation is here on the Redcliffe Peninsula, and there would be so many people reading this who would have their own horror stories, so in explaining my own dire situation you're not on your own but I am able through this book highlight corporate greed which was everywhere "In the fear of Missing out" in the days of low interest rates and even brick houses only 30 years old here in Scarborough Qld were bulldozed to subdivide as the keeping up with the jones mentally had taken over here as it's an affluent suburb of Qld Australia. I would assume that most in this the real estate industry would have been vaccinated to have done their inspections and you have already read how it can affect their "Thinking" and also maybe a lack of empathy so you might find anyone who is heavily vaccinated might not be the nicest people walking around? in fact be wary when dealing with them and that they could discriminate against you if you are unvaccinated.

The Federal and State Governments and local councils really do not care and if we talk about all the money they are wasting on Submarines (Federal) or the Local Sutton's Pavilion (Council) here in Redcliffe Qld with security guards and with people sleeping in cars near there while the local councils seem do absolutely nothing. They will discriminate against the homeless by waking them up late at night and give them fines and their will be a Wellness Camp it be near a train line I use the word "Livestock" a lot but that is all we are so think smart and be smart because there songbook is Agenda 2030 its only 6 years and 7 months away and its looming fast. Families with children getting dressed for school out of cars in 2023 when all that money was wasted on lockdowns which helped create this total disaster. Which was always pre-planned, vaccinated or not vaccinated does not really matter there coming for all of us because they think they can. The wellness camps are not "Holiday Camps" and some stay idle here in Qld with all the wasted money spent on them while a pile of chook manure and her state government will go down in history for what they truly are "Evil Beyond Words". Sadly, this homelessness will get so much worse, and we are only just hitting the tip of the iceberg because the interest rates are not stopping, and it always was one of the Plandemic Agenda's. New Zealand, US, and the UK have higher interest rates currently and we are heading that way as planned, the RBA chief has so much to answer for with his statement that they will not go up till 2024. But I am not going to sit on my hands because we need to make them accountable, so again to all of you facing similar upheaval and being traumatised and being made homeless and especially those living on the street, which must be a major nightmare, because in reality we are all one foot away from the gutter. I hope this chapter makes you realise you are not on your own and if you do have children then the problem is exacerbated 10 fold, so until it happens to you do please understand and that if you're vaccinated it will be a double whammy due to you having no innate natural immunity" so you might not survive long as a basic head cold could kill you as winter looms here in Qld. For the rest of us stay strong, all gather around as one big "'Pure Blood Tribe" as our strength is in our numbers. The latest figures in March 20th 2023, are the ranks of Queensland's homeless are growing and a new report released today found the number of homeless has shot up more than 20 per cent in five years that is almost triple the increase nationally. I have personally experienced 17% interest rates when I bought my farm in Winkleigh Tasmania in 1988 and could go back there, the wheel always turns full circle, but I really pray not. Supply and demand will dictate as the dynamics of this region is very elderly if the agenda 2030 works as planned there are gonna be a lot of empty properties as foreclosures hit. There are already a lot of uncontrollable balls in the air but the juggling act for the teetering sector is about to become a lot tougher over the next 12 to 18 months. Inflated construction costs that are likely "not coming back anytime soon" and "nowhere near enough" skilled labour to deliver.

The report, from Queensland Council of Social Services (QCOSS) and The Town of Nowhere campaign, predicts more than 220,000 households in the state will not have affordable housing within 20 years. In Logan, Beaudesert and the Gold Coast, 10 percent of households are homeless, or living in unaffordable housing. You don't have to look far here in Redcliffe, opposite the blue water square shopping centres where there are people sleeping on the pavement in doorways and if you venture out in parks and there is no place that is immune from this epidemic of homelessness with new tents pop up everywhere.

The homeless rate has risen by 8 per cent nationally since 2017, according to a report's author, University of New South Wales. In Queensland, it's gone up by 22 per cent and in regional Queensland, the increase is "even more dramatic", up 29 per cent in four years, he said. "In Brisbane rents are up by well over 30 per cent since the outbreak of COVID," Professor Pawson said. There are a lot of people making statements like QCOSS CEO Aimee McVeigh who said the report shows the scale of the state's housing crisis. "There are about 300,000 Queenslanders currently experiencing housing insecurity. The National Rental Affordability Scheme (NRAS) is starting to wind down for some people on rental arrangements, with the last subsidised rental properties set to exit the scheme in 2026 and while this is happening Ms Palaszczuk the Labour premier said caps on rental prices were also being considered but could not provide more detail with the idea to be discussed at a housing summit next Tuesday. Pilachook you have created this total shambles with your draconian state mandates, and the Olympics is very high on your Agenda and it is not hard to work out why we are in this sorry state. Another thing that is exacerbating the homeless problem is the so-called rain bombs, Moreton Bay Regional Council "Rain Bomb", which have impacted residents. We are all aware of these man made disasters. I bet the pilots are at overtime rates and how do they sleep at night taking their "Blood Money".

Work was to assess the over 2,000 properties of these disastrous bio engineered weather events, the latest hit which hit our region on 23th February 2022, and here we are well over a year later some properties are still not repaired like 6 units on the beach at Scarborough Qld and you have to feel for their owner's.

Where I live the Moreton Bay Council it is the 3rd largest council in Australia, and there is a big Agenda here and that is Agenda 2030, and we are all being geared for a Smart City with Comrade Flannery in charge because all the cameras and the 5g they are installing and please don't be conned by some of these vaccine lovers as they do not have your best interests at heart. You're all seeing the demise of this great region, the roads, the homeless and all the small businesses going to the wall and the council does not and never did care, the councillors you will never see them only unless they are touting another money wasting exercise. The aboriginal community is doing tough here as I already mentioned and will "The Voice " represent them as Anal Albo has vaccinated most of them and they will comply and do as they are told to do.

The Aborigines are very disillusioned and one I have met many times is John, an elder for Scarborough Qld, who is doing a doctorate in Psychology when I met him in a rat infested house that has since been pulled down. The Voice "is the first of three sequential reforms proposed by the Uluru Statement. The others - treaty and truth - respectively call for a treaty between the government and Indigenous people, and for "truth-telling about [Australian] history". It is all a pandemic illusion distraction as they divide and conquer all who buy into the lies. But remember we all actually have a "Voice" so lets drain this swamp once and for all. The money they are wasting trying to save trees at Scarborough beach when with a bit of foresight, they could have prevented that and they will have to knock them down anyway, that money could have been better used to help the disadvantaged, but the rich ratepayers of this area carry a lot of weight, and most are compliant to the agenda. But I am one of the lucky ones as I can move off grid and stay in my truth, but I really feel for so many people and some of them are my friends, who have elderly parents, and young children in schools who are between a rock and a hard place and just can up and leave and my thoughts and prayers are with you all. So where will the homeless situation be in a few years? I really dread to think.

Redcliffe Peninsula is a peninsula located in the Moreton Bay Region LGA in the northeast of the Brisbane metropolitan area in Queensland, Australia. The area covers the suburbs of Clontarf, Kippa-Ring, Margate, Newport, Redcliffe referred to as Rothwell, Woody Point and Scarborough. Redcliffe Peninsula is home to over 55,000 residents over its total area of 38.1 km2 (The peninsula is relatively flat with few areas rising more than 20 m above sea level. The Redcliffe Peninsula was occupied by the indigenous Ningy Ningy people. The native name is Kau-in-Kau-in, which means Blood-Blood (red-like blood). The area's first European visitors arrived on 17 July 1799, aboard the Norfolk, a British colonial sloop commanded by Matthew Flinders. Flinders explored the Moreton Bay area and landed at 10:30 a.m. at a location he called "Red Cliff Point", after the red-coloured cliffs visible from the bay, today called Woody Point. Redcliffe peninsula has a humid subtropical climate. I focus on where I was living until recently Scarborough Qld, from 2021 census people 9,178 Median weekly household income $1,336, interestingly the Median monthly mortgage repayments $1,907 and the Median weekly rent $350 there are a few clues and that rent figure and the mortgage payments because since that survey we had 11 interest rate increases so a lot of people must be under mortgage stress especially on rental properties. I will use my "crystal ball" and predict that the interest rates will not stop as they are planning it that way. Supply and demand will dictate as the dynamics of this region is very elderly if the agenda 2030 works as planned there are going to be a lot of empty properties as foreclosures hit.

The food bank here in Margate Qld is getting up to 50 new people a week and to entertain us in their wisdom this very out of touch Council have engaged an International "Drag Queen" at are local Libraries with the morality going down the toilet shame on you all and it's time to remove them we surely deserve and need better. Today 26th April 2023 I asked the local rangers the question: do you book travellers or homeless $280 for sleeping in your car through no fault of your own. Yes, unless you registered homeless you are likely to be fined welcome to another of the smart city initiatives. If you do not pay the fine then your vehicle will likely be wheel locked and then you are on the slippery slope to their wellness concentration camp you have been warned to think smart. The council needs to raise revenue to pay for the International drag queen who is booked to perform her skills in the local library to your kids. That's how out of touch they are in morality; it is a total disgrace to vote them all out. Time to vote some pure bloods in to show them how it's done properly. Let's drain the swamp in our own region enough of their dictatorial communism.

List of employers NOT requiring their employees to get vaccinated - WTF!?
1. The White House
2. Congress & Staff
3. Supreme Court
4. NIH
5. FDA
6. CDC
7. WHO
8. Moderna
9. Pfizer BioNTech
10. U.S. Postal Services
+ Covid Test /Lab Industries
+ All Illegal Immigrant Invaders
+ Countless Hidden Elite Figures

Red Flags!!
Wake up..

They do not do as we are told to do and there on the slant to oblivion as we on to them your politicians councillors do you really think they seriously took that poison are they that dumb when they were aware of the plandemic agenda.

Chapter 22

Nikola Tesla Inventions

A lot of you are aware of his inventions and how the elite could not ever have them coming out for obvious reasons. We all can relate to this genius, a critical thinker and one of us so to the NWO and the elite he might have died poor but lived as a Hero and we recognize him and his achievements, but we don't and will never recognize any of you for the simple reason everything you touch you Poison. "They laughed at me in 1897 when I told them about the Cosmic Ray. Fifty years ago, they attempted to discredit my discovery of the rotating magnetic field and my system of power transmission by alternating currents. They called me crazy when I predicted the radio and when I sent the first impulse around the world, they said it couldn't be done." Nikola Tesla. So let's look at this more thoroughly because Nikola Tesla was a genius inventor who created some ground-breaking inventions and Tesla had worked with many big names and companies in history and some of his ideas were considered so very far advanced for that time. Tesla is often featured in science fiction television shows and movies so let's shine a bright light on some of his most notable inventions and explore some other commonly asked questions about the man and his life. Nikola Tesla was born and raised in the Austrian Empire, Tesla studied engineering and physics in the 1870s without receiving a degree, gaining practical experience in the early 1880s when working with telephony and at Continental Edison in the new electric power industry. In 1884 he emigrated when he was 28 to the United States, where he became a naturalised citizen and worked for a short time at the Edison Machine Works in New York City before he struck out on his own and the Tesla Foundation has estimated that Tesla held a total of over 300 patents across five continents but it must be born in mind that. Many of these patents were for the same inventions. So, in looking at this genius's work and **Alternating Current**, this all began, and what ultimately caused such a stir at the 1893 World's Expo in Chicago and a war was levelled ever-after between the vision of Edison and the vision of Tesla for how electricity would be produced and distributed. This division can be summarised as one of cost and safety: and the DC current that Edison had that was backed by General Electric, he had been working on was costly over long distances and produced a dangerous sparking from the required converter (called a commutator). But Edison and his backers utilised the general Dangers of electric current, to instil fear in Nikola Tesla's alternative of Alternating Current and as proof, Edison sometimes would electrocute animals in his demonstrations. So consequently, Edison gave the world the Electric Chair but simultaneously maligning Tesla's attempt to offer safety at a lower cost, which Tesla responded by demonstrating that AC was perfectly safe by famously shooting current through his own body to produce light.

This Edison and Tesla, GE-Westinghouse feud in 1893 was the culmination of over a decade of shady business deals, stolen ideas, and patent suppression that Edison and his financial interests had over Tesla's inventions. When we look at this hero and you all reading this about the small guy taking on the big guys who is the better man, well the one with the most money is often not and if you ever were to and go play Texas Holdem, basically it's hard to win when you are playing against industries that own everything including "The System" because simply they will not let you WIN and can't let you because it's all a big game to them. Money simply is the route of all evil, but it is better to die poor in a grave alongside that rich guy who was "Brought" and you really were the better "Guy'" because you truly lived and could never be "brought". Yet, despite everything it is Tesla's system that provides power generation and distribution to North America in our modern era of course Nikola Tesla didn't light himself but he did invent how light could be harnessed and distributed so Tesla had. developed and had used fluorescent bulbs in his lab some 40 years before the industry actually "Invented" them. At the World's Fair, Tesla took glass tubes and bent them into famous scientists' names with effect creating the first neon signs, and it is also his Tesla Coil that might be the most impressive, and controversial certainly that the tesla coil is something that big industry would have liked to suppress as the concept that the Earth itself is a Magnet that can generate electricity. which is electromagnetism and so by utilising frequencies as an transmitter and all that is needed on the other end is the receiver very much like a radio, electromagnetic and ionising radiation was heavily researched in the late 1800s, but Nikola Tesla had researched the entire gamut including everything from a precursor to **Kirlian photography**. Which has the ability to make a life force which is is now used in medical diagnostics, this was a transformative invention of which Tesla played a central role and what we understand is now called an x-ray and like so many of Tesla's contributions that stemmed from his beliefs that we need to understand the universe is virtually around us at all times, but and we really need to use our minds to develop 'real-world devices' to augment our very innate perception of existence.

Let's look at the invention of the **Radio**, that Guglielmo Marconi was initially credited with and most still believe him to be the inventor of radio to this very day, but the Supreme Court actually had overturned Marconi's patent in 1943, when it was proven that Tesla had invented the radio years previous to Marconi. Radio signals are just another frequency that only needs a transmitter and receiver, which Tesla demonstrated in 1893 during a presentation before The National Electric Light Association and frequency and the actual misuse of it will be to the detriment of mankind as they plan this with their Agenda & 5G. So he is a genius well ahead of his time using frequencies in a very good way and in the year 1897, Tesla had applied for two patents but are you very surprised that in 1904 the U.S. Patent Office reversed its original decision and awarding Marconi a patent for the invention of the radio, possibly influenced by Marconi's financial backers in the States, who included Thomas Edison

Andrew Carnegie. The Court actually overturned Marconi's patent in 1943, when it was proven that Tesla had invented the radio years previous to Marconi. Radio signals are just another frequency that only needs a transmitter and receiver, which Tesla demonstrated in 1893 during a presentation before The National Electric Light Association and frequency and the actual misuse of it will be to the detriment of mankind as they plan with their 2030 Agenda & 5G. This also allowed the U.S. government among many others to avoid having to pay the royalties that were being claimed by Nikola Tesla. Moving on to what we now have that is referred to as **Remote Control**, this invention was a natural outcropping of radio, and was the first remote controlled Model Boat. Which when he demonstrated it in 1898 it was utilising several large batteries and radio signals controlled switches, which then energised the boat's propeller, rudder, and scaled-down running lights, by using a small radio and transmitting control box, he was then able to manoeuvre a tiny ship about a pool of water and even flash its running lights on and off and all without any visible connection between the boat and controller. Indeed very few people at that time were even aware that radio waves even existed and Tesla, an inventor often known to electrify the crowd with his many creations was yet again pushing the boundaries, with this remote-controlled vessel, although newspaper headlines chose to focus on the use of Tesla's device as a wirelessly controlled torpedo, his plans for this invention were not wholly aimed at warfare and In a 1900 article from Century magazine, Tesla described it as a moment of self-realisation, seeing his own mind and body as an automaton, reacting to external stimuli and situations. He then stated that contemporary automatons were simply using a "Borrowed Mind," and responded to orders from a distant and intelligent operator. Tesla also believed that one day we may be able to endow a machine with its "Own Mind," where it, too, can act on environmental stimuli of its own accord and when asked about the boat's potential as an explosive-delivery system, Tesla retorted, You do not see there a wireless torpedo but you see there the first of a race of robots, mechanical men which will do the laborious work of the human race and this is a big part of the 2030 Agenda, to replace you and me with these robots and also why the Illuminati regard us as bottom feeding livestock to be controlled and culled when need be. This exact technology was not widely used for some time, we now can see the power that was appropriated by the military in its pursuit of it in a remote controlled war, and of course radio controlled tanks which were introduced by the Germans in WWII, and developments in this realm have since slid quickly away from the direction of human freedoms.

The **Electric Motor**, and Nikola Tesla's invention of the electric motor has finally been popularised by a car that as his Tesla name and while the technical specifications are way beyond the scope of this summary we can say that Tesla's invention of a motor with rotating magnetic fields could have would have freed mankind much sooner from the stranglehold of Big Oil and how many wars have been created using this big oil and the need for it and understanding simple things like the Germans gun oil froze but the Russians mixed their gun oil with a gasoline that gave it another ten to twenty degrees of cold to operate in makes a huge difference. His invention of the electric motor in 1930 succumbed to the economic crisis and the world war that followed, but his invention had fundamentally changed the landscape of what we now take for granted with industrial fans, household appliances, water pumps, machine tools, power tools, disk drives, electric wristwatches and compressor to name just a few. Moving on to **Robotics**, Nikola Tesla's very enhanced scientific mind led him to another idea that all living beings are merely driven by external impulses, he stated: "I have by every thought and act of mine, demonstrated, and does so daily, to my absolute satisfaction that I am an automaton endowed with power of movement, which merely responds to external stimuli." So, the concept of the robot was born but an element of the human remained present, as Tesla asserted that these human replicas should have limitations and rightly so, namely growth and propagation but Nikola Tesla unabashedly embraced all of what intelligence could produce and his visions for a future filled with intelligent cars, robotic human companions, and the use of sensors, and autonomous systems. Limitations of robotics is certainly not on the minds of the powers that be have in mind to day and even with the human mind nothing is going to be sacred when they hijack yours as they have certainly hi-jacked so many in the last 3 years using the power of Television and this has not even started yet and sadly the future for most is looking very grim.

Next we must look at the **Laser**, yet again another of Nikola Tesla's inventions which was the laser and must be one of the best examples of the Good and Evil bound up together within the mind of mankind as lasers have certainly have transformed surgical applications in an undeniably beneficial way but they have also given rise to much of our current 'Digital Media" and the digital media has throughout this C19 Pandemic which was always simply a Plandemic because the global community has depended on digital media and social media platforms on a tremendous scale to ensure safety? Safety, what a total joke that was with the media outlets having done all they can to "debunk" the notion that Ivermectin may serve as an effective, easily accessible and affordable treatment for Covid-19. But our calls for this wonder drug Ivermectin to be used have met with a wall of resistance from healthcare regulators and a wall of silence from the media outlets as unfortunately most reporters are not interested in telling the other side of the story and in actual fact are paid to spread miss-information and basically miss-truths and those of you who bought into it and why you really need to switch the TV off because it did really coarse Covid-19. But so effective has Ivermectin been that in some of countries that have really benefited the most from its use are Mexico and Argentina, but some people are still completely unaware of its safe existence and here in Australia we all watched the media calling it "Horse Paste" and how many of you watched this travesty then in disgust decided that day to turn off the TV for good, and when that happens is truly a liberating day. There have been teams of up to twenty three researchers in many countries that have reported after nine months of looking for a COVID-19 treatment and finding nothing but evil failures like Remdesivir "we kissed a lot of frogs" that "Ivermectin was the only thing that worked against C19, and its safety and efficacy was astonishingly "blindingly positive," and that researchers concluded it reduced C19 mortality by up to 81 percent. Ivermectin has already been approved as a C19 early treatment in more than 20 countries. They have included Mexico where the mayor of Mexico City, Claudia Scheinbaum, said that the medicine had reduced hospitalisations by as much as 76%. The government of India, the world's second most populous country and also one of the world's biggest manufacturers of medicines has also recommended the use of ivermectin as an early outpatient treatment against C19, in direct contravention of WHO's own advice. Moving on to Australia on March 9, 2021, AHPRA the (Australian Health Practitioner Regulation Agency), and what a complete joke they truly are and according to a 2011 publication, Australia is the first country in the world to have a national registration and accreditation scheme regulating health practitioners to our detriment. We have all seen Dr. William Bay from Qld in his legal fight against AHPRA starting in 2022, and they have without doubt become a Stasi-like enforcement arm of the Australian Government. It has also devoted itself to purging every health practitioner in the country who dares to take a stance that is at odds with the decrees of the Covid bureaucracy National Boards threatened doctors who made any statements that "undermined public confidence in the vaccine rollout" with regulatory action and why? Because according to the TGA, if people were to gain access to Ivermectin it may cause vaccine hesitancy throughout the community and the United Australia Party rightly asks these Questions: Clive Palmer paid for 37 million doses of Hydroxychloroquine (HCQ) and donated it to the Australian public.But when it arrived in Australia, it was all destroyed by the Morrison regime and Clive Palmer also donated $1 million to fund a trial into HCQ but the TGA shut it down and it since been accepted that early use of HCQ could have saved thousands of people, but as readers here know, if there was a cheap useful treatment for Covid available, other expensive, barely tested, risky new drugs would not be given an Emergency Use Authorization, thus threatening to kill a $200 billion dollar cash cow. So, getting rid of safe competing drugs is just a part of the business plan for Big Pharma and they would be letting down their shareholders if they didn't lobby like hell to make it happen and the media were complicit in all of this.

So to the Australian Government why did you let this travesty **happen to your own people**? We all understand the real reasons why and Agenda 2030 just keeps rolling on, but be warned Governments Worldwide more people are waking up to the truth. So back to the Digital Media and information and communication technologies that have facilitated productivity and critical information flows are also the means by which false content and polarising narratives have been amplified, all too often distorting healthy public discourse and impeding the effective implementation of public health initiatives. This is by no means a new challenge that public health, political, electoral and social institutions are now being forced to confront. Just like the COVID-19 pandemic, the developing conflict in Ukraine offers another example of the widespread diffusion of competing and often erroneous narratives propagated globally by diverse actors during times of crisis and another based on misinformation and with this leap in innovation we have also crossed into the land of science fiction from Reagan's "Star Wars" laser defence system to today's Orwellian "Non-Lethal" Weapons' arsenal, which includes laser rifles and directed energy "Death Rays.With dyslexia I sometimes go off in a tangent and to you readers I hope you get my drift!

Moving on to Wireless Communications and Limitless Free Energy, and the two are very much linked, as they are the last straw for the powerful elites as what good is energy if it can't be metered and controlled?

Free wireless communications, but it also meant that aside from the cost of the tower itself, the universe was filled with free energy that could be utilised to form a world wide web connecting all people in all places, as well as allow people to harness the free energy around them. Nikola Tesla was dedicated to empowering the individual to receive and transmit this data virtually free of charge. But we did not understand the ending to that story until now? so what is the linkage 73 years after the FBI seized nearly Two Trucks of papers of one of the world's most famous inventors, the Federal Bureau of Investigations released the documents to the public and those batch of documents made available through the Freedom of Information Act also reveal Tesla did not die on January 7, 1943, as previously believed, but a day later on January 8 and Tesla was way ahead of his time. He envisioned a bright and positive future for mankind, as he patented and created hundreds of technologies that no one before had envisioned, or had dared to imagine Tesla's like UFO Antigravity Technology. We know that Tesla was all about free energy and alternative power sources and despite this, the methods and design of Tesla's revolutionary vehicle is believed to match the description of people who witnessed disk-shaped flying objects, or UFO's. It is believed that Tesla's UFO had 'eyes' made of electro-optical lenses, arranged in quadrants, allowing the pilot to see everything. Screens and monitors are placed on a console where the browser can observe all areas around the vehicle, and Tesla's Amazing invention included magnifying lenses, which could have been used without changing positions.

The evidence of such a vehicle can be found in an interview between Nikola Tesla and The New York Herald, from 1911 :"My flying machine will have neither wings nor propellers. You might see it on the ground and you would never guess that it was a flying machine. Yet it will be able to move at will through the air in any direction with perfect safety, at higher speeds than have yet been reached, regardless of weather and oblivious of "holes in the air" or downward currents. "It will ascend in such currents if desired.

It can remain stationary in the air, even in a wind, for a great length of time.Its lifting power will not depend upon any such delicate devices as the bird has to employ but upon positive mechanical action." As explained by Tesla himself, the Earth is "like a charged metal ball moving through space", which creates the enormous, rapidly varying electrostatic force. Then there is Tesla's **Death Ray**, prior to the release of the declassified documents by the FBI, many people argue that Tesla's Death Ray was just another conspiracy as previously, it was believed that Tesla's Death Ray did not exist, and the FBI claimed for over a decade that none of their agents had ever investigated Tesla's papers, nor was the bureau in possession of any of them. But after the FBI published Tesla's files, we have learned that among the published files, a letter addressed to J. Edgar Hoover, the first Director of the FBI, and highlights the importance of an article in which Tesla speaks of the death ray and its 'Crucial Importance' for future warfare and it was recommended that Tesla constantly remained under constant surveillance in order to protect him from 'Foreign Enemies' who may also have an interest in the secret of such an invaluable instrument of war and defence with free energy, and wireless electricity and with the help of funding from JP Morgan, Tesla successfully built and tested the famous Wardenclyffe Tower. This structure was a massive wireless energy transmission station which, according to Tesla, had the ability to transmit wireless power across great distances so Tesla saw the Wardenclyffe Tower as the beginning of a massive free energy project and Tesla wanted to use the tower not only to transmit free energy but to send out messages, telephone calls across the Earth. Since the direction of propagation radiates from the earth, the so-called force of gravity is toward earth and his theories were based on the Idea that our planet had the ability to conduct the signals so using a number of different towers, Tesla could have made the idea work. But as we have learned through history, the idea of 'Free Energy' isn't really welcomed by big corporations as why would they ever give free energy to the masses when you can make the masses pay big time?

So eventually, Tesla's funding was cancelled, and the tower was destroyed, along with Tesla's ideas of a world powered by free energy.When looking at Tesla's Oscillator, this device was an electromechanical apparatus patented by Tesla in 1893 and the device was popularly known as Tesla's Earthquake machine after the European inventor claimed that one version of his device caused an Earthquake in New York in 1898 so today we have similar incidents like the recent Turkey earthquake as BioEngineering weather events which will happen more frequently as they blame it on climate change and the need for the lock-down 15 minute cities you all being played as they the elite play everyone they can and in other words, the device could allegedly simulate earthquakes, which meant it could be and is weaponized. We conspiracy theorists are convinced that Tesla's technology was later further developed and is being used by HAARP which is an acronym that stands for High Frequency Active Auroral Research Program and the technology can affect weather patterns, cause earthquakes, disrupt electronic communications and affect the 'Brain waves in people' and. is a very secret military program. We actually know very little about it and what we do know is quite technical and very difficult to understand and what I hope to do is to take a little of the mystery out of haarp so that you might understand what our governments worldwide are doing and how his technology could affect you. The technology for haarp was actually invented by Nicola Tesla about 100 years ago and understanding that it works by sending radio waves into the ionosphere in order to move the jet stream and affect the weather patterns and when using these radios waves are directed into the earth; they can also cause earthquakes. 250 One of the tell tale signs that an that an earthquake or tsunami was caused by a haarp is that the sky will glow with a lavender hue right before it happens and also the Russians have a haarp that makes a noise like a woodpecker when it is activated, and these radio waves are like sound waves and we are all familiar with an opera singer that hits the high note and can shatter a glass so haarp works in much the same way, the beams are projected either out into the atmosphere to move clouds or the jet stream causing rain in one area and a drought in another or right down into the earth crust causing vibrations that can trigger an Earthquake. So naturally any area that already has fault zones is especially susceptible and furthermore, not only does haarp affect the weather and cause earthquakes but it can knock-out electronic communications which could be devastating alone but it also can affect people directly because haarp can cause people to think that they are hearing voices, affect their moods and it can also render aggressive populations harmless. Haarp works by heating up the ionosphere so when this does occur it then causes holes in the ionosphere allowing harmful radiation from the sun onto the earth and the NWO totally understand and get how radiation is such a powerful weapon truly to them. What can result from this is anyone's guess but I'm really sure it won't be any good so the reasons why I have **highlighted Tesla in this Chapter** and some of his inventions and we will very likely will see more of these events like in 2023. Speculations about HAARP triggering the recent massive earthquakes in Turkey and Syria have surfaced on social media and sadly the 7.8-magnitude quake earthquakes have left more than 3,800 people dead and thousands injured, and it is not the first time haarp has been accused of causing an earthquake. NBC News reported that in 2010, Venezuelan leader Hugo Chavez had claimed that haarp or a program like it triggered the Haiti Earthquake.

We will move on to what is Tesla's **Futuristic Aircraft** in addition to creating devices that could potentially be used as weapons, and structures that could offer Free Energy to the world, Nikola Tesla also worked on electrically powered airships that, according to reports, could transport passengers from New York to London in around three hours and these aircraft were not ordinary vehicles as they were supposedly able to harness energy right from Earth's atmosphere and would have had no need ever to stop and refuel. But why have aircraft that make use of free energy, if billions can be made by selling it?

Drones in 1898 More than a hundred years ago, Tesla invented Drones so everyone who thinks that drones are actually a product of recent technologies, you would be very wrong because it was called Tesla's **Telluamton** and think about that is that the government had this technology in their possession for over a hundred years, so naturally it raises a number of questions. Is it possible that they adopted, further developed, and used 'drones' more than half a decade ago? because anything is possible with them. "Be it known that I, Nikola Tesla a citizen of the United States, residing at New York, in the county and State of New York, have invented certain new and useful improvements in methods of and apparatus for controlling from a distance the operation of the propelling engines, the steering apparatus, and other mechanism carried by moving bodies or floating vessels, of which the following a specification, reference being had to the drawings accompanying and forming part of the same "The invention which I have described will prove useful in many ways. Vessels or Vehicles of any suitable kind may be used, like life, dispatch, or pilot boats or the like, or for carrying letters, packages, provisions, instruments, objects, or materials of any description, for establishing communication with inaccessible regions and exploring the conditions existing in the same, for killing or capturing whales or other animals of the sea, and for many other scientific, engineering, or commercial purposes; but the greatest value of my invention will result from its effect upon warfare and armaments, by   reason for its certain and unlimited destructiveness will tend to bring about and maintain permanent peace among nations." While we discussed something similar in Tesla's UFO, the truth is that he went beyond flying objects and in an unpublished article of Man's Greatest Achievement, Tesla outlined his Dynamic Theory of Gravity saying that 'luminiferous ether fills all space' and Tesla said that the ether is acted upon by the life-giving creative force. The ether is thrown into "infinitesimal whirls" ("micro helices") at near the speed of light, becoming ponderable matter. Then, the force subsides and motion ceases, matter reverts to the ether (a form of "atomic decay").

Mankind can harness these processes, to Precipitate matter from the ether and create whatever he wants with the matter, and energy derived-alter the earth's size, control earth's seasons (weather control) to guide earth's path through the Universe, like a spaceship and cause the collisions of planets to produce new suns and stars, heat, and light originate and develop life in infinite forms not only did the so called Illuminati produce new suns and stars, heat, and light originate Industrialist-Banking Cabal) steal this "aether physics"-technology, they also changed the "human knowledge of physics", replacing the knowledge of this aether-cosmos with Einstein's theories, now promoted everywhere.

To name a few **benefiting from this theft**, they were J P Morgan (Banking, Energy, Railroads, US Steel) Edison & General Electric Oil & Energy, Railroads, Aviation, War Industrials, Banking) Rockefellers (Oil, Banking, Nazi connections through IG Farben) Rothschilds (Banking, Oil & Natural Resources had connections to Kuhn Loeb & company through Jacob Schiff) Ford motors Motors, War Industrials) Brown Brothers Harriman & Co (Banking, Shipyards, Railroads, IG Farben) Du Ponts (Chemicals & War Industrials. **Poisoning the whole world** with these vaccines is not really a first and has been done before and by the chemical PFOA, formerly used in the manufacturing of DuPont's Teflon, a lot you might remember there Teflon frying pans that nearly everyone had in their kitchen and even here in Australia, but it was Dupont and the chemical Perfluorooctanoic Acid (PFOA) that was used in non-stick Teflon pans up until 2015, and has since been linked to many diseases such as breast cancer, prostate cancer, liver tumours and reduced fertility. This chemical was found to build in people's bodies over time and so daily use was eventually seen as an unacceptable risk. Teflon has also been linked to giving people short term flu-like symptoms and headaches, known as polymer fume fever and this is due to the gases released when heating the frying pans.

Manufacturers have said this isn't possible due to the 375C temperatures the pans undergo when they are made, but many still report feeling unwell especially with even the new pans so buyer beware and these fumes are also very dangerous to birds, as they breathe rapidly. Also, many people are still using non-stick pans even after they have become damaged and begin to 'flake off' and you really don't want to be eating plastic in your food as that has been linked to so many health problems. It might not be an immediate health risk swallowing a tiny amount of non-stick coating every day, but when it's best to minimise your possible risks why wouldn't you? Teflon has now been reformulated since the 2015 restrictions, but there are still concerns about the chemicals used. Considering it took over 40 years and manufacturers are not always transparent about what is in their coating the "safer" replacement could be just as harmful if not worse, DuPont began phasing out the use of PFOA (also known as C8) in 2005, after it was revealed that the company had for decades covered up the numerous health risks associated with the chemical so this revelation led to a record $16.5 million fine being levied by the EPA, and a $300 million class-action lawsuit filed by residents living near a West Virginia DuPont factory, after being poisoned by the PFOA that had contaminated the local water supply. PFOA is part of a family of substances known as PFCs (perfluorinated chemicals. There is an interesting movie 'Dark Waters' it's a 2019 American legal thriller film directed by Todd Haynes and written by Mario Correa and Matthew Michael Carnahan. This story dramatises Robert Bilott's case against the chemical manufacturing corporation DuPont after they contaminated a town with unregulated chemicals and the brave actions of a good guy to expose this and aside from causing cancer, PFOA has also been linked to hormone disruption, heart disease and other serious health problems.

President Obama declassified some of the CIA files, including those relating to scientist and inventor, Nikola Tesla. Their existence had been denied for decades but why were they hiding "In the Interest of National Security" any but by hiding this technology "For National Security "reasons has possibly cost humanity trillions and trillions of dollars and wrecked the health of humanity and of the planet. Sadly, Nikola Tesla died in New York 1943, the world seemed to forget him after he had spent most of his money, Tesla lived in a series of New York hotels, leaving behind unpaid bills and what a travesty that this great man had to leave this planet not really understanding the genius he was about to become and Tesla died a broke humanitarian. Tesla did what he did for the betterment of humanity, to help people have a better quality of life, and people have commented that he never seemed to be interested in monetary gain and a possible downside of that was he never seemed to have enough money to do what he needed to do.

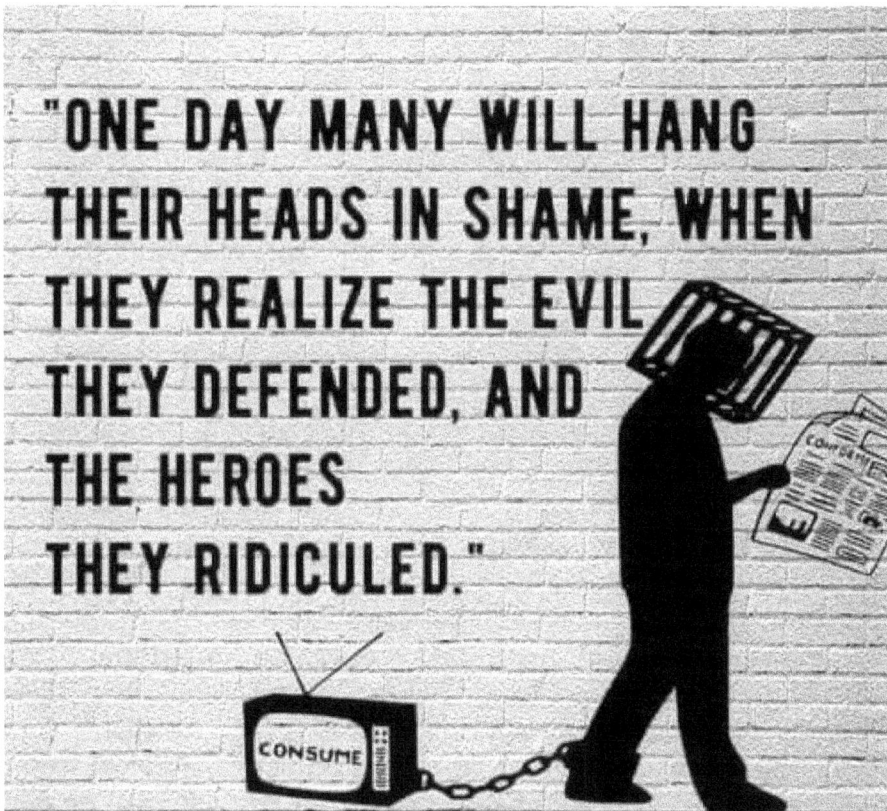
"ONE DAY MANY WILL HANG THEIR HEADS IN SHAME, WHEN THEY REALIZE THE EVIL THEY DEFENDED, AND THE HEROES THEY RIDICULED."

Chapter 23

Businesses That Did Not Discriminate

When the Lockdowns started in Australia in 2021, it was very hard on all of us the Unvaccinated (The Pure Bloods). We were the new Jews, the new unclean deemed a danger to humanity and ourselves because of the miss-conceptions that we were not protecting ourselves and others. This has since been proven to be all based on lies created by the drug companies and Governments, who were all in on this World Genocidal Plandemic Agenda. But sadly, a lot of businesses brought into this Agenda and had the signs as they had to abide by legally regarding checking in, but some regulated it to such an extent they were sending all of us they regarded as the unclean a message, and any of you reading this who did that shame on you. In an earlier chapter you would have already read about how "The Mon Como" which is a major hotel here in Redcliffe Queensland, and the incident and the assault on Martina Batovska on January 11th, 2021, which affected her so much that it ended in tragedy of her falling to her death aged 40. There is a police report of that assault on her by one of the managers, which I lodged at Redcliffe Police Station a few days after her death. Mon Como was very much involved in policing the mandate laws very vigorously and a few of you reading this would have your own stories of this establishment but at least we can vote with our feet. But how many other people also suffered similar assaults, and, discrimination, we all have seen the footage of arrests of business owners who would not buy into this tyranny with the divide and conquer by the powers that be because they could, which will be a stain on them forever. Another business that should hold their head in shame is the Two Dollar Charity Shop, Sutton Street, Redcliffe. This draconian business was mentioned to me a lot as a "Bad Egg". I was physically removed from this store even though I had mentioned I had a mask exception by the different barista clown and all I wanted to do was buy a coffee.

One friend of mine Lee was charged in this store by the Redcliffe Police and the stress caused him heart issues. He is 70 years of age and in 2022 the police dropped the charges. It's a total travesty that things like this are allowed to happen. It was total madness due to the owner's lack of training of some of her staff in basic human kindness. It should be highlighted that some businesses were dictatorial and Un-Australian and interestingly as we have long memories we do not support them anymore and since then some have struggled. But this chapter is to mainly highlight the ""Good Guys"" businesses that just treated everyone equally with respect and dignity in my hometown on the Redcliffe Peninsula, and also Sandgate, that I frequent on my bike rides and that I was personally able to live my life as normally as I needed and to them all I salute you and thank you. So, these are the places I frequented the most in those manic days of lockdowns, mask wearing and checking in.

OASIS CAFE Oasis On The Esplanade | Redcliffe QLD | Facebook

Without doubt it is one of my favourites and it is owned by Steve and Zooki and I am proud to call them my friends. They treated me during lockdowns and today with respect and love and they are thriving, as I think most normal citizens noticed their passion to treat us all equally. An added bonus is that their food is superb.

 Salt Shop | Redcliffe QLD | Facebook

 Another coffee shop that was very nice to me in the lockdowns and for that thank you.

Cafe Bohemia Sandgate | Brisbane QLD | Facebook

When I ride over to Sandgate Qld I often pop in here very funky and Sandra also very special.

Mary's Cuppa and Treats | Facebook(1)

This is my favourite place to go as it's so well done and great service with a smile .Mary the owner is a pure delight.

73 & Baker Lifestyle Pantry (facebook.com)

Yet another great place I sometimes visit.

Drift Coffee Company | Scarborough QLD | Facebook

So many great places in Scarborough and this is worth checking out.

Bazil&Co. Cafe and Bakery | Bazil&Co. (bazilandcobakery.com.au)

Yet another great place in Scarborough with superb food.

Cafe Diversity

Paul & Suzzane kindly wrote this please feel free to pop in for a coffee and cake deal of $10 or just to say hello. When we bought this business many moons ago we did not expect to be Government Policemen and to stop and prevent customers entering our establishment & refusing to take their order because they chose not to inject themselves with an untested vaccine. I don't intend to be negative but & tell you the whole story of forced mandates & lockdowns and policing, 1 person every 4 metres, enough said. I do believe we live in a beautiful country and Cafe Diversity has one of the best views of the ocean and sea breeze in your face as you hopefully enjoy one of these perfect meals. All of us Aussies have a safe country and enjoy our lives together with beautiful people and a fine example is the Rainbow Man hair and harmonica in hand with an aura to match. Be kind, be friendly & smile a lot to your fellow travellers as we spin around the universe at almost 5000 miles an hour kind regards Paul and Suzzane.

Simply Organic Hair | Redcliffe QLD | Facebook

My hairdresser and simply the very best.

Made by Me Designs | Clontarf QLD | Facebook

One of the great crystal shops and has lots of shungite.

Kezzy's Emporium | Redcliffe QLD | Facebook

Another great shop is an Aladdin's cave. **This book** will be stocked here. One of my very favourite shops with so much great energy in there. Check it out and with all of these businesses please use Cash.

Ironwood Cottage | Brisbane QLD | Facebook

This is a must visit as everything you will need mentioned in my detox chapter she will have and the owner really switched on to be able to help you.

WWW.innerbalanceph.com

Go meet Karyn. If you need help with Royal jelly balms you also find her at the local markets.

There would have been so many more shops and businesses that I did not get to who also were very kind and respectful to you all in these manic days of lockdowns that must go down in infamy all created for the damage we are all now seeing and if you complied you brought it on yourself. One local business that was kind just went bankrupt and the owner said we took two vaccines to not go broke but gone broke anyway. They seem fine so hopefully they both dodged a bullet, and they got the placebo and best wishes to them.

Chapter 24

The Damage That Mandating Did

We all heard the stories of friends and family members who would never ever take these vaccines, and some had to pay a very heavy price in losing the jobs that they loved, and some have family members they loved because they do not believe and think we are conspiracy theorists who have ostracised them. So, this chapter will feature a few true stories of normal people and their stories. But what is a Conspiracy Theory, is an explanation for an event or situation that asserts the existence of a conspiracy by powerful and sinister groups, often political in motivation when other explanations are more probable. The term generally has a negative connotation, implying that the appeal of a conspiracy theory is based in prejudice, emotional conviction, or insufficient evidence. Three years on everything we had predicted as 100% come true and now people are dropping like flies, so what was the catalyst to cause that? Well simply it is the vaccines they are and never were that anything but a Bio-Weapon, created for the results they are getting currently, and the Plandamic is working just great for all the ones behind it worldwide, how many pensions do they not have to pay for anymore, the elderly and that is some of you reading this if you over 65 are the first intended lot of casualties, then aboriginals, disadvantaged and disabled. If you are working and have a use then your use by date will be deferred depending on how much you comply but the more jabs you take will be your ultimate catalyst, and as this tragedy unfolds it is going to get so much worse. If you are not awake today after over 3 years of being lied to, sadly you probably never will wake upland if you have spent 3 years trying to wake up your friends and family members as it is unconditional love and you are still wasting oxygen and they will not detox or help themselves then have a Plan B. We will not give up on any of them and I will do it by stealth and if you got an ice maker put in the detoxes and most important NAC and Colloidal Gold for a start and camouflage it very well with orange juice If they drink it then you might over a period see an improvement in them, things like they seem more energetic, less tired and not yawning so much and little things you will have noticed like this give you clues that they're not as well as they pretend to be, they're not going to admit to their mum, dad, sisters, brothers and their friends that maybe they made a big mistake and what is worrying them. No one likes to be wrong especially family when they have ostracised you and treated you badly and now they understand you were correct all along. The guilt they will be feeling will be very painful to some, especially if they do not let you see your grandchildren or treat you like you were a pariah.

I will try to keep my own story brief and from day dot I knew in my heart this Covid-19 was not what it seemed, and then I have tried to speak out at common law events to warn people of what is coming, I wrote about it in my book 'John Warren Our Soul Music Journey's in 2021, and I was hoping to write a manuscript for a movie from the chapter in one of my books about Marc Bolan, which would have meant me flying to Sierra Leone, to interview Gloria Jones, she was the singer of the original version of The Soft Cell, hit 'Tainted Love'. and that never happened as I would not get on any aeroplane at this moment in time, and likely never will. I then tried to help Kelly Guenoun in the federal election in 2022 and we had hoped that would turn things around but because of the voting system that never was going to happen. My family members around the world in the majority complied and had this vaccine. It was their body their choice, but I wished they studied it more before they had put it in their bodies. The fact they did not saddens me and I have also lost so many friends, because I am a conspiracy theorist Truth Seeker. I spent so much time and energy on the Soul music scene and enjoyed being around like-minded people until this Plandemic Agenda hit the world most lovers of Soul music and especially in a genre called Northern Soul are from the ages 60-80 yrs old, some started at the Twisted Wheel in

Manchester in the 1960's, and most of the rest attended Wigan Casino Casino and the Blackpool Mecca and were some nicest people you would ever meet but sadly most would become compliant sheep. Especially here in Australia and I became ostracised and "I walked Away" from their sheeple droppings but have they learned the hard way with some on their 5 clot shot's them passing away in droves some might say they are old, but trust me what has caused it is this vaccines. If you had 3 vaccines or more you might very well be next, unless you really try to fix the damage they have caused your bodies and hopefully any reading can try to fix the damage as hearing they passed away too soon is very sad. So, all the soul venues around the world and especially here in Australia who treated us badly are a disgrace to the soul scene and you did not "Keep the Faith" and that shame should be on you forever. You all know who you are but cannot waste my time on you. I have tried interviewing ordinary people who are my friends and most are given pen names but all these stories are true of the effects the mandates did to some The Pure Bloods.

Today I interviewed a passionate man I'm A Centrist Moderate in Redcliffe Qld. He is aged 65 and he has had a few mental issues due to this total Plandemic, before it he was very active in the community in Mens Sheds' and had formed relationships for over 10 years. You might be aware men's sheds are often ex retired and then do the Mens Walks. Due to the dynamics of age and intellect most are vaccinated, and some are on stab number 5. I am aware there have been more than a few heart attacks among them, but it will not be because of the vaccines in their eyes. Well due to my mate not conforming and not getting vaccinated his friendship with the "sheeple" has gone forever and we often find that we are a danger to them. The lad is a diamond ultra intelligent and very switched on and I am proud to call him a mate and when reading this mate, you will be fine, it's their loss not yours. He is still involved in the Burpengary Mens Shed Moreton Bay Safe Communities which is very well run and I have attended myself as so many freedom fighters go there.Well done to all the team who run it. They have had so many guest speakers. Back to my mate's story he is also a big supporter of Pauline Anson's One nation Party, and has been involved in Politics for over 40 years with mostly freedom parties like the Liberal Democrats. He spoke that the local elections here in the Moreton Bay Region, and that be followed up by the Qld State Elections will be very instrumental in what happens especially with regards the 2030 Agenda, because he agrees with me that we are on a knife's edge and the 90% reduction in population might happen. We both agreed that this Spiritual War is an end game especially if we were to lose which we will not, he agreed the next 2 years will be very daunting for all and I am also preparing to go off grid as myself. The countdown of this book is my final goodbye as my gut feeling is that a smart city looms. My mate also mentioned he might buy a boat as there are several freedom fighters who live on boats, and some live at Scarborough Marina.

We talked about Gold and Silver and also, he wanted to get a little amount as Silver is well undervalued as a hedge when this house of cards falls as it will and as they plan it to. He was aware and spoke how much the media played in all of this and of course how they will continue to do so as propaganda will keep this illusion going a lot longer. He said people are waking up that is true dependent on how unaffected they are with this poison that is in their body's. Fear is everywhere, interest is not stopping anytime soon and he is very aware of China and their intentions on becoming the number 1 power and there is no coincidence that their military might not be as vaxxed as you are led to believe. He believes China could invade at some point and I think a lot of Australians must be aware that high vaccination rates make us very weak in the scheme of things and the USA sure will not help as it can look at the Ukraine and weapons alone are not going to help us. I think he spot on with a lots of his views sadly but we are realists as more information is coming out daily that this pandemic agenda was always a scamdemic played on most of you and there are no winners.

The lady I interviewed next, let's call her 'Daisy'. She is 49 years of age, and she grew up on a farm in country Victoria not far from the Golden Valley. She was used to a life of not having much and her family meeting a lot of their needs from the land, including having a good supply of eggs, meat, goats milk and others. Her Mum used to spin wool for clothes, from the sheep they sheared. I also did that in Tasmania, so we had a lot in common.

Daisy left home at 17 and started her first degree then moved up to live in Queensland as she always had a desire to live in a warmer climate, hence her living here in Queensland. I had met Daisy when working with the Australian party in the 2022 elections. So, I asked Daisy what the impact of the last years has done to her, and she said, before this Plandemic she had worked at Yourtown for 7 years. Most of her career at yortown was in Kids Helpline working shift work as a telephone/online counsellor and online facilitator for a peer support program called Circles. Kids Helpline offers support and counselling for children aged 5 years - 25 years.

She was a remote worker, working fully at home prior to the pandemic. Kids Helpline at that time, employed over 230 staff with many staff working from home. She supported young people who were struggling with gender disorientation, eating disorders, mental health issues, grief, bullying, Internet cyber bullying, domestic violence, suicidal ideation, self harm, rape, sexual abuse, relationship difficulties and breakups. The list as you could imagine was endless. Daisy loved her job and wanted to stay working there for the rest of her life.

During the pandemic she worked as a remote worker at home and many staff were requested to continue to do this to protect staff members from contracting covid. After a while staff were instructed to come in to work in the office one day per week. This occurred when the organisation started to formulate a vaccination policy, and informed staff there would be a survey to consult with staff about implementing this type of policy.

During her work with the children counselling and in the peer support forum Daisy began noticing things on a level of frequency she had never seen before in her clients. In the past she'd occasionally speak to clients or notice in the forum of clients feeling unwell or struggling with chronic health issues, however with the rollout of the covid vaccinations she noticed an increase in the frequency of physical complaints brought up by the children and discussed in the forum.

Children complained about constant headaches, brain fog, nausea, fainting spells and hitting their head after fainting, dizziness, being more forgetful, aches and pains that were unexplained, being more forgetful, fatigue and sleeping more often than they used to, migraines and nosebleeds. She was talking to children and young adults who had 1-2 vaccines of Pfizer or the other vaccines, and who had been vaccinated encouraged by their parents but there were also a lot who had done it without parental consent because of peer pressure. This is an important point as with cyberbullying and the pressure of your friends you can make choices that you wouldn't otherwise make or that can be harmful for your health.

Daisy had noticed that many of the other staff considered being vaccinated as a badge of honour and encouraged the vaccination programs in the forum and in their sessions with clients. They were encouraged to support the children to comply with the vaccination program for 'the good of everyone', even though as a counsellor they were usually encouraged to support the rights of clients to make their own choices within their lives and encourage self determination, as well as not putting their own opinions on to clients.

This all went out the window when the vaccines were introduced.She noticed a big difference in staff attitudes towards children and adults who were making a choice not to be injected with the covid vaccinations and she felt like she had to keep her own status a secret as a lot of the staff expressed discriminatory attitudes towards those who had not been vaccinated. She also found the sharing of private medical information odd as this was usually something that was kept private. Daisy said she had to be on her guard and that I could only imagine would have a mental impact as people in a normal scenario these types of choices were usually respected, and please remember her work colleges are all counsellors. Daisy worked part time, so she kept her mental health healthy by lots of self care and supportive people around her, as well as connecting with nature regularly to keep herself grounded.

The Company line on vaccinations was that getting a covid vaccination was 'the right thing to do' and this mandate is still in place at the publishing of this book, even though many other organisations have dropped these mandates. When her company was formulating their policy to implement the mandate, they conducted a staff survey on views and for the first time a survey was not to be done anonymously. All staff's names were connected to their feedback. Only a third of the staff completed the survey and the mandate was implemented based on 75% of a third of staff saying yes to a mandate at yourtown. Daisy had noticed a great change in her work place environment since the rollout of the vaccines including, lots of coercion, a toxic work environment and she started to not feel safe.

Prior to the plandemic she and her work colleagues worked harmoniously together, and it was very supportive of everyone and their health choices. With the pandemic and the rollout of the vaccines, this all changed, and staff were mandated to comply with being vaccinated with an experimental provisionally approved new vaccine. With the pandemic and the rollout of the vaccines, this all changed and staff were mandated to comply with being vaccinated with an experimental provisionally approved new vaccine.

Daisy was sacked from her workplace for not being injected with a covid vaccination and removed from her role as a remote counsellor.

She was required to send back her work laptop and was not allowed back in the company building. A year later as this is being written, Daisy who now works with the public daily and still has not contracted covid. Family members who are also not vaccinated have not contracted it either, even working daily with the public.

Daisy now runs her own business. She has had to go without a lot in the past year and still doesn't have an income. Her husband still supports them both, while she builds up her business. She still misses her previous work at Kids Helpline supporting children and wishes she could be there for them, especially those who have no voice or rights and no one to advocate for their rights. However, if she had to make the choice again, she would make the choice to be sacked from this workplace.

She would prefer to be poor and in good health and be able to be there to support her family, rather than be experiencing the ongoing fear that she could 'die suddenly' or be suffering from an adverse reaction from having a covid vaccine. She is also very grateful that she could help protect some of her family from having these vaccines and that they are in continued good health as well.

Daisy also commented about the ongoing impact of shedding from the covid vaccinations and working in the public since being sacked from her workplace, she used to experience daily headaches, brain fog, migraines, eye strain, forgetfulness and aches and pains that would ease by the following morning. Her health is generally good, with no issues so these symptoms were new to her. I gave her a shungite necklace that she wears every day at work and she has other crystals near her in her business and she deserves every success as she is one of the best people you could ever wish to meet , bless.

Today I got to interview a man and a women who are Jehovah's witnesses and the both delightful honest and usually when trying interview someone of faith the temperature tends to drop over my thought processes especially over life after death but both these today had lost mothers and other loved ones so they seemed open and less judgemental even though they both had 4 vaccines and apparently all Jehovah's witnesses are jabbed and reconciled to that fact quoting the bible. On the Jehovah website J.W. Org, No. Jehovah's Witnesses are not opposed to vaccination and we view vaccination as a personal decision for each Christian to make. Many of Jehovah's Witnesses choose to get vaccinated. We seek quality medical care and appreciate the many advancements of medical science to reduce the risk of serious illness. We are grateful for the commitment and dedication of health-care professionals, especially in times of crises. Jehovah's Witnesses cooperate with public health officials. For example, since the COVID-19 pandemic broke out, Jehovah's Witnesses have continued to publish reminders in hundreds of languages on this website, encouraging adherence to local safety guidelines. These include the importance of physical distance and of following regulations on public gatherings, quarantining, hand washing, and the wearing of face coverings as well as other practical measures required or recommended by the authorities. We seek medical treatment because we place a high value on life Acts 17:28. "Witnesses avail themselves of the fact that vaccinating is something for personal decision." them with their health problems. They love life and want to do whatever is reasonable and Scriptural to prolong it. "The Watchtower, July 1, 1975 "Jehovah's Witnesses gladly accept medicine and medical treatment. They want to maintain good health and to prolong life. In fact, like the first-century Christian Luke, some of Jehovah's Witnesses are physicians. Jehovah's Witnesses certainly appreciate the hard work and dedication of those who provide medical care. They are also grateful for the welcome relief from illness that those individuals provide. "The Watchtower, February 1, 2011.

For me reading all of the above is confusing so you don't accept blood transfusions but sit on the fence regarding vaccinating children so your child could die for your beliefs yet you then vaccinate your child for a cold the logic of that is mind blowing but to be fair the penny turned as I would predict most pure bloods would not accept blood transfusions. I have met and talked to some very lovely JW'S who are kind and loving. We should not judge them all as we are all perfectly-imperfect and only god can judge us.

Regarding blood I also took this from their website. Myth: Jehovah's Witnesses don't believe in medicine or medical treatment Fact: We seek the best possible medical care for ourselves and our families. When we have health problems, we go to doctors who have skill in providing medical and surgical care without blood. We appreciate advancements that have been made in the medical field. In fact, bloodless treatments developed to help Witness patients are now being used to benefit all in the community. In many countries, any patient can now choose to avoid blood-transfusion risks, such as blood-borne diseases, immune-system reactions, and human errors. Again, I find this bothersome and borders so contradictory that the vaccines are no different in the sense they do change one's DNA and the blood is affected by poisons like Graphene Oxide to the point you'll never be the same again. I asked this couple other questions and they showed me a video of their meetings which was very slick, no pressure to donate and in the service, they have a Q & A session. I noticed how well dressed they always seem to be wearing their Sunday best. I asked them about Ukraine, and I got the usual brainwashed answer that most who are vaccinated tend to repeat but I find no point in pushing their buttons. Interesting though Jehovahs don't believe in voting which again I find very confusing. Some comply with vaccines yet will not try to change the world by voting and I also asked them about Freemasons, and they had no thoughts on that topic. Interestingly though they seem to understand the TV is something to switch off. So if I was to attend a church I would and will make a visit. Love and blessings to all.

I next interviewed an Ex-Airline Stewardess a beautiful lady who has been greatly affected by this Plandemic like so many who lost jobs they lost, and let's call her ''Eyes '' because she has the most beautiful eyes, I have ever seen in any other human being I have met and she is from a far, far off world of another planetary system. About 18 months ago in 2021, I was riding my bike playing my harmonica on a Sunday, when the lady with the eyes stopped me and we got chatting and connected on a Spiritual level.

She was working as an airline stewardess for Alliance air and was really struggling because of their mandating policies and also because she was an active freedom fighter. One day after I only known her for only about 2 months I bumped into her again and she looked so very radiant and also very happy because she was pregnant which always was one her dreams, but that pregnancy which should have been one the happiest moments of her life at aged 41, was overshadowed by the policies of Alliance Air and her industry in general, so the risk to her baby boy would be put at risk if she had ever got vaccinated which she would never ever do anyway.

New research published in the New England Journal of Medicine inadvertently revealed that as many as 82 percent of pregnant women who get "vaccinated" for the Wuhan coronavirus (Covid-19) end up suffering a miscarriage n its Entitled, "Preliminary Findings of mRNA Covid-19 Vaccine Safety in Pregnant Persons," the paper contends with its words that there are "no obvious safety signals among pregnant [women] who received Covid-19 vaccines." However, a table published as part of the study shows that the vast majority of pregnant women who get injected never end up delivering a live baby. The study specifically looked at the mRNA (messenger RNA) jabs from Pfizer-BioNTech and Moderna, which are the two most widely administered Chinese Virus injections in the country. Deceptively, the research makes a more prominent claim that and the way the paper is presented makes it seem like there are no problems with the injections.

278

It takes a careful eye to look more closely at the data, which is what one British oncology researcher did to come to a much different conclusion. "The researchers inexplicably subsumed the first trimester spontaneous abortions before, and including, 20 weeks into the completed pregnancy and losses as a whole 104 [miscarriages] out of 827 pregnancies," she reportedly wrote to two prominent British doctors." However, since the aim was to discover whether Covid vaccination had any adverse effects in the different trimesters, the NEJM papers' authors should have deducted the 700 women who were not actually vaccinated until the third trimester from the total through.

So much trauma as "Eyes" suffered from anxiety anyway, it is part of her body makeup as a lot of you reading this would relate to and empathise with her and that condition. The baby boy was born healthy and is currently 10 months old, he is a very bonny lad and is totally free of all vaccinations and I already mentioned we feel that vaccinating babies is a rabbit hole you should not go down. When you see this bonny lad, let's call him "Hope" he is so full of life but calm and sees everything and is extremely spiritual and it is very possible he came back into "Eyes" life as her son for a reason that becomes clear as the years progress because they been together before and she very aware of that. On a very rare occasion I meet someone like "Eyes" who I quickly understood I have met before but such a long time ago, going all the way back to Cadiz Spain in 1510, and this present life with eyes is number 3, and we always be friends on a platonic level as there is no chemistry in this timeline but I do love her dearly, and when you meet soul mates like this, it is for "Life" and you will not and cannot cut the cord even if you wanted to. Unvaccinated mothers and unvaccinated children who are so very lucky to have been born to parents with high principles should not ever be discriminated against for their moral beliefs, but they are because the Queensland Government does discriminate, so let's look at this important topic and highlight mothers like Eyes who are truly intellectual and very savvy about this. US evidence shows that the

Centres for Disease Control, the Department of Health and Human Services and the National Institute of Health refuse to conduct any study comparing the unvaccinated child to his and her peers. While HHS is legally obligated to conduct safety studies every two years and report to Congress in accordance with the 1986 National Childhood Vaccine Injury Act, it was admitted in a 2018 court ruling that none of these vaccine safety studies were ever conducted over a thirty year span can you believe that and the very obvious reasons why they will not do studies there are culpable because they are aware of the real truths. This Medical Fraud has enabled the rise of a predatory vaccine industry and a growing number of recommended childhood vaccinations. However, as childhood vaccinations increase, the health of American children has not improved in the past thirty years and respiratory infections are rampant. Visits to the paediatrician have skyrocketed, with chronic health issues becoming a normal way of life for many and a whopping 54 percent of children and young adults in the U.S. now suffer from chronic illnesses that lead to life-long pharmaceutical prescriptions. This such an important topic especially considering mRNA poison is currently put in all vaccines and another reason anyone reading this should not do this to your newborn. I have other friends who have taken this stance and even my85 year old mother Lillian (Lil) in Rushden Northants, was not vaccinated as a child and to my grandfather who left way too early in his50's, you are a legend x because although my mother has had multiple cancers over many decades she is still with us thankfully, so is there a linkage of her longevity and that she was not vaccinated as a child I truly believe so. Ten-year studies have found that unvaccinated children are healthier in several metrics and enjoy 25 times fewer paediatric visits and also a new study published in the International Journal of Environmental Research. It's not really " Rocket Science" if you got a modicum of savviness about innate childhood immunity. As the rate of vaccination increases, so do chronic health issues such as asthma, allergic rhinitis, respiratory infections, eczema and a host of other health problems. The study, titled, "Relative Incidence of Office Visits and cumulative Rates of Billed Diagnoses Along the Axis of Vaccination" shows how childhood vaccination causes an increasing number of paediatric visits and an influx of diagnoses. The research followed 3,300 paediatric patients for ten years and was conducted at Integrative Pediatric, a paediatrics practice in Oregon run by Dr. Paul Thomas, M.D and during this very important study, Thomas's paediatric practice prioritised the parental decision process and followed the informed consent doctrine of the American Medical Association.

This plan allows parents to stop or delay vaccination if vaccine injuries were present and not every child processes vaccine ingredients in the same way; conditions like eczema, developmental delay, allergies, or autoimmune conditions are typical signs that their body is unable to process the vaccines. Dr.Thomas's practice contained the perfect mix of children who ranged from being unvaccinated to partially vaccinated to fully vaccinated per the CDC's guidelines. So, the study also found that the unvaccinated child shows fewer signs of respiratory infections and fewer fevers at well-child visits. It is very surprising to me that the unvaccinated child required twenty-five times less paediatric care over a ten-year span. The CDC pushes **for 70 doses of 16 vaccines** on a child before they reach the age of 18. Please stop and think about that and try to change your thinking as you've been totally played. Children who did receive 90 to 95 percent of the CDC-recommended vaccines for their age group were about 25 times more likely to see the paediatrician than the unvaccinated group.Vaccinated children (with a family history of autoimmune issues) suffer more compared to their unvaccinated peers and an important feature of this study was Dr. Yehuda Shoenfeld's work, which singled out a predisposition to vaccine injury called autoimmune syndrome induced by adjuvants so if there is family history of autoimmunity. Children who get vaccinated are more likely to suffer from ear infections, asthma, allergies and skin rashes, when compared to the unvaccinated who also share the same family history of autoimmune issues.

The aluminium adjuvant and the other various chemicals in the vaccine may turn on the genes that enable autoimmune issues and the family history of disease is important in determining whether vaccines should be used in the child. Vaccinated children are up to six times more likely to suffer from anaemia, allergies, sinusitis and asthma and the most concerning aspect of the study was the rise in chronic health issues among the vaccinated children. The vaccinated were also 70 percent more likely to suffer from various respiratory infections compared to the unvaccinated so do the vaccines. Vaccinated children face a 3,000% increase in allergic rhinitis and no ADHD in the unvaccinated but as vaccination uptake increased, ADHD and behavioural issues increased. Strangely, a quarter percent of the vaccinated were diagnosed with infections that the vaccines were supposed to prevent, including chicken pox or whooping cough and you are very likely going to find a similar pattern in children who **had 3 mrNA poisons.** A slight uptick in chicken pox and whooping cough was observed in the unvaccinated, but they all recovered and gained lifelong immunity to the infections. Predictably, there were no cases of measles, mumps, rubella, tetanus, hepatitis, or any other vaccine targeted infection for the children who were vaccinated and surprisingly, there were also no cases of these infections in the unvaccinated during the entire 10 year study period.

This brings up the question: **Are vaccines even necessary, or do they impose a burden of unnecessary harm to children**? As there all mRNA poisons in them all soon. So back to the story of 'Eyes' because she and her son and so many like her are being discriminated against on the basis of a moral objection that they do not as the research proves that vaccinating children is not prudent and has been proven not to be safe.   But the Australian Government in November 2015, the federal parliament passed Social Services Legislation Amendment (No Jab, No Pay) Act 2015, abolishing the right to conscientiously object to vaccination for the purpose of eligibility to certain benefits provided under A New Tax System (Family Assistance) Act 1999 (the Act).

The law took effect on 01 January 2016, and living here in Queensland Australia, the law applies to early childhood education and care services in Queensland providing: Long day care, Kindergarten, Family Day Care, Outside school hours vacation care and Limited hours or occasional care, which is absurd so a mother has no incentive to work at all when the fees for her child negate that incentive to work which is putting an unnecessary burden on all those motherland greatly impacts their self-worth and their mental health.

In concluding 'Eyes' story which some of you reading this and who were pregnant during this Pandemic, and also left jobs that you loved with all the uncertainty that entailed and it put a burden on you financially and mentally, all over a cold the Australian Governments and all World Governments should hold their heads in shame. I hope to watch Eyes and Hope evolve in the years ahead and if I was younger I would take her home to meet my mum. So, we have to empathise with these brave mothers and fathers, who are trying to do the correct thing for their children and that is to maintain their innate natural immunity.

The next lady wrote this herself and many thanks and we will call her "Bohemia" .I suppose the earliest 'Omen' I had that something like this was going to happen was in about 3rd Grade. Our elusive School Principal entered the classroom, on one of the only 2 occasions he did so. I expected he had some sort of important announcement to make & was quite confused when the only thing he had to say something mumbling about the Rockefeller's, the need to control the population, Eugenics, & somewhat conversely, that: it's quite normal for old people to die of the flu, you know!? almost, as if to say 'Remember that. What on earth was he talking about? Fast forward 40 years, like a ticking time bomb, I have remembered that. So, this probably contributed towards my inner knowing that it was all fake from the beginning.

This, together with the fact that I had started watching Max Egan and 'the Crow house' about a year prior, when the phone suddenly switched itself on to his show in the middle of the night. I had never even heard of him or the show before. 2020 Lockdowns were 1st enforced in Victoria after only about 3 deaths Australia-wide, all of whom were around-about, or over the average age of life-expectancy. (Remember that Pandemic means excess-deaths, & Australia had the lowest death rate that year for about 16 yrs., not to mention the regular flu-deaths, which far outweigh these numbers, had totally disappeared.)

When restrictions first hit me in QLD, I was studying remedial massage and I knew I would quit if I ever had to get the jab but felt torn with the mask-mandates and of course, masks weren't going to help prevent any virus, even if it were a real threat. I knew this, as the air we breathe doesn't exist in a vacuum so what I breathe in-you-breathe-out...etc. ad infinitum..masks are just diversions to divert the air around, as we still have to breathe .however, try explaining this to anyone & see where you get. I was the outcast once again, even so I did comply with the masking for the most part.had so many obstacles in my career-life, I just felt I had to do everything I can to make this work & give it my best shot & pray jab mandates don't come into the massage industry. Earlier, I had been studying Acupuncture & was almost finished, when it was decided that I could not receive any more student allowance and I had appealed this decision in the Administrative Appeals Courts, to no avail. However, they would give it to me if I studied Remedial Massage, which would greatly extend the remaining study period & expense to Govt so try and work that one out. This is just further proof that the Government does not make sense, or care about you, if you need anything and it I had to quit the massage course anyway, due to frozen shoulders & other health issues, and going back acupuncture is out of the question now too, with AHPRA requiring the jab & restrictions on free speech with Cancel-culture also seemed to be creeping into many arenas, including the College I was at, which ha forbidden teachers to talk to me, and additionally had spies following me around, all over fabricated issues, where my side of the story was refused to be heard, so I could hardly expect any assistance from them over this. As proof, I had attended rallies, APHRA would be able to deregister any potential Acupuncture licence at any time and I never did the QR codes, or mask wearing in public, although I sometimes wore a scarf. Twice I was thrown off a bus for non-masking, which is really a black mark on the Hornibrook bus lines, who left me in isolation at night, when I would have been the only passenger on the bus & easily been able to social distance. I'm not against anyone wearing a mask if they really want to, but feel for me, besides not getting enough oxygen, it's also giving others the impression that there's something to worry about.

Clearly, by now people should be able to see that it's the un jabbed & unmasked who are remaining more immune to covid? If it were so deadly, there could have been outbreaks after any one of the hundreds of protests to occur throughout the country, & never once did this happen. The media would have been all over this. But brainwashing is in effect & I personally know 2 people who have been on life-support after the jab & refuse to acknowledge any possible link and It's just heartbreaking. Double-standards also abound, as my mother was forced to get the jab to see my step-dad in a nursing home, which even-so, she was only able to do through a wall of Perspex. Then, at Christmas everything was suddenly alright & they were allowed contact & to be taken out for the day and as Robert F Kennedy Jnr. says the virus now has a calendar & a diary. lol!

Next day, back to the old rules...no end to the tyranny. The event that may have made some difference is at the protest outside of Premier Anastacia Palaszhuck's office at the height of the QLD lockdown, or rather, on my way there. We were not allowed over 8km from home and walking down the eerily quiet main streets, I saw 2 people I recognised from the protests.

She was ok with the police, as she had a mask exemption, but he didn't, so was taken into custody. They asked me about my lack of mask & I just said that there was no virus and naturally, I can't remember the total conversation, but it went something like this: The policeman (huffily): "Do you think that the world is flat, too?" (You must laugh!) me: "That's got nothing to do with anything policeman: (more huffiness) me: "Because I'm not a Dr, & I'm not following Science, right? That's why? Ok, so can you explain to me how you know that there's a virus? Since you're not a Dr either? A very long silence from me: " because the Govt. told you, & the media told you, right!?...that's how you know? Where is this coming from then, in the Govt.? From the CHO and she's a GP. She's not a virologist, or an Immunologist, or an Epidemiologist. She's just a GP. Which doesn't matter, but where is she getting the information from? Who knows? because she hasn't told us, & she will not be telling us, either. Why not? maybe because there is no evidence? If this were a real pandemic, this would have been one of the very 1st things she would have told you.In the meantime, there are (I will need to find this number) Drs & scientists who have signed a petition to say there is no pandemic. I can show you now, as I have it on my phone.

He declined to look at the petition, I expect because he wasn't allowed to, and I went on to give evidence by Dr Dolores Cahill & Geert Vanden Brosche, who are top in their virology fields. I could have also mentioned the Canadian High Court verdict only a few weeks earlier that declared that a virus cannot be proven to exist, but I had probably dropped enough truth bombs and to his credit the police officer did seem to be listening, unlike so many people, & his manner was not at all like the psycho riot police we are used to hearing about, mainly from Melbourne. Although he didn't say much, or give many clues to emotion, he did seem taken aback that there would be doctors with a totally different view. Months earlier I had gone touring police stations & dropping off info on "cops for covid-truth", as suggested by Max Egan.

As for the media, they will only tell you what the Govt. tell you, they censor all doctors opposing the agenda, & there's a lot of them, i said." A media which only gives you the Government position is the 1st sign of a totalitarian Govt." I believe it was John F Kennedy who said that they let us go not too long after I asked if I'm under arrest several times, but no response. The other girl made quite an impression, quoting a lot of the Australian Constitution to the officers & that mandates are in fact not the law and way to go!

Our Constitution is really under attack. Not too long afterwards a news clip showed a reporter asking Health Minister Young just one question where she got all the pandemic info from & she wouldn't answer. I feel very honoured to be asked to contribute to this book and one thing I find sad is the lack of cohesion & support at times. Some people won't talk to you because you couldn't make it to one protest or wearing a mask at one stage. Tricky was mad at the other guy for being detained that time (his second arrest), when he was only doing what he thought was right by resisting mandates, as encouraged by Tricky himself. So, what is the issue? I feel your pain lass but be proud you stood tall and the common theme amongst all of us is that we will never ever be defeated, and we have come this far.

I would like to thank my friends for letting me interview them as I have so many more who have been greatly affected by this calamity that should never ever happen and we will never forget all those responsible and there will come a day of reckoning as justice must be served. We also pray it will never happen again and we just want to be left alone. This what are corrupt media does not show the real reality of this Genocide and all their reporting is biased towards basically "Evil" as the people who control them are exactly that. So if you work in the media take along hard look in the mirror because you are complicit in genocide so you wages are "blood money".I would never ever let mainstream media interview me because you edit it to look favourable to your cause and there is nothing good about any of you and hopefully we will get to hold you all to account cameramen reporters it does not matter this Plandemic could not have happened without you. Shame on you. There a bit good news a honest reports are out there Rebel news and this new one starting in May 2023 The Aussie Wire Introduction - YouTube

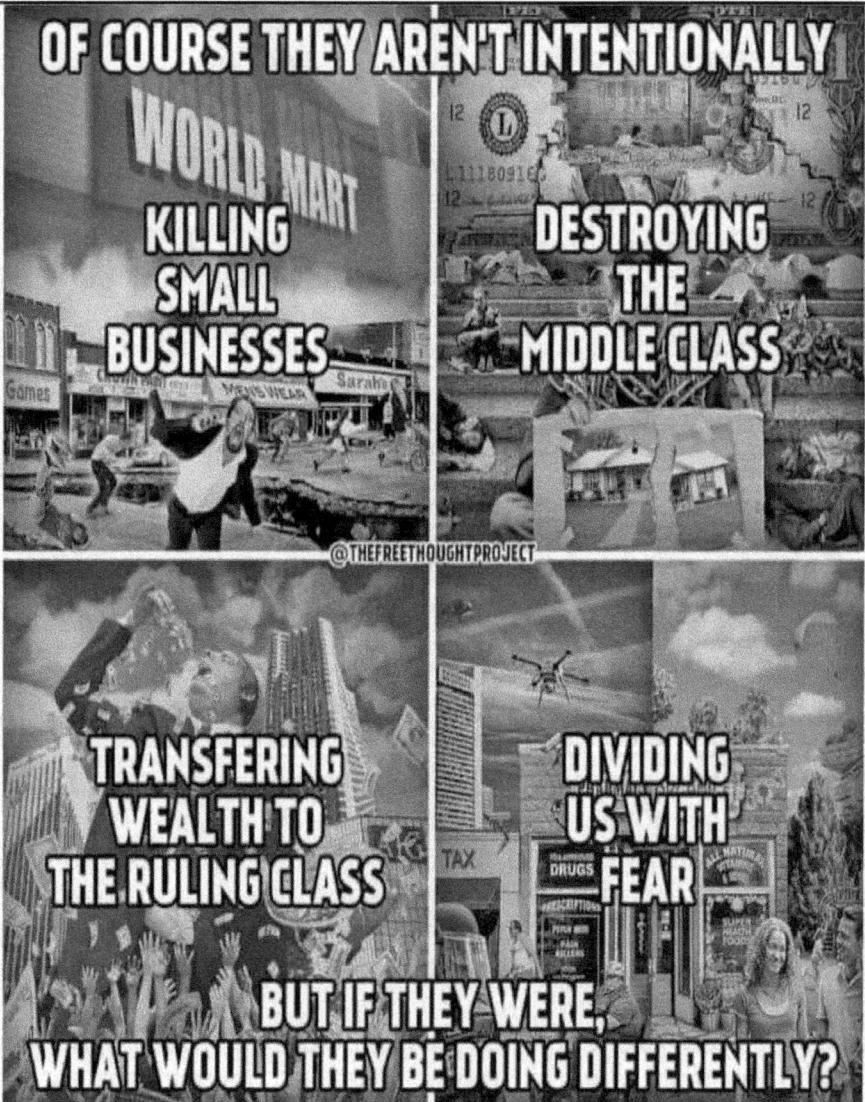

Chapter 25

Kelly Guenoun

I never expected to jump headfirst into politics, yet one warm Spring Day in October 2021 I was presented with an opportunity by email that spoke to me on so many levels. I applied and left it up to the universe to decide if I was to be chosen or not. We had just been through some of the most brutal conditions imposed on us by an overreaching government at both State and Federal levels. We had been marching in the streets and there was an overwhelming feeling that surely they wouldn't be putting more restrictions on us. They did in the form of vaccine passports and lockouts for anyone who didn't participate in the world's biggest fraud. Ahead of us we were facing segregation, medical apartheid and a whole host of discriminatory measures that were incredibly illogical and raised more questions than there were answers. Some may say it was a calling, whatever you call it, there was no doubt in my mind that I needed to stand up and be the voice of the people. I knew I had the backbone to do it and I knew that I wouldn't be scared off by the bullies in the political arena and the Labor thugs who use their union members to stand over a female to try to intimidate and scare you into submission.

Everything I had been through in my life had prepared me mentally, emotionally, and physically for this and I wasn't going to be silent. Ahead of us we were facing segregation, medical apartheid and a whole host of discriminatory measures that were incredibly illogical and raised more questions than there were answers. Some may say it was a calling, whatever you call it, there was no doubt in my mind that I needed to stand up and be the voice of the people.

I knew I had the backbone to do it and I knew that I wouldn't be scared off by the bullies in the political arena and the Labor thugs who use their union members to stand over a female to try to intimidate and scare you into submission. As a mother of eight children, I had my last child whilst there were restrictions. To say that it caused inconvenience is an understatement. I couldn't get doctors' appointments, scans, or most of my ante-natal care due to the restrictions.When I finally managed to get an appointment to get a referral to the hospital, I was approximately 27 weeks pregnant.

At one stage I thought I would be giving birth on the side of the road doing my own caesarean section with a blunt plastic knife from a takeaway shop. It was stressful and made the whole pregnancy feel harder than it needed to be. But I fought hard to have my husband with me during the surgical delivery and afterwards I made sure that my husband and all my children would be allowed into my room to visit. Put it this way, if they didn't allow them in, I would have been walking out post caesarean section than have my family denied this special moment in time with their youngest sibling.I had completely let it out of my mind about my political candidate application because I never expected to hear anything back from it.

However, while unpacking the car at a holiday apartment in Coolum Beach, the call came in early December 2021 to say that I was successful in being selected as the Federal Candidate for Petrie for the United Australia Party. I was over the moon about this as I knew I could reach out to so many people to try and help them find a way to get back to living their lives, working again because so many had lost their jobs or were forced to take leave all because they made a decision not to partake in a medical experiment. More importantly, it was about reconnecting our community again. A lot of people felt isolated, lost and not sure what to do next about their situations. Being around like-minded people helped so many get through it.I had formed a Facebook group which had almost a thousand members in just a few weeks. Initially, it was for businesses who opposed the vaccine passports and mandates. As a business owner myself, what the government was asking was complete and utter rot. None of it was science based because when you questioned the science they tried to deflect or distract with something else to keep you from uncovering the real agenda. The government expected businesses to jump through ridiculous hoops just to stay open otherwise they would face visits from police, health officers and have threatening letters sent stating that they had to comply or be shut down. With the sudden increase in members to my Facebook group, along came the censorship and what we all refer to as Facebook jail. I suddenly found myself being muted.

The leader of our political party was booted from Facebook and went to Telegram so that he could continue having a voice and trying to make people aware of what was going on in the echelons of parliament. Censorship became their tool to silence us. Anything that was labelled misinformation and disinformation we knew was too close to the truth and that this was their way of shutting it down. We were interfering with their narrative and they needed almost everyone to believe this false narrative so that they could push the medical experiment on everyone. The name calling by mainstream media was done to discredit us, to make us appear as fools, uneducated, anti-vaxxers, tin foil hatters, conspiracy theorists. The list was endless.What they (the elites) didn't count on was that there would be a large number of us who would adapt and find ways to get the message out. We were flexible, adaptable, unbreakable. They could bring their worst and we would still get back up and keep up the fight. This is why you apply to become a political candidate when you have a newborn and a house full of kids while also trying to run a business from home. I saw the world as I knew it turning into a tyrannical dictatorship and knew that fascism was alive and growing in this country and we had to fight back against it or be lost in it forever. I wanted my children to know the life that I grew up in and experience life for themselves in an unrestricted way. I want their children to grow and live an amazing life with all the freedoms to experience life. This is why you stand up. This is why you give every waking moment of your life to this. This is why I did it. For my family and for yours. I may not have won, but I gave it everything I had and I will never regret doing it.

When you have an active interest in History you immerse yourself in enough books, videos, and historical articles to know as much as you can about set periods in time. When all the mandates first started, it immediately brought a feeling of DeJa'Vu and reminded me of what I had read and what the Stormtroopers (SA) did in Nazi Germany and throughout Europe. They went door to door, business to business ensuring that fear was instilled in all and that everyone complied. They gave fines, they gave orders to shut businesses, people were arrested for being inside a business without a vaccine passport or not wearing a mask. Who wouldn't be scared? You would be surprised that there were a number of business owners here in Brisbane and many others around the country and around the world who refused to be intimidated.

We all came together because they were trying to destroy our livelihoods and the lives of workers everywhere.You must understand that it is a warrior's spirit within us that makes us stand up and not fear what they are threatening to do to us. In my mind, nothing is worse than losing your freedom to trade and make an income, your freedom to choose, your freedom to travel, your right to medical care without discrimination. It is a hill I would stand on again and I will fight to retain all those rights and freedoms with tenacity and determination to win. It is in our constitution that those rights should be protected – but they still managed to convince people that these mandates were legal when they weren't. They were in direct conflict with our constitution. If you know your rights, you never need to live in fear. The virus that they tell you will kill you if you don't wear a mask is far smaller than the holes in your mask. What does that mean?

It means you may as well go about living your life because unless you plan on living in a bubble for the rest of your life, that face nappy isn't doing you any good. I know this from over 20 years in allied health, listening to many lectures on PPE and infection control. It was one of the biggest lies in history to make you fear dying so that you would comply.My suggestion to everyone is to know history so that it cannot be repeated. We cannot allow the atrocities of the past to be our future. We cannot allow elitist grubs to call us "useless eaters" and think that they can wipe us out with fake food shortages, power outages, and planned hardships. They will try it and they will keep trying it.

They have tried to kill off our most elderly citizens because they are abundant in knowledge and can pass down natural health tips, and age-old methods for preserving, storing, and preparing for hard times. We have to prepare ourselves as best as possible because the worst is yet to come and these evil agendas cannot be allowed to win.I only hope that I can be proven wrong. Being right about the things that have happened has been bittersweet and I can only hope that the rest of the people continue their journey to becoming awake. Never forget what they did and if you get a chance, stand up, speak up and fight for your rights, and for the future generations to come. If we don't stand up now then they won't have a future with rights and freedoms. Never forget the road of the past because that is the same road to your future.

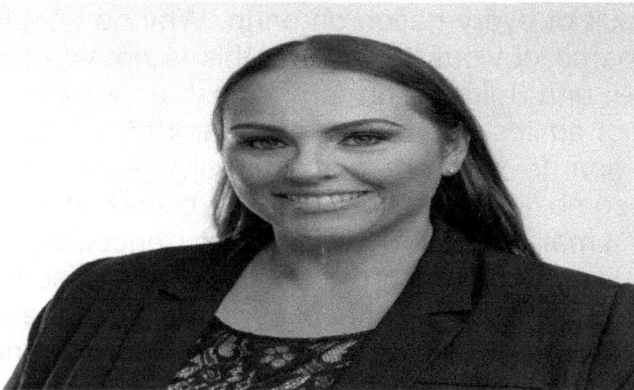

Chapter 26

Alan Walker

TIMELINE OF EVENTS THAILAND

At the very outset of what we shall call the "covid era" the media in Thailand went all in with a full thronged attack on reason, understanding and common sense. It was clear that orders were coming from elsewhere. At least it was clear to those who had the nouse and sense to see through the obfuscation and deliberate confusion, spearheaded by the Bill and Melinda Gates foundation and the World Economic Forum and carried out by their foot soldiers in Thailand. The government spread fear and confusion, often changing rules and regulations, as if at a whim. So how did the deception and the enforcement of unworkable protocols built on nefarious ideas manifest itself in Thailand? Well almost from the outset the media were obsessed with creating the greatest fear and panic imaginable and even to this day many citizens are utterly terrified of the invisible enemy which they imagine is lurking around every corner just waiting to get them. It is so sad to witness the pathetic sight of swathes of people masked and forlorn. The visible smiles erased from their faces and the creeping darkness of their soul became more and more evident. So, the same question may be asked of them which I ask of every nation on earth. Why do people not see, what seems obvious to us, that this is nothing but deception smoke and mirrors on an almost unbelievable scale. The land of smiles has become the land of faceless, almost soulless hoards who are going through a slow but sure process of zombification. There are tiny chinks of light, but they are small indeed. The most encouraging development is the creation of a group on the Telegram social media app which informs the citizenry of pertinent articles and news stories they may use to wake their friends and neighbours.

Reports which have been sadly but inevitably excluded from the local mainstream media. How I hope with every atom of my body that a tiny spring will become a stream and develop into a river of such force that all resistance to truth will be swept away in its inexorable wave. So let us return to the topic under consideration, the development of the narrative in Thailand and the response of the public. As everywhere else the Thai media misinformed the public about everything. They were told from the beginning that the virus was so unpredictable that it could kill half of the population unless the public unquestioningly obeyed the dictates of the government and that masks would stop the virus was presented as a fact.

So, here we are a full three years into this most extraordinary event, or rather series of events which has overtaken humanity, brought people into bondage, closed down businesses, caused people to distrust the government, and produced a great and fundamental divide in society between those who see and those who do not see. The unvaxxed have been subjected to the most bizarre scrutiny from those who are trapped in the matrix. It is almost as if they have become merged with some non-human force causing changes in personality, subtle at first, but more pronounced as time goes on. How many of us have lost friends, some of whom it feels have stabbed us in the back.

We have been betrayed by our icons, people we respected for decades, for example notable musicians and songwriters, Bob Dylan, Joan Baez et al. How can I speak? Consider the fact that many of the events of today have been foretold in the most unlikely ways and in the strangest settings for example various episodes of the cartoon series "The Simpsons" have foretold in precise detail many of the details of the pandemic, and yet the writers of the show right ow are totally on board with the satanic agenda and support the rats in power regardless. What short memories people have. What has happened to their souls? I have watched with extraordinary sadness as media figures previously appreciated listening to have, one by one, succumbed to the web of lies. Interestingly years ago, I used to quite enjoy (in a weird kind of way) watching documentaries about Nazi Germany and the rise of the evil regime. I wondered how it had ever happened and I asked myself the question as to how I would have responded had I been around in the 1930s during the rise of Hitler. Would I have gone along with the propaganda and the deception that was so prevalent at the time? Would I have found the strength to stand up against it and to stand for truth? I think we now all have the answer to that question. It is my conviction that those who have gone along with this horrible disgusting deception would have gone along with Adolf Hitler had they been around in Germany at that time.

Those of us who saw through this from the very beginning can be rightly proud of ourselves. There has been a plus side to the situation over the last 3 years. friendships have been and are being forged which will last for eternity. People have found a unity of heart with others in very far off parts of the world and the knowledge that they are part of a genuine brotherhood and sisterhood which cannot be destroyed or maligned by forces of evil who would try so to subjugate us and bring us into tyranny which would be akin to taking on the role of an animal under a cruel owner. The government spread fear and confusion, often changing rules at regulations, as if at a whim. From then on they relentlessly terrified the population with extreme and deceptive messaging of fear about the "virus" with their endless threats of enforced hospitalisation, and worse. Those precious few who did not buckle under the pressure faced severe trauma. Those of us who from early on saw that the emperor had no clothes, have had to cry many tears inside. The effect on businesses all over was simply horrendous and now that tourists are starting to return, and the place is busy there is a lot of talk that the economy has rebounded and that all is well. What they do not see however is that there were winners and the losers were the many who went out of business due to the lockdown and the winners were those who then bought up the businesses at fire sale prices.

The tourists just see the streets full of businesses, but they do not see the numerous stories of human tragedy behind the many closures. I saw firsthand the long lines for food and the terrible poverty that resulted.I have mentioned earlier about winners, however no one who took the jab was ever a winner and no amount of money would ever convince a sound mind to put the liquid into their veins. But sound minds seem to be in short supply right now.

Still the brainwashing continues, and the news media is relentless in trying to keep up the fear even now when we know so much more and when we are well aware that almost everything we were told was a lie. Still the coercion continues and the ostracising of all who have a different opinion and people are still thrown off buses for refusing to wear a mask. It is amazing but true that the vast majority of people in Thailand are totally terrified of covid and many of them, I fear, will wear masks at the least for the rest of their lives. Here is a recent article from Thai PBS and it illustrates just how brainwashed people are, but they are still pushing the fear.

The Thai Ministry of Public Health is closely monitoring the spread of the new XBB.1.16 COVID-19 sub-variant in India. It has not yet been detected in Thailand, according to Public Health Permanent Secretary Dr. Opart Karnkawinpong. In Thailand, 150 new COVID-19 cases were reported between March 19th and 25th 2023, averaging 21 new cases a day. 30 of them are suffering from lung infections, 19 require ventilators and six people have died. He said that all the deceased were aged 60 or over, had a chronic disease, were pregnant women or weighed over 90kg. Most were not vaccinated or received their last vaccine dose more than three months ago. The Public Health Ministry has launched a long-acting antibody combination (LAAB) treatment for high risk people in shelters for the elderly, the bed-ridden and kidney patients requiring dialysis, adding that LAAB can help lower the mortality rate.

Dr. Opart said that COVID-19 is tending towards becoming a seasonal disease, like flu, which spreads during the rainy season. Hence the need for the Public Health Ministry to adjust its monitoring and preventive measures. There is some good news from Thailand. A top Thai doctor Dr Sucharit Bkakdi is at the forefront of the fight against the vaccines. He said there is nothing subtle about how ineffective and dangerous the so-called "covid-19 vaccines" are. He maintains the lying and criminality involved in their promotion is absolute and severe. The profiteers and perpetrators of these coerced injections should, he believes, all be imprisoned immediately, and any and all authorization for emergency "vaccine" use should be stopped.

Dr Bhakti shared these views with The World Council for Health on March 14th, 2022. Dr Bhakti continued and described the essential mechanisms of harm from the covid injections. He warns us against them in no uncertain terms, and with no regard for the enemies he's made among the most wicked people in the world: the perpetrators of the Covid-19 crimes against humanity. Dr Bhakdi describes the dangers to our fertility and the very real danger that these injections may decimate the human population. Breastfeeding dangers for infants, and the risk for genetically modifying our offspring before they are even conceived are very real. He also includes advice for pathologists to reliably detect the covid-injection induced spike protein and autoimmune disease processes, both on live patients' biopsies and on autopsies. This is very important; without proper tissue preparation the very direct harms and deaths from these injections are being ignored. Justice requires evidence; and in this case evidence requires proper microscopic staining techniques. As Dr Ryan Cole has said "You cannot find what you are not looking for." Prof Sucharit Bhakdi has published over three hundred articles in the fields of virology, immunology, bacteriology, and parasitology. He has received 11 scientific awards as well as the Order of Merit of Rhineland-Palatinate.

From 1990 to 2012, Prof Bhakdi was Editor-in-Chief of the journal Medical Microbiology and Immunology. Dr Bhakdi is such an intelligent and calm person; it takes a severe situation for him to choose such an aggressive stance against big pharma and their cohorts, in defence of all of us. Thanks, and blessings to Dr Sucharit Bhakdi.

Lockdowns have really hurt people in Thailand. It was clear from the beginning that they would, or at least it should have been to their mental health. They have hurt the populace by inflicting real isolation, they have made mental health worse, played a part in the overall decline in health, kept the dying from their families, and added to the anguish of bereavement.They have taken away livelihoods, and led to more domestic violence, especially here in Thailand and they have hit the poor the most. They have put people off getting medical help and made long medical waiting lists worse. There is more drunkenness and people are losing their minds. Who knows in the long term how many will die due to lockdowns, the jabs and 5g along with the media have tried to scare people to death to just go along with the lockdowns. Established moral standards underwent a similar upheaval and depriving people of the opportunity to be with loved ones during their final days and hours was now the right thing to do, even as thousands of care home residents and hospital patients died lonely, frightened and confused.

The task of evaluating lockdowns, of identifying and responding to matters of importance, posed a distinctive challenge. Lockdowns profoundly disrupted the very frameworks of values, commitments, concerns, projects, habits, expectations and relationships relative to which the significance of unfolding events is more usually grasped; established moral standards underwent a similar upheaval. Then there were all of the usual routines, through which we encountered the little things that mattered to us during the course of our daily lives: the walk to the shop; morning coffee with a friend; the journey to work; regular visits to an elderly relative.

Children were prohibited from seeing their friends, confined to their homes (which, for many of them were small flats with no outdoor space), allowed out no more than once per day (for exercise, not play!), with significant risk of serious harm in the guise of mental health problems, neglect, abuse, impaired social and emotional development, and loss of educational opportunities. Women had to give birth without the support of partners, family members or friends, leaving many of them traumatised. The unthinkable became not only acceptable but obligatory and then there were all of the usual routines, through which we encountered the little things that mattered to us during the course of our daily lives: the walk to the shop; morning coffee with a friend; the journey to work; regular visits to an elderly relative.

On top of this, many of those projects that gave people's lives short- or longer-term meaning and structure were lost, suspended, curtailed, or substantially altered—getting married; starting or developing a business; studying for a university degree and graduating; doing one's A-levels; visiting relatives overseas; training to be a pilot; and participating in community groups. Privation of this interpersonal and social scaffolding exacerbated the challenge of evaluating lockdowns. They not only disrupted our value-systems; they also made it more difficult to interact with others in ways that would otherwise help us to make sense of things." Hence, the significance of lockdowns could not be assessed relative to an established background of values, as they involved the profound and pervasive disruption of that very value system. For many of us, the resultant predicament amounted to an all-enveloping experience of disorientation, a feeling of having lost the ground beneath our feet, the structured, habitual context within which we used to think and act. Losing life structure in this way, and experiencing it as lost, is not simply a matter of "putting things on hold" and resuming them at a later date or of removing things that can later be adequately replaced as there is so much that can never be recovered or replaced.

One respondent to a survey of pandemic experiences (in which I was involved) wrote the following: Human beings are not objects that can be stored away for a while, remaining unaltered until they are re-activated. Human life is a process of pursuing meaningful life possibilities, which fit together as parts of a larger, temporally organised pattern. Many of us experienced not just the suspension, but the irrevocable loss of possibilities that were profoundly important to us. For some, this involved losing whole networks of goals and values that were central to the structures of their lives, to who they were and to who they aspired to be.

There are certain possibilities that cannot be taken away from someone while leaving their identity intact. For instance, being a musician may be more than just something that a person does; it may be central to the kind of person they are and also to their sense of being a particular, distinctive person. As other survey respondents wrote: "terrible grief and mourning for my lost 'life'""; "grief over the future life that is no longer likely to be available"; "I feel a great sense of loss over things which have given me pleasure and confirmed my sense of self throughout my life. They're absent now and may not return soon, if at all (singing in choirs, performing, rehearsing)". A full appreciation of the costs of lockdowns needs to somehow factor in and evaluate the cost of depriving people of their social identities in this manner, inhibiting their ability to be who they are and pursue possibilities central to their lives.

Double Disorientation

For many of us, the task of weighing up the pros and cons of lockdowns thus involved evaluating policy measures so extreme that they disrupted the very fabric of our lives.It is important, though, to acknowledge that lockdowns are far from unique in this respect. A sense of having lost one's moorings is common to many other experiences of upheaval,associated with the likes of bereavement, loss of long-term employment, breakdown of a relationship, and diagnosis of serious illness. There are also other disorienting events, such as natural disasters and political instability, which similarly affect whole societies and cultures. However, two further ingredients were added to the disorientation of lockdowns, making them quite distinctive. First of all, lockdowns further deprived us of our usual resources for comprehending and navigating disorienting situations. When faced with a loss of much that we took for granted, most of us turn to other people for guidance and support in making sense of things, reassembling a coherent evaluative framework, and working out how to proceed with life. Friends, relatives, colleagues and professionals can play a variety of different roles in this regard. Privation of this interpersonal and social scaffolding exacerbated the challenge of evaluating lockdowns.

They not only disrupted our value systems; they also made it more difficult to interact with others in ways that would otherwise help us to make sense of things. Even when we did get to see others, social distancing, masks, a perception of conversation-partners as potential virus carriers, and a consequent awkwardness and distrust frequently impeded interactions. A framework of values was eroded and partly replaced by a virus-centric alternative. "Not so!", one might protest, "We could do it all online". But we really couldn't and in working through something in person, making sense of it together, acknowledging and negotiating disagreements together. We experience the pauses, the moments of hesitation, the subtle interplay of expression and gesture, the awkward smiles, the searching for words, the gradual confessions, the crystallisation of initially inchoate ideas. All of this helps to generate dialogical space, open up new possibilities, and enable the recognition and consideration of alternative perspectives. It is not replicated in Zoom meetings, and it is a far cry from the "gifs", "memes", stylized interactions and rampant confirmation biases of social media. In this way, lockdowns further compromised the ability to grasp, think through, and evaluate the implications of lockdowns.

It amounted to a sort of double-disorientation: we were deprived of resources that we would otherwise draw upon so as to evaluate and respond to disorienting events. The second factor that further impeded our ability to weigh up the harms and benefits of lockdowns was the widespread and persistent tendency to identify the effects of lockdowns with the effects of the virus. In the deluge of monothematic media coverage and messaging that replaced the richness of our social world, "due to contestable policy decisions taken in response to Covid" was abbreviated simply to "due to Covid" or "due to the pandemic": it is the virus that has eroded the values we hold dear and so it is the virus that now demands all our attention and concern. (Try typing "due to Covid" into Google and scrolling through the first few hundred hits.)

The incontestability of the existence of the virus and the deaths caused by it became wedded to a contestable political response, conferring upon the latter an illusory impression of inevitability and authority: Covid did this to us all. In this way, when the various harms of lockdowns were acknowledged and contemplated in any detail, they were presented as necessary harms, rather than reasons to question a contingent political response. The combination of these factors helped to facilitate an abstract, partial conception of what was at stake, curiously dislodged from previously established and far wider-ranging values, commitments, cares and concerns.

Nevertheless, a shared narrative constructed during the lockdowns remains deeply entrenched, a new bedrock for some people. Supposedly liberal, democratic countries have thus impeded their citizens' abilities to think and act responsibly and critically, to contemplate the impact of unprecedented and destructive policies in relation to a shared pre-established sense of what is important to us all and why. A framework of values was eroded and partly replaced by a virus-centric alternative. Of course, restrictions have now been lifted within the UK, at least for the most part, and in many other countries too.

While there remains any prospect whatsoever of further lockdowns, the development of a comprehensive cost-benefit analysis that reflects our values as a society and somehow factors in the cost of what has been done to individual and shared value systems remains an urgent task.

Because I wanted to get a Thai perspective on what it is like to be the only dissenter in a large group of people, I turned to someone with whom I am very familiar. My former wife. The questions and her answers follow: Were you aware that the biggest ever study into masks completed in January 2023 showed no positive effect from wearing them? No, we hear nothing like that in the Thai media, we only hear about how good the vaccine is and that we should take it to protect others. We have never heard anything about anyone dying from the vaccine or that masks do not work. What do your friends or family think about your thinking about the jabs/masks? They do not understand me and they believe everything they hear on television and they do not believe anyone has died from the vaccine.

Are you aware that the Thai government is seriously considering making it illegal for any foreigner to live in Thailand without taking the jabs? What do you think about that? Well, this is simply disgusting. There is nothing more to say and are you aware that the World Council for Health and thousands of doctors want these jabs banned? I am aware but most people would not be. Did you know there is a vaccine injury fund in Thailand and the government has already been forced to pay out compensation to many families of people who have died after taking the jab? I had no idea. So yes as the respondent indicated, there is an almost total ignorance of the fact that there is a vaccine injury fund. This is something so vitally important for every citizen to know and yet they have no idea. What kind of insanity is this? How can anyone not smell a rat in the light of all this? Well, there is the old saying that when they move their lips, we can be sure that they are lying.Well, I guess with the availability of modern technology and the many different modes of communication now available we can extend the imagery, for the lips no longer need to move. Every written word, every piece of big pharma research, every article written by those who were in acquiescence to the cult is a lie. Not just a lie, it's a lie of monumental order. We can never really know what has gone on in the minds of some of the main perpetrators of this horrendous deception. When did evil take root in them? We can ponder these issues until the prevails come home. What's one thing we know for certain, it pains us greatly to say it, is that evil has taken root. in them. The effects are there for all you can see. and this is not a pretty sight. The reality that we live in and somehow come to terms with is more bizarre than any episode of our favourite fantasy or science fiction series if I had presented all that has happened in the last 3 years in the form of a script to a Hollywood studio, they most likely would have rejected it for being far-fetched.

The fear which has been planted into the hearts and minds of the Thai population is palpable. There are those who of a certainty will wear the mask until the moment that they die; they're all those for whom any number of booster shots is acceptable. Yes, there are those paralyzed by fear. The size of anybody holding up the baby's arms to be vaccinated is truly abhorrent. God bless the little ones, and God bless all of us you have realised that we are in a fight, I'm not exaggerating. It is a fight for the whole future of humanity. Covid was a scam and we knew it from the start they wanted the juice inside us so it could attack our heart.

They went to get it in their droves, they stood for hours in the rain. They wanted the juice inside us so it could attack our brain. They rolled up their sleeves at anti-vaxxers and they went wild. They wanted the juice inside us so we could have no children. Ahern, Sunak and Biden we know what's in your head you want the juice inside us and ninety percent dead. Murdering scum that is their name Global genocide that is their game. We put you on notice we know we will win. For this there is no game and we will never give in. Bless

Chapter 27

The Future

Having got this fair in reading my book I trust you have **received some hope** and that it is not the end game for all of you, we all have choices, and everyone must walk in their own shoes, there is no right or wrong when walking your own spiritual path and the lessons you were here to learn. Some of us are more aware than others as we were born with spiritual gifts and awareness and also have very powerful guides, who will not let us stray from the straight and narrow, but we are all Imperfect - Perfect. This chapter will be a mixed bag because when I started this book over 3 months ago, things have since morphed even more and the evil that runs this agenda knows no bounds, to the depths of their evilness and Surveillance will be a key component for them and Big brother is everywhere and it will get so much worse Worldwide, and where I am living in Moreton Bay Qld, they will use any excuse and they think we are daft because Moreton Bay is leading the way to develop new CCTV technology to identify koalas, and help to keep them safe around roads. Comrade Mayor Peter Flannery, said the tech innovation was developed in partnership with Lone Pine Koala Sanctuary, the State Government's Daisy Hill Koala Centre, and tech company Sapio. "We're training Council's CCTV cameras to identify koala movements across the region, so we can activate warning signs near roads when they're there and also better inform the design and location of our fauna crossing infrastructure," he said. Public safety (Closed circuit television cameras) is popping up everywhere. Koala movements, when did you last see one, they are like us. Human Livestock are an endangered species and people like Comrade Flannery will lie and tell you anything because he is paid to do that. You only have to look at the devastation Moreton Bay Council has done to the region in their power hungry rate creating developments, but there is no stopping the push to make us lose the lovely identity we once had. We are told that public safety is been identified as a high priority for action within the Moreton Bay Regional Council and key to this notion is that community that maintains liveable places, community infrastructure and promotes social connection will lead to an improved quality of closed circuit televisions cameras in a range of public places and buildings throughout the region. The cameras help to create a safer environment and reduce crime levels by deterring potential offenders and helping in crime detection and closed-circuit televisions cameras in a range of public places and buildings throughout the region. So, reading all that rubbish, **do you feel safer?** Well, I do not because the police are basically non-existent and if you report a problem you are simply wasting your time, they do not have the resources and manpower because the mandating of vaccines took a heavy toll and lots of the "Good Guys Left" including some of my friends and others have gotten sick due to the vaccines, maybe also due to the heavy use of **Wi-Fi in patrol cars** and police stations.

Again, Comrade Flannery and other councillors we don't buy into agenda as the real reasons for your gearing Moreton Bay Qld, which is the 3rd largest council in Australia, is for a 'Smart City Tag' they love us to be one the first in world and if you don't cotton on to their aim as it's already happening in front of your eyes Big brother is everywhere here, and all the 5G towers popping up is only the start.

Smart City outcomes, so no hiding their Agenda and it sure is not about protecting Koala's. You also notice even though the homeless situation is well recognised they lock the toilets at night and also put up barriers that they lock at night to keep out people who are sadly living in their cars and I mentioned they starting booking them if you not homeless registered some too proud to do that and then when they cannot pay their fines they put aSper immobilisation device to your vehicles. But remember all these dictatorial actions are by vaccine sheeple who will pay the price for the stupidity of their actions and putting vaccinated poison in their bodies.

There is a big agenda going on here and even Blue Water Square Management, a shopping centre in Redcliffe Qld have the rainbow on their window and they are so confident they are winning this spiritual war and that will be their downfall. So, stand up and fight peacefully that we all had enough of the actions of some very uneducated, possibly corrupt people who get paid very well to do a job they are not doing they must Go, and we will Win.

SMART DUST Nanochips and smart dust is a dangerous new face of the human microchipping agenda and are the new technological means for the advancement of the human microchipping agenda. Due to their incredibly tiny size, both nanochips and smart dust have the capacity to infiltrate the human body, become lodged within, and begin to set up a synthetic network on the inside which can be remotely controlled from the outside and needless to say, this has very grave for our freedoms, privacy and health implications, because it means the New World Order would be moving from controlling the outside world and our environment society, to controlling the inside world which is your body.

There are different forms of controlling of humanity and history is filled with examples of societies where the people were sharply divided into 2 categories which are the 'Rulers and Slaves' and understanding who you are is so important because this be your likely future and in the distant past, the slaves were usually kept in place because the Rulers had access to and control over their resources, such as money, food, water, weapons and other necessities of life and the control of our environment. In recent history, control was implemented not only by monopolising resources but also via propaganda control of the mind and having read this book you should have a basic understanding of how they going to plan to achieve all of this and it has manifested itself in many ways, like the caste system in India where you must remain in your position on the hierarchical ladder for life, the royal bloodlines in Rome, the Middle East and Europe who also claimed an inherent and divine right to rule.

The centralization of power in Nazi Germany and Soviet Russia during the 1930s where a single autocrat or a very small committee decided the fate of millions, also in the West especially in the US with the advent of specialised mind control techniques that were refined by the CIA. It is a heavy topic which is worth studying much more, Monarch Programming is a method of mind control used by numerous organisations for covert purposes and the project itself is a continuation of the CIA's MK-ULTRA, a mind-control program and the methods are unspeakably brutal and sadistic, monarch programming begins early in a monarch slave's life as they are taken "as infants and traumatised using electroshocks, drugs, sexual abuse, mind games, and hypnosis in order to force the mind to split and create an alternative personality to deal with the pain. The victim imagines that someone else is being tortured and the mind is forced to split. Each personality or alter, as in 'alternate personality' is then programmed and trained to perform specific tasks and missions as given to the NWO controllers is unheard of power to remotely and subconsciously influence people without them ever knowing, including the ability to create sex slaves and sleeper assassins.

The Smart Agenda is basically synonymous with the UN Agenda 21 or Agenda 2030, and the smart grid is synonymous with the IoT (Internet of Things) which is also going to use the new 5G network to achieve its desired saturation levels and in a fundamental way, Vaccines, Gmos, Bioengineered food and Geo-Engineering are all connected, as they are delivery systems whereby this miniature technology of nanochips and smart dust is planned to be inserted into all our bodies. Some chemtrails contain smart dust motes which readily infiltrate the body, communicate with other motes in your body, set up their own network and which can, unfortunately, be remotely controlled. Even if you are fastidious about what you eat and what you expose yourself to, it is difficult to see how you can avoid breathing in a mote of smart dust, that was dropped on you by a plane spraying chemtrails so if we do not all fight as one today, then there will be no future tomorrow it might sound like science fiction, but this is are horrific reality and with nanochips and motes inside your body, the NWO criminals can combine the IoT smart grid with brain mapping, and other technological information in their attempt to pull off their ultimate end-game 2030, and to remotely influence and control an entire population by overriding and programming all the thoughts, feelings and actions of the masses. While this kind of technology can be used for the benefit of mankind, like many things today, it has also been weaponized and the existence of smart dust forms a massive threat against the sovereignty of every human being alive. What we are up against is nothing less than the attempted technological possession of humanity and the nanochips will also be pushed using peer pressure, encouraging people to get in the game out of social conformity. Like so many other governmental programs, the chips may initially be voluntary before they will become mandatory, there is already a segment of society that is willingly chipping itself using tattoo ink and recently, a company in Wisconsin introduced such an internal system and began encouraging its employees to get chipped. Although it was not mandatory, it reported that about half of them, 41 out of 85, stepped forward and chose to get chipped. The human microchipping agenda is really the same thing as the transhumanist agenda to turn all of mankind into a machine which will ultimately mean becoming not superhuman but subhuman, but it can never replace the spirit of consciousness inside of you, which is your true power if you are aware and don't get chipped. This chapter must be a reality check as to be forewarned is to be forearmed, but it can drop your vibration if bought into the fear as it has always been about fear and total compliance.

Whistleblowers standing up comes with inherent dangers but that's all fear based and living without fear does set you free to achieve more than most in your life's journey. Dr. Kary Mullis had been a constant thorn in Big Pharma's side then he suddenly died in 2019, just months before the plandemic started.

The late Dr Kary Mullis, inventor of the PCR "test," has been blowing the whistle on Fauci and Big Pharma for 30 years. Inventor of the PCR Technique, Dr Kary Mullis, About Anthony Fauci: He's Not a Scientist and Doesn't Understand Medicine. The PCR Testing Scam: According to Its Inventor, Dr Kary Mullis, the Technique CANNOT Be Used to Detect Viruses and these whistleblowers are the saint's of the future and understanding they would properly pay the ultimate price in their own demise. There are so many that have paid the ultimate price over the last 3 years, too many to mention but what choice do they all have when there is a position to really.

Horse Racing I have been interested in this industry for over 50 years and had some amazing wins and have been banned by a few bookies in Australia, and the UK, and I also was a Brisbane Turf Club member for 15 years. But this industry like many has been a total disgrace with the mandating of not being able to venture onto a racecourse due to not being vaccinated. The horse racing industry has very big web sites like Racing.Com and the constant advertising of going to get vaccinated and aligning themselves to this Agenda was a disgrace with Trainers, Jockeys, Strappers and Owners who all were all put in a position they should never should have had to do, and that was get vaccinated to keep their jobs call me cynical, but I bet there are more than a few people connected in the industry who would have managed to get a placebo but you gotta feel for the little guys who did not have those contacts and got the real juice. Headlines like this were the norm, Victorian racing industry will mandate vaccinations against C19 for all staff and people involved with horse racing by the end of November 2021, and the industry consultation has found 67 percent of staff were already fully or partially vaccinated, and the mandate will affect trainers jockeys, race day officials, and other staff, so to Victorian racing and all the Racing clubs in Australia shame on you, and please do not forget what they did. Statements like this Bendigo Jockey Club CEO, Aaron Hearps said it was a progressive move by Racing Victoria "I think it's ultimately to protect the safety and well being of all the participants," he said.

.Aaron Hearps you should hold your head in shame, and will you say sorry to those who have received Jab injuries after your mandates. Trainers and jockeys as well like Bendigo horse trainer Josh Julius "As an industry participant, I think the majority have been doing the right thing and will keep doing the right thing to make sure we can keep going." sorry Josh you needed to grow some testicular fortitude there was no right thing you poisoned yourself. I am doing this for all the people who did not want to do this and all who have left the industry which they loved. How could you be so naive and so plain dumb? Another scandal is that Political donations from gambling agencies that facilitate betting on horse racing have skyrocketed, totalling almost half a million dollars a year, new research shows.

Data shows yearly donations from these gambling companies increased from $9,900 in 2010-11 to $473,161 in 2019-20. The industry made a total of $2.7m donations in the decade, largely via Tabcorp and Crown Resorts, which owns the online betting company Betfair Australia who incidentally have banned me successful punters are not very popular. The Liberals accepted $1.3m, Labor took $1.1m and the Nationals received $229,000.

But let's highlight a Sporting Hero and they are in all sports and some like **William Pike** reading his journey, also had his hands tied very tight by the power's that be and he will not and cannot wilt so Pike and other unvaccinated riders can ride at meetings of crowds less than 1000, with Racing and Wagering Western Australia dithering on an industry wide policy pending the Western Australian government's implementation of the "Safe Transition" plan on February 5 2022, when borders were reopened and that date was a D-Day for Pike. From Carry A Gun at the once a year track Norseman in March 2002 to Material Witness at Pinjarra Pike had won 2871 races, but has yet meant so much more to Western Australian and Australian racing.

He has a cult following the "Pike in the Last" mantra could have been an epitaph until this, he is renowned for getting losing punters out on his last ride of the day. A feared opponent with a glittering CV and five consecutive seasons of more than 200 winners are just one. Now Pike had not only placed his career in danger with his personal decision not to be vaccinated against Covid, but his heroic public stance in doing so is alienating him from an industry that has afforded him his opportunities, though yes one that he has given so much back to. Let's remember he donated his 2020 Perth Cup trophy for auction to raise money for bushfires appeal as one example fine example and the fallout already includes, as I understand, the loss of his lucrative social media contract with TAB touch, but it is his potential personal loss as much as the industries and its fans that will hit harder. We are aware that jockeys are a split-second decision from disaster, as we saw in Melbourne Victoria, recently with serious race falls injuring some of the best jockeys in Australia.

So supreme sportsmen like William Pike who are ultra fit and want to remain and not be vaccinated had their careers often decided by unfit, fat non-jockeys and do you not find that the recent falls of so many supreme Jockeys like Jamie Kah, Craig Williams and Ethan Brown ect, who I wish the best too, was it because of the absurd workloads? but also combined with the jockeys who are vaccinated? Which would be most? who might not have the same amount of split decision thinking they might have had before they were vaccinated? Interestingly, Willie Pike could ask Jamie Kah, Ben Melham, Mark Zahra and Ethan Brown about the consequences of their actions in breaching stupid community Covid protocols in the infamous Airbnb saga and the impact it had on them missing the spring racing carnival and beyond, their is rebel in us all and how draconian was the racing industry, it was always going to be proved that it was a crock of shite and we all see how the people in power like Boris Johnson and his cronies partied while you were controlled. But it wasn't only William Pike who wasn't allowed at Ascot racecourse on Perth Cup day there were others like William Smith or William

Jones who couldn't go either, or simply anyone who had not met government mandates to be double vaccinated at that time. "The mainstream media has a way of twisting words and leading up to this, I didn't want to comment," he told the journalists from Freedom Media WA. I wanted to make sure I had my story straight and they (the media) went and posted things anyway, Pike said he chose Freedom Media WA to share his story because he liked their work and you I all will be aware of the media's roll in this genocide so good on you Willie Pike. "I wanted my story and my reasons to be told factually, so I turned to you guys, because I know you have a reputation for that." He thanked some police and nurses who had "walked away from their jobs" in paving the way for in his words giving him the courage to "Stand My Ground" Other Australian sportsmen went out on their own terms as Carlton's Liam Jones retired his AFL career when he didn't want to follow AFL vaccination policy. The NRL had not at that time mandated double vaccination, yet the Bulldogs split with John Asiata over his refusal to be vaccinated.

On the global scale, World No 1 tennis player Novak Djokovic vaccination position was when weeks out from the Australian Open where all players must be vaxxed and comes back to Australia and wipes the floor of them winning the title easily "Pure Bloods Freedom Forever" and it's also worth noting that polarising NBA star Kyrie Irving is yet to lace up for a game then due to his vaccination stance.

 William Pike you an absolute hero when tarnishing a well-earned reputation, but he knows that, and again, will face the obvious consequences from his own volition yet he talks of legacy." I want to leave my children are in a better position than I was in, doesn't necessarily mean money, it probably means more education and that doesn't mean pen and paper education, if I can give them more street smarts than I had, that's where I'd like to head things," he said. "If you like me, you like me, if you don't you don't, that's how I am." Pike will remain well liked, racing survived but was poorer without him, but he back doing what he does best and Pike will remain well liked, racing survived but was poorer without him, but he back doing what he does best and recently won another big race in 2023 Champion WA jockey William Pike booted home a record-extending 11th WATC Derby (2400m) winner when Sydney raider Awesome John outclassed the locals at Ascot on Saturday.

Social Media. Ex-CIA agents who are deciding facebook policy like Aaron Berman as Aaron identifies himself as the manager of "the team that writes the rules for Facebook", determining "what is acceptable and what is not." Thus, he and his team effectively decide what content the platform's 2.9 billion active users see and what they don't see. Aaron was CIA. until July 2019, when he left his job as a senior analytic manager at the agency to become senior product policy manager for misinformation at Meta, the company that owns Facebook, Instagram and WhatsApp. In his 15-year career, Aaron Berman rose to become a highly influential part of the CIA and for years, he prepared and edited the president of the United States' daily brief, "wr[iting] and overs[eeing] intelligence analysis to enable the President and senior U.S. officials to make decisions on the most critical national security issues," especially on "the impact of influence operations on social movements, security, and democracy," his LinkedIn profile reads and none of this is mentioned in the Facebook video, a lot of you reading this like myself have had month after month of bans because they fear us, the little people who can hi-jack their agenda. Facebook has recruited dozens of individuals from the Central Intelligence Agency, as well as many more from other agencies like the FBI and Department of Defense. These hires are primarily in highly politically sensitive sectors such as trust, security and content moderation, to the point where some might feel it becomes difficult to see where the U.S. national security state ends and Facebook begins. In previous investigations, this author has detailed how TikTok is flooded with NATO officials, how former FBI agents abound at

315

Twitter, and how Reddit is led by a former war planner for the NATO think tank, the Atlantic Council, but the sheer scale of infiltration of Facebook blows these away because Facebook, in short, is utterly swarming with spooks.

The Voice would give advice to parliament on matters that are important to improve the lives of Indigenous Australians. For those who are not aware we still do not know the date that the referendum will be run, but it will be on a Saturday after September, because the joke is that our prime minister says otherwise it risks clashing with several sporting grand final weekends. It will be the first referendum in many people's lifetimes. Millions of Australians who will be eligible to vote in this poll were too young, or not even born, when the last referendum was held it all part the pandemic agenda you induce them with money to take poisons that will kill then pretend you care Mr Anal Albo and divide and conquer the rest of all Australians but the real Agenda is this the secret 'agenda for the Voice' has been allegedly left behind at a Canberra cafe fuelling fears Australia's and divide and conquer the rest of all Australians but the real Agenda is that the secret agenda for the referendum gets up and fears Australia's way of life will be turned on its head if the referendum gets up. The alleged 11-point agenda apparently found by a member of the public and handed to One Nation Senator Pauline Hanson, outlines various 'opportunities' to pursue should the Voice to Parliament be enshrined in the constitution. They include Indigenous job quotas, a takeover of Australian beaches and national parks, and a recommendation that First Nations people be granted first choice of all public housing. The alleged 11-point plan sent to Senator Hanson recommended First Nations people be granted first choice of all public housing and reverting beaches and national parks to 'ownership of the Mob that traditionally inhabits the area'. Non-Indigenous Australians who use those beaches or national parks would subsequently be charged a fee, which would generate revenue for Indigenous owners, according to the alleged document. This week April 2023 some Aboriginal elders went from South

Australia to Canberra to be heard and found nobody to see with these clowns are politicians who are out of touch there is no "Voice"

Your Pets We all love our pets, and they are truly man's best friend, and I would trust them over nearly all humans and most of you reading this would agree? And this initiative is sadly coming and there is no end to what they plan for all of us, and nothing is sacred. The WEF wants to slaughter millions of pet cats and dogs to fight climate change and the World Economic Forum has recently launched a controversial new initiative that will have animal rights activists up in arms, because the WEF is now calling for millions of cats and dogs worldwide to be slaughtered in an effort to reduce the "carbon pawprint" they produce as a result of eating The WEF, which has ordered mainstream media outlets to begin pushing the narrative, wants to introduce an international policy that would require the majority of pet owners to euthanize their animals. Most of you who were compliant and took their poisons into your arms and breathed in their toxins and prepared to eat their injected meat and bugs and happy to let you children also be injected and poisoned will you ever Wake Up? This is end game for all there is no real winner, if you are not in the 1%, even leaders like Anal Albo are not or Pilachook here in Qld might think there because they are very delusional and are going to be in for a shock when their puppet strings are severed and they hang out to dry, that day for them all is looming fast and they must start to press the panic button at some point, they are corrupt and obsolete. I notice Labour wins NSW and the Labour party controls every state except Tasmania, but It's all an illusion there all in on this, and they will sit on their hands as this great country goes down the toilet, when watching them in the senate, when there is an important vote that affects mankind they are noticeably absent. But a change is going to come as it only takes a few brave people to rock their boat as the brave French citizens and the farmers in Holland have shown us, KTF because as Doctor William Bay correctly screams out we will WIN simply because we are the 1% and always will lose to the 10% as

We hold the high moral ground as we understand the Art Of War Sun Tzu. The devil will not save them or any of you complicit in all this tyranny as you will be accountable.

China and Taiwan Many point out the semiconductor production in Taiwan, which could certainly be the main reason, but there is strong evidence to suggest that US biological activity in Taiwan is the reason for escalation. The US does fund biolabs there, and not just some, but a lot, according to the US NIH, there are 1,251 microbiology labs on the island of Taiwan and keep in mind Taiwan is roughly the size of Maryland and one lab of particular importance is the BSL-4 lab in Taipei, which has conducted research, and notoriously reported leaks on C19.85+ people reportedly exposed to C19 at their lab via rodents. I'm not sure exactly how many of the 1,251 biolabs the US funds, or which non-government entities are involved, but the US political and militaristic interest in Taiwan would suggest that they have assets on the island they do not want to fall into the hands of China. And given the DNC's track record with Ukraine, we can deduce whatever the Deep State is doing in Taiwan is not for philanthropic purposes. The US' actions indicate they expect China to move into Taiwan soon, and China's demands toward the US suggest that China also intends to move into Taiwan, and they don't want the US supplying weapons to Taiwan. So, it appears that the Deep State has another proxy country in Taiwan, and they are desperately trying to prevent it from falling into China's hands. But they must know this is folly. We could arm Taiwan up to their necks, it's not going to stop China, the 2nd most powerful military on Earth resistance is futile and will only cause unnecessary death and destruction. We have been waiting for the next domino to fall in Taiwan and tensions continue to rise. How will the Western world continue to deny US/NATO biological malfeasance in not just one but two proxy countries. How can the US propaganda machine deny allegations from not one, but two of the other world superpowers? So, can the nations of the world support the West as the allegations and evidence continues to stack up?

They cannot hope to win as China will move in, and given China's vast militaristic superiority to Taiwan, and the relatively small geographical ground to secure, if and when China moves into Taiwan, I would expect it to move significantly faster than the Russian Special Military Operation in Ukraine. Welcome to WW3. Hollywood and Western media made us believe WW3 would feature uniformed armies, nuclear bombs and Continental kinetic warfare. In reality, we got globalist infiltration, proxy wars, biological weapons, and weaponized mass propaganda. But make no mistake, this is WW3. The landscape of what we as humans recognize as "warfare" has simply evolved and Bioweapons research and attacks have been the West's modus operandi for the last 70 years at least and most relevant to the current situation were numerous mysterious outbreaks of illnesses in countries bordering on Russia such as Ukraine and Georgia. Another reason is that on the front line of the superpower struggle between the United States and China, Taiwan has fashioned a defensive masterstroke. It has become indispensable to both sides. In dominating the fabrication of the most advanced semiconductors, the giant Taiwan Semiconductor Manufacturing Company Ltd has captured a technology that's crucial to the cutting-edge digital devices and weapons of today and tomorrow. TSMC accounts for more than 90% of global output of these chips, according to industry estimates. Both superpowers now find themselves deeply dependent on the small island at the centre of their increasingly tense rivalryFor Washington, allowing an increasingly powerful China to overrun TSMC's foundries in a conflict would threaten U.S. military and technological leadership. However, if Beijing invades, there is no guarantee it could seize the prized foundries intact. They could easily become a casualty of the fighting, severing the supply of chips to China's vast electronics industry. Even if the foundries survived a Chinese takeover, they would almost certainly be cut off from a global supply chain essential to their output. My crystal ball tells me the next two years are going to be very tough for all, they come too far to give up. They are coming after all of us as they need a distraction at the moment and all because Donald Trump exposed the reality of power in the US and the globalist 'elite' who hold on to it at all costs, that we get rubbish like, former US President Donald J. Trump is to be arrested, his mugshot will be taken, his fingerprints taken, and he will be reminded of his 'Miranda rights' to legal representation and to remain silent. This is all due to the actions of a prosecutor, Alvin Bragg, who despite what fact-checkers say has benefited professionally from the financial largesse of socialist billionaire George Soros. In 2021, Bragg was elected as the New York County District Attorney after Soros poured millions into a political action committee that went and spent some of those funds on campaign efforts and voter turnout activities for Bragg seeks to bring Trump down over 'hush money' paid to a pornographic film 'actress' and former stripper who claimed she had an affair with the former President. In the UK Australian journalist Julian Assange has languished for 1450 days in a jail cell of a country that isn't his, and is set to be extradited to sit in another jail cell of a country that isn't his, while he awaits trial in a courtroom of a country that isn't his. If he's found guilty by that foreign court, he faces up to 175 years in jail: an effective death sentence. For what? Exposing war crimes, the Australian Government is a joke, and he has proven to be on the right side of history. They do not help him but to all of us he is a "Proper Aussie Hero" Free Julian Assange. Trust nobody and learn from history, think outside the box, prepare and plan, and remember the ones who want 2030 are only 1% and have Satan, but we have about 10-15 % who all fight to the death and we have God. So, they lose and we win. The book is coming to a close and I end with this as it explains your future no "Crystal Ball" from me just their blatant disregard for anything that we regard as sacrosanct, but we have news for them the NWO you will lose and in the generations, to come this "War Cry of Freedom" will come to pass. So, what does "The Future" hold for all of us? Well let me talk about my own backyard because here as I have already mentioned we have a high rate of compliance in taking these poisons which will have a very big detrimental effect on them mentioned we have a high rate of compliance in taking these poisons which will have a very big detrimental effect on them and sadly their families. So we all are going to be affected at some point in time depending on their current comorbidities and age. No wage growth, everything rising mortgages, rents, food, fuel, electricity etc: and people will have to tighten their belts a lot more does not augur well and factor in that Australia has one the world's highest rates of credit card debt all this "pay wave " crap as most "wants it now" which is a total recipe for disaster. So, the book journey ends on May 4rd 2023 and just spoke to another local business. He mentioned to me we took 2 vaccines to stay open but we went bankrupt anyway sadly that was always part of the agenda's plan.All my life I have kept a buffer with a rainy day bank account. It is not really rocket science to hold some back for that "Disaster Moment" I truly feel for my children, yours and your grandchildrens. Latest jab injuries which I included in my last book and now have risen to from 21 February 2021 that the World Health Organisation had 102,000 reports of COVID vaccine adverse drug reactions on its ᵥvigiaccess.org database. This week the number passed the 5,000,000 mark. Let me repeat this because it is hard to believe. According to WHO's own data, more than 5,000,000 people are suspected to have been harmed by the COVID vaccines. The exact number today is 5,026,245 people, including tens of thousands of deaths and this calamity has only just started and we the real figure would be many more times that. The future looks extremely grim as politicians have kicked the can down the road."kicked the can down the road Time for a "reset" a government for the people "The Survivors". There is an old UK show called "The Survivors" and lots of clues in regards to the future. So, I suggest to all think smart and bat smart and don't eat cricket flour or anything intended to "Kill you Up" I already predicted where I am currently living will be a Smart City very soon and it's time to get out of dodge. I suggest picking your friends wisely and enjoy every day to the maximum.

Finally, the last 3 years have been the hardest on the Unvaccinated and the loss of jobs which we loved. I was planning to make a movie manuscript in Sierra Leone Africa of one of my book chapters which would have been a blockbuster musical documentary that Netflix would pay megabucks for. But that will never happen as I never fly there in the current financial climate and the risks that entails. The unvaccinated have been treated despicably by some of their family members and treated like vermin all because they are deemed" Conspiracy Theorist's". Even though 3 years on and we have been proven to be correct in our thinking, that level of totally unacceptable behaviour continues to this day. I have spoken to so many people that this is happening too. Children, Grandchildren and friends they loved all their lives, spoiled, gave them anything and in return they now treat them like "Total Strangers". This common theme is that the vaccinated brains are being hijacked by these poisons and "They are not the Same People" they were before they did what they did. But with unconditional love please stay very strong and walk in "The Light". Please note not all vaccinated act in this despicable way, maybe they got "Lucky and Got The Placebo.

I would again assert that I have done research from different countries and reviewed data and have personally talked with people about their experiences with the vaccines to arrive at what I am covering in this book and I done my very best but expect flak from some mostly men who are total Narcissists and Egotists "I Will Never Pick up Your Rubbish" The colouring of my hair began with the rollout of the so-called vaccines. The colours are my way of expressing concern for our world and as a child a rainbow represented a wonder of the world. I create a rainbow of colour in my hair to highlight the issues the world is currently facing. The rainbow has been hijacked for nefarious purposes and is aligned with ideology of which I am not associated with.

Disclaimer: The information in this book is not medical science or medical advice. I do not have any medical training aside from my own research and interest in this area. The information I publish is not intended to diagnose, treat, cure or prevent any disease, disorder, pain, injury, deformity, or physical or mental condition. I just report my own results, understanding & research.

Acknowledgements. There are so many, and I am bound to miss some people out as this book has really made me brain dead but not a zombie. It's been some journey like being on a runaway train I could not or would want to get off till it was finished. Thanks to other writers, to my family for their support and to my editor Robert who has always been there for me, to Steve who did the cover much love to you. Finally, to all my friends who showed their support there will not be another book but this might get revised in the future. I did my best and hope you find some things thought provoking and finally there is Hope all we need is God and each other. Thanks to the beautiful people who gave me the artwork. Love and blessings to every one of you. Finally thank you to all who supported me over the last three years and hopefully the book helps a few of you and thanks for purchasing it and reading it and reviewing it accordingly. **Since publishing in May 2023** a lot has happened so I will update my book. It was no surprise that libraries world wide banned this book. I donated it to my local Moreton bay library but it did not fit criteria yet books teaching children anal sex are appropriate. The purchasers of books should hold their head in shame. Qld state library put my donated book in the rubbish bin there so scared the truth coming out as it will and they're in panic mode and all will be held to account. Amazon, well they will not let me promote my book. Its shadow is banned so the sales are non-existent, not one in the USA and they have this book in the absurdist fiction category and we were number 18. Book shop's world-wide have it online Barnes and Noble (USA) Target (USA) Foyles (UK). Available worldwide on ebay, amazon sadly not reporting sales so being robbed to be expected. I have just advertised in the latest light newspaper.

Chapter 28
Book Update-November 2023

Since I published in May 2023 a lot has happened and brick by brick we are knocking their edifice down and they're in panic mode. Me and a few brave ladies have been protesting weekly through the Redcliffe markets every Sunday for several months and then we stand outside the war memorial which is full of freemason signs on the wall like **codes, tomfoolery and secrets**. We are followed by security which is to be expected but the reaction by the general public is very heartwarming. The signs we carry with messages like keeping cash alive, saving the bees, vaccine injuries, no more lock downs and mandates seem to resonate with most people. Early in October 2023 the local police raided my old address and I feel for the man living there who was woken up at 10 pm with torches and banging on his front & back door they wanted to interview me as they have other locals for speaking out, freedom of speech is dead in Prison Australia that is how fearful they are of the truth coming out. The current level of people taking the booster is well under 2% in the USA as most are realising the vaccines were what we predicted a bio-weapon but you have to feel for anyone who succumbed to keep food on the table and sadly the fear is kicking in for them as I get told since I had the booster I have not been well. But when you understand the detoxes available you can try to get the poisons out of your body and in all honesty I would suggest all reading this to detox daily and do a parasite cleanse regularly. The vaccination of our children is not stopping with teenagers having their Gardasil vaccine recently here in Qld. It has been 13 years since the U.S. Food and Drug Administration (FDA) supplied fast-tracked approval for Merck's Gardasil vaccine promoted for the prevention of cervical cancer and other conditions attributed to four types of human papillomavirus (HPV).

The agency initially licensed Gardasil solely for 9- to 26-year-old girls and women, but subsequent FDA decisions now enable Merck to market Gardasil's successor the nine-valent Gardasil 9 vaccine—to a much broader age range 9 to 45 years and to both **males** and females. As a result of Gardasil's expanding markets not just in the U.S. but internationally, the blockbuster HPV vaccine has become Merck's third highest-grossing product, bringing in annual global revenues of about $2.3 billion. However, Gardasil's safety record has been nothing short of disastrous. Children's Health Defense and Robert F. Kennedy Jr. has just produced a video detailing the many problems with the development and safety of Gardasil. Why give Gardasil to males who do not have a cervix? The reason for that is obvious.

You have to avoid all vaccines and injectables including the dentist's anaesthetics, the dies for tests and obviously things like botox and naturally blood transfusions. There are unvaccinated doctors out there so network and find who they are as they help you in times of emergency, not all doctors are evil as portrayed.

I have added this to my protocol for what it's worth, it ties in with what another friend sent me this week and a man he knows who got his very high PSA reading down to zero in a few weeks. If you know anyone with cancer or other debilitating disease. This actually works and thank you "lifesaver" for providing this piece.

PARASITES ARE IN HUMANS HORSES, FOALS, COWS, CALVES, SHEEP, GOATS, DOGS AND CATS I would like to draw your attention to the following. After a year and a half of research, I found out that most of the diseases that people and animals suffer from are caused by parasites. My research started with gathering information about Lyme. My dog had contracted Lyme from tick bites and was very sick of it. The vet told me it was the borrelia bacteria. But this is not correct. They are not bacteria, but parasites. So the vet's remedies didn't work.

After thorough research I found out that it concerns parasites. I came across this on a forum in which a woman told us that she was cured of Lyme disease and how she did it. Now you will be wondering how many parasites there actually are. At first I thought about five or ten species. After much reading and studying, it turned out to be hundreds of thousands of different species.

There are even parasites that are themselves carriers of parasites. Single-celled and multicellular parasites. Many types of parasites are not even known and that is because the species present in humans and animals also cross with each other.
All people and animals have parasites in their bodies. Over time, these will cause all kinds of physical problems. Doctors treat symptoms but do not solve the problem. I will share my knowledge with you from now on.
Everyone knows people who suffer from Cancer, Osteoarthritis, Lyme, Alzheimer's, Migraine, Cysts, HIV and AIDS, etc. All these diseases are related to and caused by parasites. Also recommended for people who have been vaxxed because the jabs are full of all parasites. With a good parasite killer you can get better. Use the Joe Tippens protocol. Preferably search via Duckduckgo. You will not often find this information on other search engines. It is also available from the horse/produce shop. Why is Fenbendazole **better than** the Ivermectin paste?
Fenbendazole is 99.9% pure. Ivermectin paste contains E171 Nano titanium dioxide. This E171 is toxic to humans and animals. The paste is difficult to introduce into animals. You can sprinkle the Fenbendazole powder over the food. It's cheaper and healthier.
Joe Tippins's Fenbendazole Protocol For Cancer: https://deeprootsathome.com/joe-tippins-fenbendazole-protocol/ Spread the word, share this knowledge and save your cattle, pets, friends and your family. I personally combine both with ivermectin and fenbendazole. Vaccine mRNA contaminates breast milk most would be aware for sometime this was always planned and going to happen as the evidence is coming out by Dr John Campbell PhD a retired emergency nurse, teacher and author - reviews a new study he says provides

"pretty conclusive proof" that mRNA from the COVID-19 vaccines migrates into breast milk, "probably for the first 48 hours after vaccination." According to the study, the breast milk of 10 of 13 women who took the vaccine tested positive for mRNA up to 45 hours after the vaccine was administered. "This is consistent with other studies, so there's no real debate about this anymore,"

I am currently working with a very astute man we will call "lifesaver" who let me add some of his findings. Since the rollout of the covid "vaccines", the immune system has come into many interviews and conversations. Senior Doctors overseas have constantly stated that you have to 'build your immune system', 'look after your immune system' no one has ever said what the immune system is or where to find it. I asked random people in the street 'where would you find your immune system?' The answers I received varied ' near your heart', ' near your stomach' ' you have to be careful what you eat because it is in your stomach. Most immune cells are made in the bone marrow of the long bones in your legs and pelvis. Some antibody cells are made in the spleen and the main antioxidant cell, **glutathione**, which maintains the immune system in good condition is made in the liver. Why the need for NAC supplement especially if you vaxxed and everyone over 65 as it depletes at 65.

I studied Anatomy and Physiology in my Nursing training and I have put together this document to introduce members of the public to the role and makeup of the immune system so that they can gain an appreciation of why diet and lifestyle play such an important role in maintaining a healthy immune system. This IS NOT a scientific document nor is it a learning tool for health professionals. It is a light-hearted basic explanation of the immune system. I have cut corners and left out complex scientific data so as to make it easier to understand for members of our community. I am also a Veteran of the Vietnam War era and on my first introduction to the immune system, I saw immediately that it was an Army, the most highly-skilled, efficient army I have ever seen.

I am going to call viruses and bacteria--foreign invaders because that's what they are. Every time you inhale a breath or cut yourself while pruning the roses, millions of foreign invaders enter the body either through the lungs or via the cut on your hand. The front line troops are already on patrol, **dendritic cells** and **Macrophages** are the radar cells, scanning the cells of the body for any sign of an invading enemy. They start the killing and devouring process. On detection of an invader, they communicate with the bone marrow. The special forces are immediately sent to the area, cytotoxic [poisonous to the cells] **killer T cells**. These cells kill everything in their path including cancer cells. Another of the special forces cells is the **Neutrophils** they arrive at the injury, block disable, spray jelly over the invaders and then sucks them up, **what a team!!** These neutrophils are special, they can travel through blood vessels and remember these vessels are full of blood under pressure. Here is where it gets interesting and I want you to think about this next time you are out in public. When you take a breath you are inhaling all the airborne microbes around you, if the wind is blowing it stirs up the soil, leaves, dry dog manure, dry bird droppings on leaves and you are inhaling millions of these on every breath. The third special forces cell is the **Basophils;** they survey and detect cancer cells, and protect the body from Parasites, Poisons and Venoms. They also eat animal dander [flakes that are shedding off cats, dogs, and birds]. You are sitting at an outdoor café, the person next to you has a dog, a mild breeze is blowing and the dog is rubbing against the table and panting. You are inhaling millions of 'flakes' coming out of and off that dog. They enter your lungs and sit in the tubes and tiny airbags at the base of your lungs the enemy is immediately detected, special forces are urgently contacted and Basophils arrive at the scene ready to consume the animal by-products. The basophils immediately detect fluid on the animal flakes" I'm not eating this, it's got piss on it". Your immune system has every type of cell to combat this problem. A message is sent to the bone marrow for the "Piss drinking cells" **Pinocytes** named by crazy scientists after the famous drink in the 60s Pina-colada -[pineapple juice, coconut milk, brandy].

These pinocytes will drink every type of foreign fluid that enters the body and the animal 'dander' flakes are coated with saliva, urine, faeces, and water. The second line of defence forces are **Monocytes** [stored in the spleen} They kill all foreign intruders including cancer cells. **Eosinophils** attack and kill parasites, nematodes [pinworm, hookworm and more], you have all seen the videos of worms being pulled out of people's fingers and ears. These cells arrive at the intruders and immediately **inflame** the surrounding tissue to set up an allergic response. There is a set of cells that follow up after the killer cells have done the job. These are the scavengers of the body **Phagocytes** they eat all the leftover roadkill. There is nothing to be alarmed about with these facts, you have been breathing your whole life and you are still alive. If your immune system is in good condition, it can kill **most** microscopic intruders with ease. The cells of the immune system are microscopic themselves so it is a big ask for these little cells to kill the venom from an eastern brown snake. The immune system needs a hand and so anti-venom is injected. Respiratory viruses if not treated correctly can become infected with bacteria requiring antibiotics. For more than a hundred years, respiratory viruses with a heavy mucus build-up were treated in hospitals with steam inhalation. It is still the best treatment. Steam inhaled hourly with menthol/eucalyptus drops instilled twice per day soothes the irritation in the throat, breaks up mucus, and kills the virus. Combine inhalation with deep breathing and deep coughing. If you regularly get infected with respiratory viruses including 'covid', or think you may have a vaccine injury, you should have your immune system, vascular system and internal organs examined. This is a list of the blood tests you need for a full examination of the above systems. FBC,ESR.Full WCC including Eosinophils, D3,T cell count,Full clotting factors and D Dimer. Ask your doctor to please copy this list as listed. If your doctor refuses to order the tests, you can take the list to Sullivan and Nick. or QML and pay $480, once you have the results, take them to your doctor and demand treatment. Something to think about: a conventional army has troops in reserve, the immune system only builds troops when it needs them, and it doesn't keep reserves.

To build up the immune system, start a worm farm, run your hands through the castings, and dig in the garden with your bare hands. The immune system will build an army to combat the invading microbes. Your immune system works best and builds when it has work to do. You can now appreciate just how fantastic the immune system is in looking after our health, every one of the front line and support troops detect and kill cancer cells, we need to look after our protectors. Eat fresh green vegetables, carrots, nuts, salads, sardines, and smoked kippers, these foods build the bone marrow, the liver and the spleen. Wean yourself off junk food, it damages the immune system.

If you continue feeling unwell or have a vaccine injury, here are the drugs needed to 'detox' your body.

N Acetylcysteine take as directed Glutathione boosts immunity over the counter purchase

Zinc [blocks the entry of foreign bodies into body cells] --over the counter purchase

High dose Vit. C over the counter purchase

Hydroxychloroquine is an anti-parasitic drug alternate

Ivermectin purchase EASYMEC 350kg from a produce farm supply

Alternate with Fenbendazole once per month Vit D3 over the counter purchase

Quercetin reduces allergic responses and boosts immunity over the counter purchase include Tumeric

Andrographis powder. 300mg daily [there are bottles of quercetin and Andrographis combined but the dose may not be high enough].

If you notice your breathing is becoming difficult, immediately chew nicotine gum or apply a patch [protects the respiratory centre in the brain]

Specific spike protein destroyer

Nattokinase enzyme buy over the counter   [caution--can lower blood pressure and increase clotting times]   50mg twice daily Bromelain 500mg once daily Curcumin 500 mg three time daily and I would suggest intermittent fasting and ingesting Colloidal Gold.

Cancer stem cell killers

Turmeric,curcumin,GrapeSkin,Resveratrol,Soybean,genistein Broccoli,Sulforaphane,GreenTea,EGCE[epigallocatechin gallate] and add Fenbendazole.

Natural Blood Pressure reducers

Garlic,antioxidants, nitric oxide relaxes muscles and dilates blood vessels thereby reducing blood pressure, Onions contain quercetin,Olives   contain   polyphenols,   Oregano   contains carvacrol, reduces heart rate, stabilises arterial pressure. Celery reduces both systolic and diastolic blood pressure.

During my years of work, I gave many lectures to both hospital professionals and outside citizens on many different clinical topics. One such lecture was snake envenomation and the effects on the human body. Snake venom is a sterile substance. I noted during many years of emergency work that not all snake bites are life threatening even from venomous snakes, it depended on a number of factors.
Some snakes eject venom before the fangs reach the person, some envenomation is superficial and not into a blood vessel [a pressure bandage stops further travel of the venom]. There are a number of snakes and spiders that not only have venom that paralyses the nervous system but it also destroys the tissue at the injection site. A small amount of snake venom is beneficial to the human body, it thins the blood. This is why drug companies use synthetic [man made] snake venom peptides in a number of common prescription drugs.

This brings me to the 'covid vax' injections. By now, you should know they are not vaccines,

The latest research from many scientists and laboratories have stated that **synthetic venom has been used from 20 poisonous snakes and 15 poisonous sea snails. [cono snails]** and placed in the vax bottles. [please read on and don't be dismissive, this document could save your life]

Phospholipase [PLA2] is an enzyme synthesised from the RattleSnake venom and used in most covid vax bottles. This enzyme destroys your Zinc reserves, destroys tissue in your internal organs and leads to multiple organ failure.

The bacteria **E Coli** occurs naturally in the bowel and in healthy people it stays there. For people with underlying health problems or obesity, E coli travels to other parts of the body.

PLA2 is taken up by E Coli and replicated in not only that bacteria but also any yeast in the body. Antibiotics cause yeast to proliferate.

Your body is now manufacturing the synthesised **PLA2** rattlesnake enzyme and this is having a very damaging effect on your internal body.

Some of the Vax bottles contain not only synthesised snake venom protein but also cone snail venom. If you have been injected with the Covid Jab, you have to presume that the injection contained one or more snake and or snail venom peptides, those peptides enter your Gut and your body is now manufacturing snake and snail peptides. Here are some effects your body may be displaying from the damage of the venom.

Holding a false belief that nothing can be changed by fact

Aggressiveness/anger
Chest pain
Confusion
Cough
Dark urine
Fainting
Forgetfulness
Change in walking or balance

Unsteadiness
Change in urine retention or output
Feeling cold
Shivering
Uncontrolled eye movement
Shaking

Information source: British medical Journal 2021 article titled 'Snake bits and Covid 19 have similar effects'
University of Arizona August 2021 "Researchers have found the mechanism responsible for the Covid 19 mortality as an enzyme related to the RattleSnake Venom. They confirmed the enzyme as PLA2.
European Commission and joint research centre in partnership with the University of Salerno Italy 18/7/20 Plasma, faecal and urine samples taken from hundreds of covid 19 deceased patients. Large numbers of blood and faecal samples taken from Covid deceased people in Italy revealed not only PLA2 but E Coli deposits all through the body.
All 36 synthesised venoms from snakes and cone snails were found in the samples. Research scientists had never seen levels of venom this high. You should immediately start talking to a Doctor who has not been corrupted by the Pharmaceutical industry or threatened into silence.

Zinc tablets to replace the zinc destroyed by the venom
Glutathione an antioxidant essential for your immune system
NAC N.Acetyl cysteine, Vitamin C
EDTA ethylenediamine tetra-actil acid
Bromelain, Aloe Vera, Resveratrol
This is newly released information and I have no doubt that more research will be conducted in the future. For a full list of snakes and cono Snails venoms watch **Dr Brian Ardis's** videos,

Cancer virus found in covid shots.

Microbiologist Kevin McKernan pioneered research on testing some of the covid vaccine vials and discovered unacceptable levels of double-stranded DNA plasmids floating around. This is DNA contamination. He found the contamination in Pfizer and Moderna vials. In Pfizer's mRNA injection, McKernan also discovered Simian Virus 40 ("SV40") promoters which are tied to cancer development in humans. He emphasised that the SV40 found is a viral piece, it is not the whole virus. However, it still presents a risk of driving cancer. We are all aware of the real pandemic which is **"turbo cancer"** and the high deaths above the normal yearly averages which is logically explained by the above and understanding when you have no innate natural immune system anymore. So much research is coming out to confirm to all of us laymen these fear's and it's beyond being tragic. Japanese Professor Murakami of Tokyo University expressed his concerns over the alarming discovery of SV40 promoters McKernan had made. He said: "The Pfizer vaccine has a staggering problem. I have made an amazing discovery. This figure is an enlarged view of Pfizer's vaccine sequence.As you can see, the Pfizer vaccine sequence contains part of the SV40 sequence here. This sequence is known as a promoter. Roughly speaking, the promoter causes increased expression of the gene. The problem is that the sequence is present in a well-known carcinogenic virus.

"The question is why such a sequence that is derived from a cancer virus is present in Pfizer's vaccine. There should be absolutely no need for such a carcinogenic virus sequence in the vaccine. Well most of you reading this will truly understand the reasons why.

Moreton Bay Where I live is the 3rd largest council area in Australia and was recently named as a city and Smart it is not with the comrade mayor and is bunch of clown councillors who continue to wreak havoc on this iconic place with there poor decisions as anyone living locally reading this will have seen them in action not doing any real good and justifying their high salaries.

334

Recenting near the wreck of the Gayandah at Woody Point they would have spent a huge amount at a guess it would be a million dollars on park improvements rubbing salt into the wounds of the people living next door who are homeless in "tent city" where up to 19 tents and which in such an affluent city should never ever happen. We need to drain the swamp on these high paid bureaucrats who are out of touch with the locals and there aims to make this another concrete jungle of highrises. We all see how overdevelopment and no real infrastructure to be able to cope with it is creating a car park when you want to drive anywhere. The homeless situation is dire here in Moreton Bay as they demolish more homes and more sheeple move here from Timbuctoo and beyond as the desire to live in a smart 15 minute city increases. I recently took 9 homeschool children aged 5-12 years of age to meet councillor Karl Winchester the children highlighted the need for the Ningy Ningy aborigines to be more recognised with more local signage but he explained the Gubbi Gubbi were here first, the poor children were confused and I just bite my tongue and the word moron sprung to mind he is about useless as tit's on a bull.

Zombism. You will all have noticed the level of zombism that is taking place among the vaccinated especially when they use those brain **EMF zapping tampon earbuds**. It is ironic that so many who exercise wear them so their body is willing but their brain is "dead". For all of us they are a danger driving their cars riding their bikes and sadly as the amount of graphene oxide near there blood brain barrier combined with the spike proteins and the vibrations are increased you will notice some very bizarre events going forword.

Late term abortions. Yvette D'ath is commonly known as "mrs death" and even when you put her name in google it comes up as death and with her involvement in late term abortions D'Ath is one of the Three Wicked Vampire Witches of the George St Cabal responsible for Trad's monster abortion law and practice in the Big Q. Big Abortion is part of the Big Bio-Tech, Big Pharma, Big Organ Harvesting Combine of the CCP.

This industry requires a steady supply of foetal tissue, stem cells and human organs. Since their Euthanasia law came into effect in Jan 2022, the Cabal and the Flying Monkeys are moving fast on the Qld population itself, not just the most vulnerable at the beginning and end of life.

Talking of death we all notice the "Jab Cab's" which a lot of us sadly refer to as the ambulances because they are extremely busy and it's so sad as many would not be in them if they had bothered to listen to us they truly are dropping like flies.

HAARP

We all see that their agenda's using their weapons on us is poisoning us through cloud seeding and the haarp is their main way of destroying area's that won't comply like Hawaii and Aculpoco.

HAARP

U.S. PATENT 4,686,605

WEAPONIZED WEATHER CONTROL

Notable quotes from patent:

- "A means and method is provided to cause interference with or even total disruption of communications over a very large portion of the earth"

- "Weather modification is possible by, for example, altering upper atmosphere wind patterns or altering solar absorption patterns by constructing one or more plumes of atmospheric particles which will act as a lens or focusing device."

- "The earth's magnetic field could be decreased or disrupted at appropriate altitudes to modify or eliminate the magnetic field."

Sadly this is just the start as they will use this weapon more and more and blame everything on climate change as they ramp up their fear and whey you are aware of all these distractions and an Agenda for them to reach their goal by 2030. For most of you reading this we don't watch their propaganda and understand the "big picture' so just stay in your high vibration as we truly are the survivor's.

Duncan Tyrrell. Brisbane.

I would like to thank Rainbow Harmonica Man for offering me the opportunity to write this article to be included in his excellent, ground-breaking book.

'An environment that is not safe to disagree in is not an environment focused on growth – it's an environment focused on control.' Wendi Jade.My first experience of the COVID-19 pandemic, (plandemic) was not from personal experience, but one played out entirely on the TV. (Tell-lie-vision.) It was horrifying. Aired footage recovered from a train station in China showed adults falling dead to the floor and being immediately surrounded by people wearing Hazmat suits. To me, the footage resembled a scene from a Hollywood movie. How convenient that the people wearing Hazmat suits were on hand when members of the public died and fell face down onto the floor. Was it staged? Were Hazmat wearers standing by, waiting for a cue to respond? My hackles were raised. Something wasn't right. Similar footage was aired every minute, of every hour, of every day. This terrible pandemic would sweep the world and kill millions if we don't follow our government's directions, they told us. 'Follow the science for your safety,' became clichéd and repeated around the globe by every news programme bulletin. 'We must stay home,' one Prime Minister insisted. Mandates, mandates, mandates. It was full on and in your face. Fear, fear, and more fear. A Behavioural Insights Team was set up by the UK government, involving behavioural scientists fully intent on making the public do exactly what they were being told. In truth, the British public were being manipulated to comply. Further teams were set up in the UK. One was simply named, the 'Nudge Unit.' Nudge theory is about denying certain choices or making other choices harder. Applied effectively, it is used to avoid having arguments and instead to manipulate people without them realising.) Borrowed from, A State of Fear, written by Laura Dodsworth. Incidentally, Nudge Units were formed elsewhere to control world-wide behaviour. The entire operation was in total lockstep.

I attended two live talk shows by David Icke in 2014, and 2016. (I would have attended a third show in 2019, but that year, David Icke was banned by the federal government from entering and speaking in Australia). The first show I attended was on the Gold Coast, and the second, in Brisbane. After the second show, I was compelled to buy one of David's many controversial books. The book I chose was titled, The Phantom Self, first published in 2016. In his book, David talks about a Plandemic in which a virus would sweep the world and a vaccine would be the only way to prevent hundreds of thousands of deaths, nay, millions. This vaccine would be deemed mandatory, and was the only way for society to return to a 'new normal.' His book is by no means a novel. I was primed and ready for this plandemic, and fully prepared when it arrived in 2020. My soul was screaming at me, telling me the entire operation was a psyop; a major propaganda exercise not seen on this scale in recent history. The rebel in me decided not to participate, and not be subjected to a totalitarian government. I decided I would not comply, and would avoid the nonsense even if it meant not being able to travel, or enter cafés and restaurants. I wasn't playing their game.

Months later, tired of fighting sheeple and fake nonsensical rules, my anxiety levels peaked. Going about my daily life without wearing a mask, I was verbally abused, which took its toll. None of the so-called directions made any sense to me. We were told we had to wear a mask while walking into a restaurant, but it was OK to remove it once we sat down. Then we had to put the mask on again if we stood to leave or use the bathroom. Why? The alleged virus would get you if you stood drinking in a pub, but would leave you alone if you sat. Bunnings, bottle shops etc, were immune to the virus, but if you step into a nursing home, gym, or church, then the evil beast would pounce, according to the government propaganda. Asymptomatic people were allegedly spreaders; unheard of, and quarantining healthy people, in my opinion, was criminal. Even the government changed their rules on a regular basis, adding to the confusion.

The entire psyop was cleverly and deliberately designed to create fear, and uncertainty. In the early days of the plandemic, every death was recorded as 'died from covid' according to government statistics and mainstream media. But less than twelve months after the jab was introduced, people were dying suddenly (SADS) and the government, doctors and the media had no idea why. Even **Yvette De'Ath**, (Minister for Health and Ambulance Services: 12 Nov 2020 - 17 May 2022,) had no idea why there were so many sudden deaths, especially in young, healthy people, including fit athletes.

Eventually, the universe and Facebook guided me towards a group of like-minded, everyday Queenslanders not buying into the planned agenda. Finally, I didn't feel so alone. A meeting in the Botanical Gardens in Brisbane was organised for the following month, which I planned to attend. As I approached the gathering, my fight-and-flight mode peaked. Skirting the crowd and keeping an eye-out for police, my anxiety levels reduced as I gingerly began to mingle. Safety in numbers. I had seen footage of police in Melbourne, Victoria, picking off individuals on the edge of a crowd. Thanks to the group, I made many friends, some of which are friends to this day.

Watching footage of police brutality in Australia, being barred from pubs and clubs, and despite belonging to a group of like-minded souls, my anxiety levels skyrocketed. I needed help, and after several months of exceptional therapy I was able to control my anxiety, and was no longer triggered by fear and confrontation. Strong enough to hold my truth, I re-joined groups, gatherings, and protests, and marched through the streets of Brisbane many times, usually on a Saturday afternoon. It was amazing to be part of a group of like-minded souls who knew that the government had overreached and was slowly eroding our freedom. (Despotism). The more we were told to stay indoors, the more determined I was to go outside. Mandates aren't law, I learned, so I felt confident that I wasn't breaking any laws. Conspiracy theories were exposed. Now, no longer theories.

One particular morning I woke up feeling empowered, and that was the day I stepped away from the false matrix created by the cabal. It was an amazing feeling, and so invigorating. I surrounded myself with love, then somehow, the zombies that thought it was their job to police me and the community, were leaving me alone. Now able to walk through the local shopping mall unchallenged, my confidence grew. I was somehow protected. With my head held high, I walked into shops, marched past staff holding out a mask for me to wear, politely saying 'no thank you,' and walking on. To be amongst almost 100% compliant souls was, to me, empowering, while at the same time, feeling sorry for them. I sent them love. Not falling for the propaganda, instead of looking for masks I looked for faces, and smiled at everyone, masked, or unmasked. People stepped aside in fear as this man, not wearing a mask, was walking through a crowded shopping mall. Fear was in their eyes whether they looked at me or not, and most of the time I felt invisible as these 'masked worriers' went about their daily ritual of handwashing, adjusting their face masks, and social distancing. Isn't social distancing an oxymoron?

Things got even crazier when 'vaccines' were first introduced. Covid injectables do not come under the vaccine definition, but that definition has since been altered to fit the agenda. (Vaccine. Variable noun: A special substance that you take into your body to prevent a disease, and that often contains a weakened or dead form of the disease-causing organism. Cambridge Dictionary.) A covid injection is an mRNA gene altering therapy using messenger RNA, not a live or weakened organism. The so-called solution to the plandemic was said to be a miracle, and deemed to be close to 100% effective at creating immunity. Natural immunity was a distant memory. Incentives to take the jab raised their ugly head, and virtue signallers posted on Facebook that they were 'Fully Vaccinated.' Those who declined the jab were banned from society, including myself. Remember the green tick on partaker's phones? Countless businesses weren't compliant, and I supported those whenever I could during those unprecedented times. '

'Flash mobs' were organised and turned up at a moment's notice when police began intimidating business owners; usually owners of cafés. The police soon left when the 'flash mob' heckled them. Many businesses refused to accept cash because they were brainwashed by the MSM into believing that cash was infested with germs and therefore would more than likely spread covid. On one occasion, I withdrew cash from an ATM and went into a shop with my newly minted notes stuffed inside my wallet. The assistant told me how much my purchase was, and when I handed over the cash, she pinched it between her thumb and forefinger. I commented on why she had done that even though the cash was fresh from an ATM, and she said it was because I had touched it. When she gave me my receipt, I took it from her using my thumb and forefinger and said, 'ewe! You touched it!' then walked away. Don't mess with the awakened.

A recognised cancer charity I was a volunteer for became problematic for me when staff and volunteers were asked to always wear a face mask during working hours. An email arrived in my inbox telling me about mandatory covid jabs for all staff, including volunteers. No, thank you. I resigned from my position, telling them I have a perfectly good immune system without an 'irreversible, invasive, gene altering, experimental medical procedure.' **(I do not know of one person who regrets not getting the jab.)** We have been close to four-years since the Plandemic began. The truth is surfacing, and politicians have stepped down from their role, using lame excuses. They, '…no longer have the energy to continue,' or '…want to spend more time with their family.' (There are no visitors allowed in Gitmo). All the 'useful idiots' across the globe have done the damage and will pay for their crimes against humanity. A virus didn't change our lives; a tyrannical government did. If you didn't know the truth behind the plandemic before reading this book, then, hopefully you will have gained enough awareness to know that the so-called virus was created for the vaccine, and not the reverse.

We are facing a depopulation agenda. As I write, the entire planet is entering a new era, and life will change for the better. I am optimistic that our new world will be filled with love, and respect for fellow man. A new monetary system, QFS, (Quantum Financial System) is ready and waiting for the plug to be pulled on the old Fiat system. Unfortunately, some will not make it into the new world, but for those that do, I'll see you in the new world we created.

Thank you Duncan my good friend for that lovely insight and it is a privilege to work with great warriors like your good self .I often talk about not sharing body fluids with vaccinated people but recently I tried a friendship with a vaccinated person and even that is fraught with danger because they are basically on a different wavelength unless their wake enough to the dangers of emfs and will continue to wear them even though you have warned them how incredibly dangerous they actually are. They also might continue to do up the nose PCR tests but we can only try until the penny hopefully drops especially when you feel a love for them.

The Future.

Weapon's and the future young people have had no self discipline training and therefore will need to join either the cadets or once attaining the age of 18 will need to join the militia if wanting to hold a weapons 'carry' licence.Initial basic training will be [four?] weeks with the AMF reserve, they will participate in physical training, weapons instruction, ethics instruction. With further training, the militia men will learn the skills to diffuse a hostage situation, diffuse aggressive confrontation, storm a building and disarm a perpetrator. Further classroom education could include trauma counselling, training them for disaster relief work and placing the militia men in a very good position for future careers in the AMF or a career in the militia. Annual training with the Reserve AMF will be ongoing with compulsory range live firing [to be determined]. Weapons will be issued on loan from the AMF and each militia man is accountable for and the maintenance of that weapon to a high military standard.

No private weapons will be permitted to be carried whilst on duty. This militia will be necessary for the protection of a free people

In the homeless chapter I mentioned my dispute with real estate Century 21 in Scarborough Qld and I tried to resolve it with the RTA but was astounded when John Eagle the property manager tried to claim $1000 damages to a carpet I had marked but it was already damaged in the entry report when I moved in 2018 so I called him a "Parasite" and they proceeded to take me to QCAT my court case was resolved in my favour regards to carpet and I received some of my bond back. So to any you reading this in similar disputes as some real estates are using this as a rort to kick people when they're already down by stealing their bond's don't let them get away it most are vaccinated zombies with no real empathy of compassion the industry needs a big broom and a massive sweep out.
The owner of my leased property **Lyndall Ketting** you are the lowest of the low. I paint the walls of your unit labour free and you try this very "low trick" but karma is a bitch as your name is in lights.

The Net Zero Scam

Here in Australia the madness continues with this manic Labour government backed by the equally mad greens. gone the days of hugging the trees there now want them cut down to install. To cope, Australia's energy market operator is proposing over 10,000 kilometres of new transmission lines, linking major renewable precincts with their proposed smart cities. The perpetrators of the net zero scam bang on about how we need to be sustainable and use renewable energy however they're prepared to destroy the environment in order to do it. The media is complicit in the scam and manipulation of the public perception as they alter weather graphics on news programs to show scary red heatwave areas when temperatures in those areas are cooler now than 5 years ago. Sweden has announced that it is scrapping the WEF's green energy targets and has declared that man-made global warming science is a scam.

Instead, the Swedish Government is shifting back to nuclear power and has ditched its targets for a "100% renewable energy" supply.

The reason why this tyrannical labour government wants to destroy farms and farmers is very obvious if only you, the so-called educated, woke up. Farmers will not be able to get insurance, use helicopters and drones to help keep pests at bay and ultimately feed us and you will be forced to eat their bugs and cancer creating foods. Time for the communal food growing allotments to come back because us the awake will buy into their agenda's.

Remember Sweden compared very well in the covid plandemic scam when they also did not buy into the lock-downs. No wonder the news media are totally silent about the data that show that Sweden's open society policy was what the rest of the world should have done, too. Numerous studies have shown Sweden's excess death rate to be among the lowest in Europe during the pandemic and in several analyses, Sweden was at the bottom. This is remarkable considering that Sweden has admitted that it did too little to protect people living in nursing homes. Unlike the rest of the world, Sweden largely avoided implementing mandatory lockdowns, instead relying on voluntary curbs on social gatherings, and keeping most schools, restaurants, bars and businesses open. Face masks were not mandated. But here in Australia the mask's are still very evident as the brainwashing of the sheep truly worked

Tavistock

Financed as you would expect by the Rothschilds, Rockefellers and the British Royal Family, the Tavistock Institute is where "the matrix" is generated. They control more than 450 of the Fortune 500 corporations which explains why so many are now requiring their employees to be vaccinated. We realise that covid is just the latest of a series of scams designed to degrade humanity, sheepilise and herd it into pens. This started in both world wars, the Great Depression, the Cold War, Vietnam, Korea, Iraq and Afghanistan. Most of what we know about the world is a lie. Everything that happens is engineered. The "news"has always been a well rehearsed and planned lie.

The abdication of free speech, fairness and any normal common sense by the mass media, medicine, government, education and law is consistent with this picture. We have been satanically possessed for reasons that most reading is very clear as light is day to see.

Rothschild is the sorcerer that these very sick people advertise their power and wealth through evil book ect, and Tavistock is his magic wand. Hundreds of US "think tanks" plot the destruction of democracy and national independence. The field of psychology is very dedicated to mind control. The Illuminati may have over-reached this time. They sent everyone to their room but neglected to shut down the Internet. It is hard to permanently enslave people who can communicate and share information instantly on a worldwide basis. Despite their efforts, the truth about the "vaccines" is out. Make no mistake, the satanists want everyone and everything you hold dear. They are going to demonise and persecute the unvaccinated because they think they can.

Monica Smit

Met her today to see her speak before she mentions this is her calling. We swapped books and I hope to break bread with her one day as she truly inspires me as a younger person and we so much need more visionaries like her.

Monica's book is called Cell 22 from party girl to political prisoner.

The Light Newspaper

We all respect and enjoy reading The Light newspaper and another publication well worth reading is Uncensored from Auckland New Zealand

Rainbow Holistic Product's

The need to detox which I do constantly having gone from having aspergilloma fungus ball which I still have and coughing up tablespoons of blood 5 years ago to know never been fitter or healthier shown by my latest blood results in the 1 percent of bloods that as normal as can be comes lots hard work, the love of god and finally natural medicines.
So I decided to make my own with tablets. The fillers are a worry and I only use Lion's Mane and Tumeric as fillers.So slowly build all these Product's
Ivermectin capsules, Fenbendazole capsules, Zeolite capsules, Bentonite capsules and Andrographhis capsules. Colloidal silver and gold spray bottles and creams and natural zinc and aloe vera sunscreens. Shungite necklaces and packets to make your own shungite water. Emf products and Emf readers.
They are in selected crystal shops and they also stock my books.

A few are.

Made by Me design's

More than your average crystal store based in Margate Qld they have a wide range of products including crystals, jewellery,holistic products,herbs and much more. They also offer workshops, events and reading's reiki and holistic therapies.
Check out madebymebrisbane on facebook or instagram or

www.madebymedesigns.com.au

Kezzys Emporium Redcliffe

Facebook click on link

An amazing store owned by a truly amazing lady.

This is the tragic story of a local man here in Qld Australia.

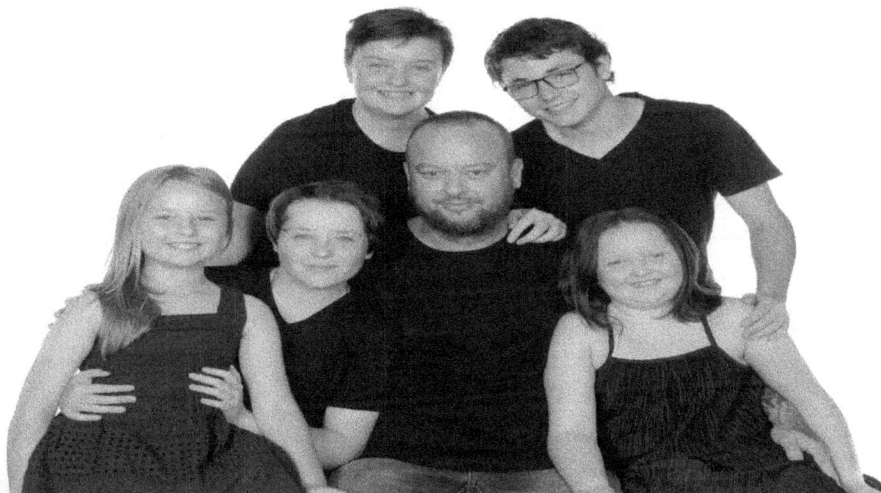

Hi everyone, I'm Lin and this is a story of losing a son through coercive government policy, shameful public misinformation and blatant lies. I tell you Damien's story as he no longer can. Damien, his partner Hannah and I had many conversations about the safety and efficacy of the injections and we agreed they were unsafe, untested and not something we would be doing unless dragged kicking and screaming.Damien had living with him and his long-term partner Hannah, five children from his previous marriage, and Hannah's two children He was father to all children equally. The children were aged between 4-17 at the time of his death. The main provider for his family, Damien was a cleaner and active in his children's lives. Unbeknown to me, he took the first two injections in order to continue volunteering at his children's school which he loved and had time to do due to the hours of his work. He had his first injection on the 18th of January 2022 and second on the 16th of February. After Damien's second he experienced violent shaking in his extremities for several hours afterwards. He and Hannah were frightened by this and decided he should not have any more, but due to a mandate requirement in applying for a new job, he reluctantly decided to get the third injection. He did not even get to start.

Damien received his booster at 10:14am on Friday 21st of October 2022. He experienced pain in his arm within 15 minutes, pain in his shoulder that evening and a general unwell feeling the next day. However, he and Hannah were relieved that he had no repeat of the shaking in his extremities. Damien got up early on Sunday 23rd while Hannah was still asleep. When she woke, she asked the kids where their Dad was and they replied that he'd gone to the toilet. Hannah knocked on the toilet door but received no response. She tried to open the door and, through the crack, saw Damien collapsed on the floor unresponsive. His collapse had knocked out a tooth and he had saliva and fluid coming from this mouth. As Damien's body was blocking the door Hannah physically tore the door apart to drag him out. Hannah asked their eldest daughter to call 000 while she performed CPR chest compressions on Damien while waiting for the ambulance to arrive. On arrival, paramedics continued with the CPR and administered two bags of fluid and four adrenaline injections in an attempt to revive him. Damien was unresponsive and was declared dead at 10.49am. His young family witnessed everything. Police were called and arrived at 11.19am and were provided with a life extinct form. Because of his sudden death at just 40 years old, Damien's body was taken to the Brisbane Morgue for investigation.

Hannah received a phone call a fortnight later from the Coronial Nurse advising that their preliminary examination showed he had an enlarged heart and heavy lungs and that it would be up to 12 months before a formal finding by the Coroner would be made. Hannah called back later and told the office that Damien had received an injection under 48 hours prior to his death. Damien's GP advised the Coroner's office that Damien had no known heart issues, no symptoms, and was the healthiest he had seen him in sometime. I have had to follow up several times with the Coroner's office to obtain all documentation completed at the autopsy. I received a copy of the written "Doctor's Notice To Coroner After Autopsy Form " listing Dilated left ventricle and heavy lungs in the Summary of autopsy findings, which differs from the Coronial Nurse's verbal report of an enlarged heart.

Does something seem wrong here? Damn right it does. I registered all the injection details in the DAEN on the TGA website around February this year as an adverse event and have had no response or follow-up whatsoever from them. I have tried to claim reimbursement for Damien's cremation through the Federal Government compensation scheme. In the claim form is a requirement to tick one of the government-approved list of medical diagnoses, none of which apply to Damien. Also required is confirmation from a doctor that the death was injection related and of course no doctor will sign that for fear of deregistration.

Damien's passing has been devastating. His youngest girls are seeing counsellors to process the grief and trauma they suffered in seeing their father dead. The children and Hannah have had their birthdays and Christmas without him and Damien has been sadly missed in family celebrations. I don't believe it's a coincidence that my son died within 48 hours of his injection and I strongly believe his death is linked to the injection. I have joined a class action to sue the Federal Government for wrongful death.These drugs should have been suspended and investigated and no-one else should have to endure the grief we have suffered.

No mother should be concerned with her child's funeral arrangements or trying to get information from the Coroner's office. No mother should have to decide where her child's ashes should go. No mother should experience the death of their child because of a medicine that was released without full testing. I have seen many stories of deaths shared on jab_injuries_australia in Instagram and these medicines should have been suspended and investigated long before Damien took his fatal dose. Damien's death will not be in vain; I will make sure of that. I will NOT be silent.

So ending this book update with the tragic story of a local man here in Queensland Australia meeting Lin her pain is truly heartbreaking and this must not be allowed to happen again to anyone. As a parent I have buried a child, bless you Ethan Elizabeth Warren .

If God deems it the book will be updated again in June 2024.

THE FIGHT FOR FREEDOM GOES ON

TO BE CONTINUED

www.ingramcontent.com/pod-product-compliance
Lightning Source LLC
Chambersburg PA
CBHW081406270326
41931CB00016B/3390